Core Approaches in Counselling and Psychotherapy

Core Approaches in Counselling and Psychotherapy is a comprehensive guide to the four main psychological approaches (humanistic, psychodynamic, behavioural and cognitive) and introduces several of the most common therapies used today. This textbook contains sufficient coverage to explain all of the most important elements of these core approaches and sufficient depth to provide a detailed analysis of the ten main therapies: person-centred therapy, psychoanalytic therapy, behaviour therapy, cognitive therapy, Gestalt therapy, transactional analysis, rational emotive behaviour therapy, cognitive-behaviour therapy, multimodal therapy and neurolinguistic programming.

The book focuses on the development of each approach and presents the associated therapy in its historical and psychological context, giving a deeper insight into the theories and clarifying the overlap between different therapies.

Presented in a unique style, with a clear layout, rigorous content and extensive online resources at www.routledge.com/cw/short, *Core Approaches in Counselling and Psychotherapy* is an invaluable asset for undergraduate and postgraduate students at all levels of study and is the ideal textbook for any degree or higher-level module in counselling.

Fay Short lectures on Social Psychology and Psychotherapy, alongside her role as Director for Teaching and Learning in Psychology, at Bangor University. She is a Chartered Psychologist with the British Psychological Society and a member of the British Association for Counselling and Psychotherapy, and has recently been awarded a highly prestigious National Teaching Fellowship award from the Higher Education Academy.

Phil Thomas is Lecturer at Coleg Llandrillo and Bangor University, where he is the Director of the counselling pathway within the Masters in Education. As a qualified teacher and therapist trained to NLP Master Practitioner level, he has a particular interest in the applications of therapy in education. He also provides counselling and supervision within his private practice.

Core Approaches in Counselling and Psychotherapy

Fay Short and
Phil Thomas

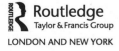
Routledge
Taylor & Francis Group

LONDON AND NEW YORK

First published 2015
by Routledge
27 Church Road, Hove, East Sussex, BN3 2FA

and by Routledge
711 Third Avenue, New York, NY 10017

Routledge is an imprint of the Taylor & Francis Group, an informa business

British Library Cataloguing in Publication Data
A catalogue record for this book is available from the British Library

Library of Congress Cataloging in Publication Data
Short, Fay.
  Core approaches in counselling and psychotherapy/Fay Short and
  Phil Thomas.
  pages cm
  1. Psychotherapy. 2. Counseling psychology. I. Title.
  RC480.S43 2014
  616.89′14—dc23
  2014005577

ISBN: 978-1-44416-728-3 (hbk)
ISBN: 978-0-415-74514-7 (pbk)
ISBN: 978-0-203-77339-0 (ebk)

Typeset in Frutiger and Joanna
by Florence Production Ltd, Stoodleigh, Devon, UK

To my mum and dad for teaching me the meaning of life and my husband for giving my life meaning.
—Fay Short

To my family for their love, my tutors for their guidance, my students for their enthusiasm. Finally, to my clients who have given me the opportunity to put my learning into practice.
—Phil Thomas

To Elaine Ward, Tina Usherwood and Keith Mathews for being willing to demonstrate their excellence on video.
—Fay Short and Phil Thomas

Contents

About the authors

FAY SHORT

Dr Fay Short is a Senior Lecturer at Bangor University and a Chartered Psychologist with the British Psychological Society. Dr Short initially worked in the field of cognitive neuropsychology investigating our understanding of our physical body – she was presented with a research award from the American Psychological Association for her work on body representation in the virtual world. After the completion of her PhD, she began to expand her research interests to explore the interaction between psychotherapy and education. She has completed two qualifications in teaching (PGCert for Further Education and PGCert for Higher Education) and a Master's in Education Studies focusing on the applications of psychotherapy in learning environments. She is a member of the Bangor Academy of Teaching Fellows and is a Fellow of the Higher Education Academy – she has recently won the National Union of Students Teacher of the Year award at Bangor University and a highly prestigious National Teaching Fellowship award from the HEA. Alongside her academic role as Director of Undergraduate Studies in Psychology, she lectures in counselling and psychotherapy and supports students through the university counselling service. She is an accredited hypnotherapist, NLP practitioner and practitioner of REBT, and her innovative work on the applications of therapeutic communications skills have led to invitations to present at conferences and public events across the country.

PHIL THOMAS

Phil Thomas is Lecturer at Llandrillo College and Bangor University. He is the Director of the counselling pathway within the part-time MA in Education Studies, Bangor University. A qualified teacher and therapist, his Master's Degree dissertation focused on overcoming test anxiety. After completing his counselling qualification, he trained as an NLP Master Practitioner and has an interest in applications of NLP in education. He describes his approach as systematic eclecticism. He provides counselling for students as part of the college counselling service, and supervises counsellors and student mentors within the student services team. He also provides counselling and supervises counsellors within private practice.

Preface

Counselling and psychotherapy have been described as a 'talking cure' and it is certainly true that these processes can offer a successful non-medicinal alternative in the treatment of depression, anxiety, psychosis, etc. But to suggest that therapy is simply a treatment for mental health issues or a crutch for the worried well is to miss the true value of this incredible process. An appreciation of counselling and psychotherapy can offer a unique insight into human nature and a deep understanding of how to connect with another person. Appreciation of the core approaches in counselling and psychotherapy can inform all of our interactions, within and beyond the therapeutic setting. Those who eventually pursue a career in healthcare will benefit immensely from this knowledge, but even those who choose a profession in the field of business or education or engineering – indeed, any field that involves some interaction with other human beings – will benefit from understanding those theories which explain human nature. Furthermore, successful application of these theories to our interpersonal interactions can significantly aid both our professional and personal relationships. There is, perhaps, no other academic area that can boast such a profound and wide-reaching effect on all aspects of our lives.

Permissions

Photograph of Aaron Beck appears courtesy of the Beck Institute for Cognitive Behavior Therapy, www.beckinstitute.org.

Photograph of Donald Meichenbaum appears courtesy of himself.

Photograph of Ulric Neisser appears courtesy of Cornell University.

Guide to the companion website

www.routledge.com/cw/Short

Visit the companion website for *Core Approaches in Counselling and Psychotherapy* to discuss a comprehensive range of resources designed to enhance the teaching and learning experience for both students and instructors.

On the companion website you'll find the following range of resources with which you can engage with the content of *Core Approaches in Counselling and Psychotherapy*.

INSTRUCTOR RESOURCES

- PowerPoint presentations for each chapter of the book
- A test bank of essay questions, short answer questions and multiple choice questions for use with students

STUDENT RESOURCES

- Chapter-by-chapter material including mindmaps, essay questions, short answer questions and wordclouds to enhance your understanding of each section
- Multiple choice questions to test your knowledge of the content
- Useful resources and links for exploring topics further
- A glossary of key terms
- Therapy in action – four videos of therapy sessions, with an assessment form and transcript for each

Introduction

This book aims to provide you with a comprehensive guide to the four main psychological approaches (humanistic, psychodynamic, behavioural and cognitive) and introduce you to several of the most common – and sometimes controversial – therapies used today (person-centred therapy, psychoanalytic therapy, behaviour therapy, cognitive therapy, gestalt therapy, transactional analysis, rational emotive behaviour therapy, cognitive-behaviour therapy, multimodal therapy and neurolinguistic programming). This textbook offers a guide to this subject for those studying at undergraduate or postgraduate level. You will find that the book contains sufficient coverage to explain all of the most important elements of the core approaches and sufficient depth to provide you with a detailed analysis of the main therapies. However, the content of the book is so clearly explained and the presentation of the book is so accessible that this textbook is also an ideal introduction for those who simply wish to learn more about this fascinating topic.

You will notice that this book is quite unique in style and format. It does not contain huge paragraphs of text. Instead, all information is presented in simple note style to improve digestion. Cognitive psychology teaches us that we cannot maintain attention for long periods of time, especially when the topic is difficult – long chapters filled with rolling paragraphs are almost impossible to understand when you are struggling with the core concepts. And it is just as impossible to resist copying these perfect paragraphs when you are trying to paraphrase to avoid plagiarism. It is far easier to read and understand short chunks of text highlighting the main points and then use this primary information as a foundation on which to build your own work. This book was written with the intention of providing lists of facts, brief explanations, clear relationships between concepts and an opportunity to quickly digest chunks of information for future use in essays, reports, exams or your interactions with others.

For further information on how to get the best from this textbook, please consult the following frequently asked questions.

HOW DO I READ THIS BOOK?

This book is designed to provide you with a comprehensive overview of the four main approaches to counselling and psychotherapy. This means that it contains a significant depth of analysis and this level of detail can be difficult to digest in one sitting. We recommend that you read this book like a magazine rather than a novel. Instead of starting at the beginning and finishing at the end, we suggest that you start by flicking through the contents of the entire book and then move backwards and forwards through the various chapters according to your own needs as a student.

You should start exploring this book by reading through the contents list and getting an overview of the focus of each chapter. This is similar to the way that you might browse through the contents of a magazine. You should then skim swiftly through each chapter in order to gain a general understanding of the material covered in that section. Again, this is similar to the way that you might flick through a magazine in order to get a general overview of the different articles. Pay particular attention to headings and subheadings within the chapters as these will often give you an indication of the key topics covered in the text. It is often a good idea to ask yourself at the end of each chapter 'What does this chapter tell me?' If you can answer this question, move on to skim through the next chapter. If you cannot answer this question, skim back through the chapter.

Once you have a basic knowledge of the general contents, return to the start of the book and begin reading chapters of interest in more depth. You will notice that each chapter starts with a set of learning outcomes. These outcomes tell you what you should be able to do by the time you reach the end of the chapter. Once you have finished reading that chapter, return to the learning outcomes and ask yourself whether you can now meet these outcomes. If not, reread the chapter with the learning outcomes in mind.

Although it is not necessary to read this book from beginning to end, the chapters in this book are set out in a specific order to aid your learning. The first chapter is designed to provide you with a basic understanding of the therapeutic process, the following four chapters each focus on one of the core approaches with an associated therapy, and the final chapter describes several integrative/eclectic therapies. After skimming through the entire book, it is a good idea to start reading more thoroughly in the first chapter. This chapter will help you to establish a basic understanding of therapy in general. It is also a good idea to cover the chapters focusing on the four core approaches (Chapters 2–5) before exploring the integrative and eclectic therapies (Chapter 6). However, as noted above, there is no 'correct' order in which you should read this book – feel free to skim, flick forward, turn back, reread and jump sections according to your own desire for knowledge. Every chapter is self-contained and can be easily understood if read independently. However, the chapters are also designed to support each other and information can often be appreciated at a deeper level if you have first read the content of a previous chapter. This means that there may be occasions when you want to return to an earlier chapter to remind yourself about a key concept and this is highly recommended to support your learning process. For example, before starting the final chapter on integrative and eclectic therapies, you might want to reread the last section of the first chapter as this defines the concepts of integration and eclecticism.

Once you have read all of the chapters, you could reflect on the whole book by skimming through the summary tables. You will notice that every section in every chapter concludes with a summary table which contains all of the content for that section distilled into a set of key words. Consider these summary tables after you have finished reading the book. Look over the key words in order to check knowledge (can you explain and expand on every key term?), understand associations (do you appreciate the links between different topics?) and revise content (can you use these words as an aid to memory?).

IS THERE A DIFFERENCE BETWEEN AN APPROACH AND A THERAPY?

There is indeed a difference between an approach and a therapy, and this will be addressed in more detail in Chapter 1. However, it is good to get a basic understanding of this distinction before starting the book.

An approach could be described as the umbrella term for all theories and concepts converging on a similar set of principles. For example, the humanistic approach includes several theories relating to the positive nature of humans, the tendency towards self-actualisation and the importance of viewing the individual as the expert on the self. Theories and direction of focus may differ between different contributors to the approach, but the key principles are usually similar. For example, under the humanistic umbrella, Rogers focuses on the concept of congruence between the actual self and the self-concept whereas Maslow focuses on movement up the hierarchy of needs, but both theorists agree on the basic principle of self-actualisation.

Therapy could be described as the practical application of an approach. Several different therapies can operate under a single approach and each therapy may apply the theories within the approach in a slightly different manner, but all of the therapies under a single approach will share a common philosophy of human nature. For example, it is argued that both person-centred therapy and existential therapy operate under the humanistic approach because the core assumptions about human nature are similarly humanistic for each therapeutic application.

DOES THIS BOOK COVER ALL OF THE DIFFERENT APPROACHES AND THERAPIES?

There are far too many approaches and therapies in existence to be able to successfully describe them all in any one book. It is also important to note that practitioners are constantly developing new therapeutic methods so there could be several new methods created in the short space of time between writing this introduction and publishing this textbook.

This book focuses on four core approaches in psychology and ten different therapies. These four approaches were selected because they are generally agreed to be the most common perspectives in psychology. The therapies associated with each approach are regarded as the most typical examples of that approach. The remaining therapies presented in the final chapter of this book demonstrate interesting examples of integration and eclecticism.

WHAT ARE THE FOUR 'CORE' APPROACHES?

The four core approaches presented in this textbook are the three 'forces' and single 'revolution' in psychology. The three forces are numbered according to their impact on the field of psychology. Behaviourism and psychodynamic theory are regarded as the first two forces because they initially dominated the field until the humanistic perspective was introduced as a third perspective in psychology. In this textbook, however, we present the three forces in reverse order (humanistic, psychodynamic, behavioural). There are three reasons for covering these approaches in this order.

First, one of the most popular current forms of therapy combines the behavioural and cognitive approaches to produce cognitive-behaviour therapy. However, although they are commonly practised together, theoretically they are quite distinct with an independent background and development. It is important to achieve a firm grounding in the theories and concepts underpinning each before moving on to explore the combined application of cognitive-behaviour therapy (the combined approach is covered in full in Chapter 6). In order to fully understand how these two approaches are integrated, it is sensible to consider the two approaches consecutively. It was, therefore, logical to reverse the three forces so that the chapter on behaviourism precedes the chapter on the cognitive revolution.

Second, the humanistic approach often forms the foundation for all types of therapy. Almost all practitioners, irrespective of their own individual approach to psychotherapy, appreciate the importance of the therapeutic relationship. All modern therapies emphasise the value of the therapist adopting a non-judgemental attitude towards the client and highlight the benefits of ensuring that the client assumes responsibility for his or her own life. These are all key assumptions of the humanistic approach so it is logical for the reader to understand the basic principles of this approach before being introduced to alternative therapies.

Third, the humanistic approach provides an excellent therapeutic foundation for student readers. We are not suggesting that students should begin with this approach because it is the easiest. In fact, the humanistic approach is arguably the most difficult type of therapy given that the therapist is required to simply be with the client without being able to rely on activities and exercises to fill the time. However, although it is not the easiest, this approach is arguably the least destructive. As with many practical skills, one can only learn how to counsel effectively by engaging in the act of therapy. Unfortunately, there is a circular problem associated with this learning requirement: we should not risk the wellbeing of the client with an untrained therapist and yet all therapists need to practise therapy in order to train. The learner therapist intending to adopt a particular approach at the start of his or her training would be well advised to begin from a person-centred perspective. Unlike those therapies which may involve interpretation (psychoanalytic) or exposure to fears (behaviour therapy), the non-judgemental and non-advisory methods of person-centred therapy are least likely to do any harm to the client. For this reason, it is logical for the reader to be introduced to the humanistic approach at the start of his or her training.

WHY DOES THIS BOOK FOCUS ON BIOGRAPHIES OF KEY FIGURES?

We would argue that people who wish to pursue a career in therapy should have an interest in the lives of others. Therapists are frequently exposed to the life stories of others and invited to explore the significance of key events, so it is logical to assume that they should appreciate the importance of how beliefs and values are influenced by life history. This appreciation can significantly improve understanding of the core approaches in psychotherapy; the reader can link biographical information to the perspectives of the key figure in order to understand the development of the approach in a historical context. It can be very difficult to understand some of the nuances of an approach without appreciating the origin of these concepts. For example, biographical details relating to the early childhood of Sigmund Freud give us an important understanding of his relationship with his mother and this context helps us to appreciate his theories relating to the Oedipus conflict. Instead of seeing a man who has plucked some apparently strange ideas out of thin air, we are able to see someone who has analytically reflected on his own feelings as a child in order to devise a theory to explain human nature. In this way, the biographies of these crucial figures help us to see how the key events in their life stories interact with the development of the theory.

We have carefully selected the biographies of those who have had a fundamental impact on the therapeutic approach. We do appreciate the significant contribution of modern theorists who may be shaping the current face of therapy, and we have incorporated many modern theories and concepts throughout this textbook. However, in terms of biographies, we have specifically focused on those who are generally regarded as the founding fathers of the approach. This focus will give you a unique insight into the original grounding of the theories in the appropriate historical and personal context.

WHY DOES THIS BOOK INCLUDE CASE STUDIES FOR EACH APPROACH?

The reader will notice that each chapter ends with a novel case study involving a client presenting with a set of concerns and a therapist addressing these concerns using the therapy discussed in that particular chapter. Since each therapy is best suited for certain types of difficulties, each case study is unique in order to ensure that the examples provided are as clear as possible. To help the reader understand the work of the therapist, the case study will start with a brief description of the client presentation, including their self-reported history and symptoms. The reader will then be provided with a description of the session and a series of questions to direct the reader towards any crucial parts of the interaction. This session can be viewed by watching the associated video content of the therapy session in action, and a full written transcript of the session is available in the online resources. Please note that these videos depict REAL interactions; although the session has been arranged for the purposes of the video and the sessions will not continue after the recording, the interaction within the session is genuine. Neither individual is acting – the therapist is a qualified practitioner in that specific type of therapy and the client is reporting genuine experiences and emotions. The case study section of the chapter will conclude with a reflective report about the session from the perspective of the client. This will provide the reader with an insight into the client experience of each type of therapy.

The aim of these case studies is to provide the reader with a real-world example of therapy in action. Unlike many other fields of psychology, counselling and psychotherapy are not exclusively academic. In order to fully understand therapeutic approaches and methods, the reader must appreciate how these concepts can be applied in interactions with clients. The best way to present these interactions is in the form of case studies and we hope that readers are able to use these examples in order to further their own understanding and practice of counselling and psychotherapy.

We would now like to end this introduction by wishing you happy reading. We hope that this textbook serves as a knowledgeable guide on your journey through the fascinating subject of human nature. Perhaps more importantly, we hope that this book will inspire you to further your own learning experience by using your newfound understanding to support, encourage and assist your fellow man. To misquote the eminent Carl Rogers, education is a direction, not a destination.

Chapter 1

Counselling and psychotherapy

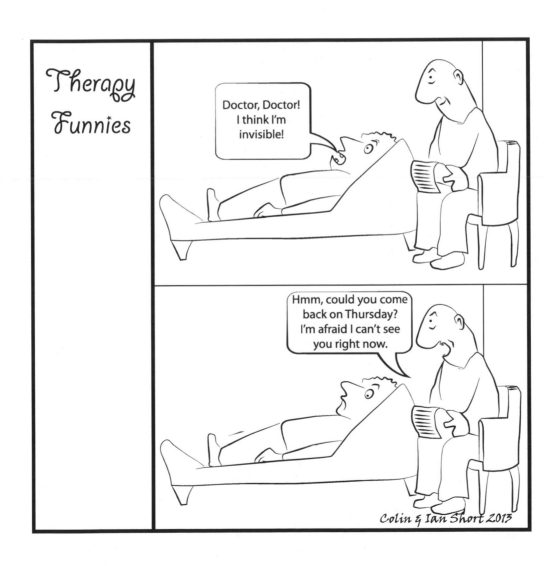

CHAPTER CONTENTS

- Introduction to counselling and psychotherapy

- Defining counselling and psychotherapy
  - Definitions of counselling and psychotherapy
  - Differences between counselling and psychotherapy
  - Career paths in counselling and psychotherapy

- Therapist and client roles in the therapeutic relationship
  - Differences between helping and therapy
  - Role of the client in therapy
  - Role of the therapist in therapy
  - Relationship between therapist and client
  - Therapy in the modern world

- Boundaries and ethics in the therapeutic relationship
  - Boundaries in therapy
  - Therapeutic contract
  - Ethical guidelines

- Appreciating diversity in the therapeutic relationship
  - Cultural assumptions in mainstream therapy
  - Multiculturalism in the therapeutic relationship
  - Self-reflection to recognise bias and prejudice
  - Criticism of multicultural therapy
  - Working holistically

- Approaches, therapies and models
  - Defining approaches, therapies, and models
  - Purist versus non-purist perspectives
  - Integration and eclecticism versus syncretism
  - Types of integration and eclecticism
  - Egan's skilled helper model

INTRODUCTION TO COUNSELLING AND PSYCHOTHERAPY

This chapter aims to introduce the reader to the concepts of counselling and psychotherapy. Key concepts such as ethical issues and sociocultural diversity will be explored in this chapter. You will also be introduced to the idea of counselling and psychotherapy as career options and provided with a clear route to becoming a therapist in the UK. It is impossible to develop a good understanding of any specific therapy without first understanding the field in general, so this introductory chapter will provide you with a general overview of the fascinating field of counselling and psychotherapy.

> ## LEARNING OUTCOMES
>
> By the end of this chapter, you will be able to:
> - appreciate the differences and similarities between the fields of counselling, psychotherapy and psychology
> - discuss the different roles of the therapist and the client in the therapeutic relationship
> - acknowledge the importance of maintaining boundaries and outline the ethical issues associated with therapy
> - appreciate the differences between an approach, therapy and model, and discuss each of these with consideration of the differing methods adopted by practitioners

DEFINING COUNSELLING AND PSYCHOTHERAPY

> ## LEARNING OUTCOMES
>
> After reading this section, you will be able to:
> - outline the definitions of counselling
> - appreciate the differences between counselling and psychotherapy
> - recognise the career possibilities in the field of counselling and psychotherapy

Definitions of counselling and psychotherapy

UK versus US

American spelling = Counseling

British spelling = Counselling

Simplicity

For the sake of simplicity, this textbook will focus on 'counselling' (British spelling) whenever the term is used. However, in general, this book will use the terms 'therapy' and 'therapist' to refer to all aspects of the therapeutic encounter.

What are counselling and psychotherapy?

British Association for Counselling and Psychotherapy (BACP) definition of counselling and psychotherapy

'Counselling and psychotherapy are umbrella terms that cover a range of talking therapies. They are delivered by trained practitioners who work with people over a short or long term to help them bring about effective change or enhance their wellbeing.' (BACP, 2013)

British Psychological Society (BPS) definition of counselling

'Counselling is concerned with the interplay between psychological principles and the counselling process and is developed by substantial reflection on practice and research. Its understandings derive both from formal psychological enquiry and from the interpersonal relationships between practitioner and the client.' (BPS, 2013)

American Psychological Association (APA) definition of counselling

'Counseling psychology centers on typical or normal developmental issues as well as atypical or disordered development as it applies to human experience from individual, family, group, systems and organizational perspectives. Counseling psychologists help people with physical, emotional and mental disorders improve wellbeing, alleviate distress and maladjustment, and resolve crises. In addition, practitioners in this professional specialty provide assessment, diagnosis and treatment of psychopathology.' (APA, 2013)

World Health Organization (WHO) definition of counselling

'Counselling provides a supportive and non-judgemental atmosphere for people to talk over their problems and explore more satisfactory ways of living.' (WHO, 2013)

To summarise, counselling and psychotherapy include the following:

Collaborative relationship between therapist and client

Client seeks to enhance his or her emotional or psychological wellbeing

Therapist seeks to provide a supportive environment in which the client can work towards seeking to enhance his or her emotional or psychological wellbeing

What does a therapist do?

Essentially, a therapist will provide support to those in need by offering a safe non-judgemental environment in which the client can explore his or her own issues

Specifically, a therapist may offer support for distinct clients and/or problems

Client groups may include:

Individuals

Groups

Families

Spouses/partners

Children

Adolescents

Adults

Older adults

Employees

Students

Problem types may include:

Depression

Stress

Anxiety

Low self-esteem

Low confidence

Poor anger management

Insomnia

Eating disorders

Addictions

Marital or relationship difficulties

Sexual disfunctions

Employment issues

Financial concerns

Prior trauma or abuse

Bereavement

Modern public perception is much more positive towards therapy

British Association for Counselling and Psychotherapy (2010a) conducted a wide-scale review of public attitudes towards counselling and psychotherapy

Meta-analysis of current research in the field followed up by a telephone survey of 1440 adults in the UK

21% of respondents had consulted a counsellor in the past

88% of respondents agreed that consultation with a counsellor might make many people happier

What happens in counselling and psychotherapy sessions?

Therapy sessions can vary depending on the orientation of the therapist, issues raised by the client, and demands of the service in which the therapy is offered. However, in general, most therapy will follow this pattern

Initial contact made by a referral agent or the client

Client registers by completing an initial written assessment (usually in the form of a questionnaire)

Client attends an initial meeting to assess his or her needs – risk assessments will also be completed at this time and further referrals may be made if the client is deemed unsuited for the specific type of therapy

Client is allocated to an appropriate therapist (may be the therapist from the initial assessment) or added to a waiting list for the next available therapist (if the service is particularly busy)

Client attends a first session with the therapist

> First session typically involves information gathering and contracting – client is invited to tell his or her story, therapist will outline important policies and procedures (including confidentiality), and relationship boundaries will be established

Client attends a series of sessions to work through his or her issues

> Each session will typically last for one 'therapeutic hour' (50 minutes)
>
> Sessions will often run once per week for an agreed time frame
>
> Short-term therapy might run for as little as six weeks; long-term therapy could run for years

If possible, client is given advance warning in the penultimate session so that the relationship can be drawn to a satisfactory close

Client attends the final session with the therapist

> Final session typically involves reflection on progress and ending the relationship
>
> Client is encouraged to consider how s/he has changed during the therapy and to think about how life will continue beyond the therapeutic relationship
>
> Both parties express their feelings about the end of the therapeutic relationship

Client is asked to complete another written assessment (questionnaire) to determine the impact of the therapy and may also be asked to complete an evaluation of the service

Ending the therapeutic relationship can be difficult

> Both client and/or therapist are entitled to end the relationship at any time if it is felt that it is no longer providing any therapeutic benefit
>
> In the ideal scenario, client and therapist agree on a set number of sessions, complete the therapeutic process within those allotted sessions, and part on good terms with a positive ending
>
> However, it is often the case that therapy ends under less ideal circumstances
>
> > Clients may seek to end the therapy if they are not ready to address issues – ending therapy can be an effective way of avoiding difficult emotional investigations
> >
> > Therapists may feel that the client is no longer benefiting from therapy but the client may be reluctant to be entirely independent
> >
> > In both of these cases, the relationship end must be carefully managed by the therapist to encourage positive closure and ensure that the door remains open for the client to return to therapy in the future

How does a client access a therapist?

There are many ways in which an individual can obtain counselling support

Referral by a GP or other health practitioner

Often the GP is the first point of contact for an individual who is struggling with his or her mental wellbeing

BACP (2010a) found that a GP or health practitioner had referred 65% of those receiving therapy

Referral by a tutor, teacher, lecturer or employer

It is possible for an authority figure to submit a referral on behalf of someone in his or her care – for example, a tutor may refer a student to the student counselling service

This is less common as most therapeutic services insist on initial requests from the client rather than a third party

BACP (2010a) found that employers had referred only 7% of those receiving therapy

Self-referral

Any individuals struggling with their own mental wellbeing can seek support from independent agencies advertised through websites, public directories, etc.

This approach carries the risk of self-referral to an inappropriate or illegitimate agency so it is important for individuals to check that the organisation is a member of a relevant governing body (like the BPS or BACP), employs only those who have been professionally trained and hold the relevant professional accreditations, and has full counselling insurance

BACP (2010a) found that 9% of those receiving therapy found a therapist independently through a public directory

Where do therapists work?

Sadly, there is a lack of employment opportunities available for those who qualify as therapists

Many students have a specific job in mind and they are pursuing a career in therapy in order to do this job

However, unless you are completely aware of exactly where you could apply for work and, more importantly, who will pay for this work, you may discover that your dream job does not actually exist

For example, some students decide that they want to work with adolescent girls who are suffering with eating disorders – however, once they qualify as a therapist, they discover that there is no such organisation in their area so there are no paid positions available with this focus

Assuming that you aim to work full time as a therapist, it is essential that you ask yourself 'who will pay me to do this job?'

Five main ways (other ways do exist but are less common) in which one can have gainful employment in counselling or psychotherapy in the UK

Care agencies

Most therapists work as paid or unpaid volunteers for organisations responsible for providing care to those experiencing specific difficulties, such as substance misuse, bereavement, etc.

Unpaid volunteering in care agencies is particularly popular with trainee therapists or recently qualified therapists working towards full accreditation with a professional body (you need a certain number of hours to gain accreditation)

Healthcare providers

Many therapists work with clients through healthcare organisations based in hospitals, general practices and community healthcare centres

88% of respondents in a telephone survey of 1440 adults in the UK felt that counselling should be available on the National Health Service (BACP, 2010a)

Education settings

Student therapists are widely available in university and college settings, and many schools now often fund a small service employing one or two therapists

Workplaces

Many large companies offer in-house confidential counselling services for employees

This recent move towards offering therapy through human resources is a positive step for therapy, especially since the BACP (2010a) survey suggests that 53% of employed respondents feel stressed by their jobs and 54% feel that the workplace should offer confidential counselling services

Private practice

Some therapists establish their own practices to support private paying clients

The BACP (2010a) survey found that 65% of respondents would be willing to pay for therapy

Legal loopholes in the UK today mean that any individual can open a practice, irrespective of qualifications or accreditation

It is absolutely essential that clients ensure that the selected therapist is qualified (at least a diploma, Bachelors or Master's degree in counselling or psychotherapy), accredited by a professional body (BPS, BACP, UKCP, etc.), and fully insured to practise as a therapist

Differences between counselling and psychotherapy

Psychology, counselling and psychotherapy

CLINICAL PSYCHOLOGIST

Clinical psychologists often work with individuals suffering severe physical or mental disorders and impairments

Clinical psychologists can be defined by focusing on the concept of the 'clinic' – it involves treatment of patients usually in a clinical setting

Clinical psychologists often work alongside medical doctors and neurologists to treat a patient population in health and social care settings (often the NHS)

COUNSELLING PSYCHOLOGIST

Counselling psychologists often work with individuals, couples or families experiencing mental health concerns

Counselling psychologists work in many different locations to support patients and non-patients in healthcare, prison, industry, education, etc.

Minimal difference in job role between clinical and counselling psychologists and many job adverts ask for either type of qualified individual

COUNSELLOR/PSYCHOTHERAPIST

At the present time, there is no recognised distinction between these two titles as both involve the same work role and accreditation process

Counsellors and psychotherapists often work with individuals, couples or families experiencing concerns and worries, or needing space to explore their own thoughts and feelings

Minimal difference in job role between counsellor/psychotherapist and counselling psychologist, although in practice it is often the case that the counselling psychologist will work with those who have significant mental health issues whereas the counsellor/psychotherapist will work with the 'worried well'

PSYCHIATRIST

Psychiatry is substantially different from psychology, counselling and psychotherapy

Psychiatrists are based on the medical model

> Psychiatrists are medical doctors with a specialism in mental health

> Psychiatrists work with patients in the health service

> Psychiatrists can diagnose, treat and medicate patients

Career paths in counselling and psychotherapy

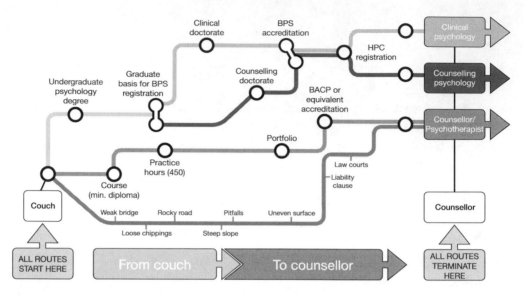

FIGURE 1.1 **Couch to counsellor.**

Important note

Please note that the information contained in this chapter is in accordance with current regulations in the UK in 2012 – please check on the websites of the relevant accrediting bodies for the most up-to-date information.

Clinical psychologist

Health Professions Council (HPC)

> You must register with the HPC to be a chartered clinical psychologist

>> Health Professions Council is the governmental body responsible for governing all protected titles

>> You must register with the HPC to use the legally protected title 'clinical psychologist'

>> Registration with the HPC requires you to submit evidence of having completed an approved course (clinical psychology doctorate)

British Psychological Society (BPS)

> You should register with the BPS to be an accredited clinical psychologist

>> British Psychological Society is the governing body for psychologists in the UK

>> Registration with the BPS requires you to complete a doctorate (PhD) in clinical psychology (accredited by BPS)

>> Highly competitive programme – usually need a BPS-accredited first-class degree and possibly a Master's in psychology

Counselling psychologist

Health Professions Council (HPC)

You must register with the HPC to be a chartered counselling psychologist

Health Professions Council is the governmental body responsible for governing all protected titles

You must register with the HPC to use the legally protected title 'counselling psychologist'

Registration with the HPC requires you to submit evidence of having completed an approved course (counselling psychology doctorate)

British Psychological Society (BPS)

You should register with the BPS to be an accredited counselling psychologist

British Psychological Society is the governing body for psychologists in the UK

Registration with the BPS requires you to complete a doctorate (PhD) in counselling psychology (accredited by BPS) or the BPS Qualification in Counselling Psychology (QCoP)

Highly competitive programme – usually need a BPS-accredited first-class degree and possibly a Master's in psychology

Counsellor/psychotherapist

Health Professions Council (HPC)

Counsellor is not a legally protected title in the UK so you do not have to register with the HPC

Anyone can work as a counsellor, irrespective of qualifications or membership of professional bodies

In February 2011, the UK government recommended a system of voluntary registration and recommended that statutory regulation of titles only be considered when voluntary registers are not sufficient to manage risk

In March 2011, the UK government confirmed that it was not its intention to proceed with the statutory regulation of psychotherapists and counsellors

HOWEVER . . .

Although it is not compulsory to hold the title with the HPC, it is recommended that counsellors and psychotherapists hold appropriate qualifications and 'volunteer' to register with appropriate professional organisations

In the absence of qualifications and professional accreditation, counsellors and psychotherapists are unable to get insurance, thus making them vulnerable to risk

British Association for Counselling and Psychotherapy (BACP)

>   You could register with the BACP to be an accredited counsellor

>>   British Association of Counselling and Psychotherapy is the governing body for counsellors and psychotherapists (no distinction) in the UK

>>   Registration with the BACP requires you to complete an accredited or equivalent course (minimum diploma level), complete 450 hours of practice in a supervised placement, and submit a detailed portfolio demonstrating reflection and continuous professional development

>   Arguably, the most common route to becoming an accredited counsellor

OR

>   Any other professional body for counselling and/or psychotherapy

>>   Specific therapies may have their own professional bodies that can offer an appropriate level of accreditation

>>   For example, the British Association for the Person-Centred Approach (BAPCA) or the British Association for Behavioural and Cognitive Psychotherapies (BABCP)

>>   These routes usually follow specific training courses for that therapeutic orientation, rather than general counselling/psychotherapy courses

>>   If searching for a professional body, students should look for those that are recognised at a national level and have their own set of ethical guidelines to which practitioners are expected to adhere

DECISIONS, DECISIONS . . .

It can be difficult to decide which career to pursue, especially since clinical psychology, counselling psychology and counselling/psychotherapy all seem very similar yet require very different training plans.

It is advisable to work backwards in order to identify the appropriate path. Try following these steps to form a personal career plan.

1. Search for your dream job as though you are ready to apply today. Consider websites, newspapers, etc.
2. Identify a job that meets your needs – look at the job description and/or contact the employer to find out exactly what you will be doing on a daily basis.
3. Once you have found an advert for your dream job, look for the job specification (may be titled 'essential/desirable requirements').
4. Identify the required qualifications for this job – do they want a BACP accredited counsellor? BPS accredited counselling psychologist? BPS accredited

clinical psychologist? Write out a plan to gain the relevant qualifications and accreditation to meet those job requirements.

5.   Identify the required skills for this job – do they want you to have good teamwork skills or communications skills or information technology skills? Think about your experiences to date and try to find examples of your abilities to excel in these skills. If you cannot identify any experiences to demonstrate some of the skills, write out a plan to gain experiences that demonstrate your abilities to excel in those skills. People often ignore these skills until they are looking for a job and then they struggle to find past experiences to demonstrate the required skills – it is better to think about these in advance so that you can begin working towards bolstering your weaker skills.

6.   Pull together your plans to set out actions for gaining your dream job!

Although this specific job is unlikely to still be available when you have gained all of the relevant qualifications and skills, you will be in a good position to find other similar roles.

SUMMARY

Counselling and psychotherapy definition: BACP, BPS, APA, WHO; collaborative, supportive, enhance emotional or psychological wellbeing; therapist offers safe non-judgemental environment to explore own issues; client access through health practitioner, teacher/employer or self-referral; often consists of 50-minute session once per week for a time-limited period; therapists work in care agencies, healthcare organisations, education establishments, workplaces, private practices

Differences: clinical psychologist (patients with mental and physical disorders), counselling psychologist (patients and clients with mental health disorders), counsellor/psychotherapist (worried well clients), psychiatrist (medical doctor with mental health specialism)

Careers: clinical and counselling psychologists must register with HPC (legally protected title) and gain accreditation with BPS (doctorate), counsellor/psychotherapists not required to register with HPC (not legally protected) but should register with professional body like BACP (diploma, 450 hours practice, portfolio)

THERAPIST AND CLIENT ROLES IN THE THERAPEUTIC RELATIONSHIP

LEARNING OUTCOMES

After reading this section, you will be able to:

- differentiate between helping and therapy
- outline the role of the client
- outline the role of the therapist
- discuss the nature of the relationship between the client and the therapist
- debate the nature and value of therapy in the modern world

Differences between helping and therapy

Therapy and helping may differ in many key areas

      Contract

      Boundaries

      Direction

      Advice

      Criticism

      Equality

      Outcome

Contract

Therapy involves a short-term therapeutic agreement (formal or informal) between the client and the therapist

Other forms of helping may not involve a specific contract for the helper to provide personal support

For example, one friend may help another friend by listening to his worries, but they have not agreed to a specific therapeutic contract

Boundaries

Therapy involves a distinct type of relationship defined by strict boundaries and a code of ethics

Other forms of helping may not involve such strict boundaries or include a formal code of ethics

For example, a hairdresser may help a client by listening to her problems, but he is not abiding by a professional code of ethics

Direction

Therapy is often non-directive (particularly person-centred), and even those approaches that involve some direction (such as cognitive-behaviour therapy) will try to promote client-led activity whenever possible

Other forms of helping will usually involve the individual being directed towards a specific activity/goal/aim, etc.

For example, a debt advisor may help a client by telling them to set up a low-interest loan specifically to reach the goal of making the overall debt more manageable

Advice

Therapy does not usually involve the provision of advice – many people experience some confusion about therapy as they may expect the therapist to act as an expert offering specific advice and guidance, but this is very rarely the case in a therapeutic relationship

Other forms of helping will usually involve the individual being given advice or guidance on the most effective way to solve a problem or achieve a goal

For example, a teacher may help a student by advising them on how to revise in order to successfully pass an exam

Criticism

Therapy does not usually involve criticism, although it can be challenging for the client

Other forms of helping may use constructive criticism to highlight areas for improvement or motivate further action

For example, a personal trainer may help a client by criticising them in order to motivate them to work harder in the gym

Equality

Therapy involves equality between therapist and client – it is essential that the relationship between the therapist and client remain equal throughout the therapeutic process in order for the client to take ownership of their own growth and development

Other forms of helping may involve a power imbalance as the helper holds more expert power than the person being helped

For example, a lecturer may help a student in many ways but the relationship is always imbalanced because the lecturer has the power to award good or bad grades

Outcome

Therapy does not have a guaranteed outcome – it frequently focuses on the self-exploratory journey rather than the eventual destination, and goals established at the start may not be the desired outcome by the end of the process

Other forms of helping may set a specific outcome at the start and the relationship may be considered a failure if this outcome is not met by the end

For example, a dietitian may help a client by instructing them to eat a wheat-free diet to alleviate allergies and this will have a successful outcome provided that the client follows the advice

Distinctions between therapy, guidance and advice (Sutton & Stewart, 2002)

Advice

> Persuasive one-way exchange involving the advice-giver offering an opinion, making a judgement or making a recommendation

Guidance

> Encouraging a one-way exchange involving the guide showing the way, educating, influencing or instructing

Therapy

> Facilitative two-way collaborative and supportive relationship that allows clients to explore their problem, understand their problem and resolve or come to terms with their problem

> Therapists should not give advice as this would result in the therapist taking control of the life of the client rather than the client learning to control his/her own life (Sutton & Stewart, 2002)

HELPING VERSUS THERAPY

Consider the following literary and film figures – each of these characters adopted the role of 'helper' in some shape or form. Do you think that these characters could be classed as 'therapists'?

> John Keating in *Dead Poets Society*
>
> Emma Woodhouse in *Emma*
>
> Yoda in *Star Wars*
>
> Albert Pennyworth in *Batman*
>
> Annie Sullivan in *The Miracle Worker*
>
> Patch Adams in *Patch Adams*
>
> Clarence in *It's A Wonderful Life*
>
> Amelie in *Amelie*
>
> The caterpillar in *Alice in Wonderland*

Role of the client in therapy

Reasons for attending therapy

Many people visit a therapist for many different reasons

> Clients may be suffering with a disorder such as depression, or have experienced a recent life event such as divorce, or be coping with a previous trauma such as bereavement, or simply be finding it difficult to make their own way through life without support

Most clients are not mentally ill and do not have a specific diagnosis

> Therapists use the term 'client' because this implies that they are accessing a service, rather than 'patient' because this implies that they have a disorder

> Client is often regarded as the 'worried well'

Clients may simply need somewhere safe to voice their feelings

> It is remarkably difficult to find a confidential and non-judgemental ear

> Many people know that friends and family want the best for them so they may find it difficult to avoid offering advice or opinions when you share your thoughts

> Many people do not want to burden others with their problems, especially since others have their own difficulties

> Many people feel that others may judge them if they are completely honest, and this is likely to be true if the disclosure presents them in a negative light

> Many people feel that others do not have time to listen to them talk (and they are often right)

> Therapy involves an hour of time dedicated to focusing on your problems without fear of judgement or future consequences of disclosure

'Counselling is a wonderful twentieth-century invention. We live in a complex, busy, changing world. In this world, there are many different types of experience that are difficult for people to cope with. Most of the time we get on with life, but sometimes we are stopped in our tracks by an event or situation that we do not, at that moment, have the resources to sort out. Most of the time, we find ways of dealing with such problems in living by talking to family, friends, neighbours, priests, or our family doctor. But occasionally their advice is not sufficient, or we are too embarrassed or ashamed to tell them what is bothering us, or we just don't have an appropriate person to turn to. Counselling is a really useful option at these moments.' (McLeod, 2003)

Carl Jung was once asked by his grandson how people coped before there were therapists and Jung replied, 'They had friends' (Spicer, n.d., cited in Sills, 2006)

High-risk clients

Most new clients will be asked to complete an initial assessment in the introductory therapy session or before attending the first therapy session

> Clinical Outcomes in Routine Evaluation Outcome Measure (CORE-OM) is a common measure for a therapeutic assessment

Assessments are designed to do the following

> Outline the current state of the client to provide the therapist with a preliminary understanding of the mental condition of the client

> Provide a measure by which the therapy can be evaluated – the client will often be asked to complete the same assessment again at the end of the therapeutic relationship to determine the impact of the therapy

> Identify any potential risk factors

Possible risk factors include the following

> Client is likely to engage in self-harm or attempt suicide

> Client is suffering harm or potential harm from another person

> Client is likely to attempt to hurt others (especially vulnerable others such as a child)

> Client is aware of harm or potential harm to others (especially vulnerable others such as a child)

Assessing the risk associated with a client can be a difficult task

> Often difficult to identify expressions or behaviours indicating genuine risk

> Client may say 'he makes me so angry that I could kill him'

>> This expression could be perceived as a flippant turn of phrase designed to exaggerate feelings of anger without any genuine intention to cause harm

>> This expression could be interpreted as a genuine threat to kill

> Client could self-harm by snapping an elastic band against the skin or making small nicks in the back of the arm with a clean knife

>> These actions could be perceived as the first steps towards more significant self-harm

>> These actions could be perceived as a way of dealing with difficulties in a non-life-threatening manner and this could prevent the client from reaching higher levels of emotional intensity and causing more significant self-damage

> In both of these cases, the therapist will need to take all factors into consideration to decide whether the client is high risk

If a client is identified as high risk, the therapist may need to implement certain policies and procedures

> Therapist may need to discuss the case with other professionals to decide on an appropriate course of action

> Therapist may need to establish some safe practice guidelines, such as not working alone with the client

> Therapist may need to breach confidentiality to report the client to the appropriate authorities

Client expectations

Managing expectations is essential to ensure that the client understands the possibilities afforded by therapy and does not expect something that cannot be delivered

Most client dissatisfaction is caused by a lack of understanding of the true nature of therapy and this could be addressed by exploring expectations in the first session

Common inaccurate client expectations include the following

'Therapy will fix/cure me'

Therapy is not a magic wand

Therapy can be highly effective in supporting the client to address his or her own problems, but there are no guaranteed outcomes

Therapy is definitely not a quick and easy fix – it will take time and effort on the part of the client

Risks associated with this inaccurate expectation are that clients will disengage once they realise that they are not being 'fixed'

Other risks are that clients are referred to the service (by doctors, family, friends, court orders, etc.) with the expectation that this will be a cure

'My therapist is responsible for making me better'

Although the therapist is responsible for many things (such as the provision of a safe non-judgemental environment), the client is responsible for his or her own self-development

Client must be willing to engage with therapy and recognise that therapy involves work during and between sessions

This causes a huge problem during enforced therapy (such as court-ordered therapy) because the individual has not chosen to attend therapy so s/he is unlikely to engage with the process

'Therapy is an opportunity to have a little chat'

Therapy is hard work

Client must strive to address life issues and this can often be difficult and stressful

Therapist is likely to be challenging during the sessions and this can be difficult for the client to accept

Therapy should certainly not be a friendly little chat designed to make the client feel good about him/herself – instead, it should be hard work on the part of both client and therapist as they seek to explore and address difficult topics

'My therapist will be on call 24/7 in the event of an emergency'

Boundaries must be established at the start of the therapeutic relationship to ensure that the client does not assume that the therapist will be constantly available

This can be very difficult in the event of an emergency

It is incredibly heart wrenching to receive a midnight email from a distraught client, but the therapist who responds by inviting the client to an immediate meeting is likely to get the same email again and again (if the client is in immediate risk, the therapist should simply call the emergency services and then relinquish responsibility for that time period)

'Therapy will make me a better person and will ensure that bad things no longer happen to me'

Again, therapy is not a magic wand

Therapy cannot make someone a better person or guarantee that unhappy events will never strike again

However, therapy can help people understand and accept themselves and help them to explore solutions to their problems

'I believe that my therapist is my friend/loves me/desires me because s/he understands me so completely'

There is a risk of romantic affection in any therapeutic relationship, as clients may be surprised by the intense feelings aroused when the therapist genuinely demonstrates an interest in their lives

It is essential that the therapeutic relationship remains professional at all times – the therapist should never take advantage of the position of power and boundaries must be constantly held in place

It is important for therapy to explore the expectations of the client in the initial sessions

It is good practice for a therapist to ask the client what they expect to do in the therapy sessions and what they expect to gain from therapy

Therapist can then address any areas of confusion or inaccurate expectations at the start of the therapeutic relationship to minimise the risk of future problems

Role of the therapist in therapy

Traits of successful therapists

Following a review of hundreds of studies into therapy, Wampold informed an American Psychological Association symposium of the critical traits associated with effective therapists (Whitbourne, 2011)

Sophisticated interpersonal skills

Sensitive cultural awareness

Ability to inspire trust in the therapist and optimism about the therapy

Willingness to form an alliance with the client by explaining the basis of symptoms and developing an agreed treatment plan

Confidence about the therapy and attention to the progress of the therapy

Flexibility to adapt the therapy to the individual

Self-insight to avoid boundary issues

Evidence-based practice and continued professional development

According to the BACP (2010b), therapists should aspire to the following personal qualities

Empathy: ability to communicate understanding of another person's experience from that person's perspective

Sincerity: personal commitment to consistency between what is professed and what is done

Integrity: commitment to being moral in dealings with others, personal straight-forwardness, honesty and coherence

Resilience: capacity to work with the client's concerns without being personally diminished

Respect: demonstrating appropriate esteem to others and their understanding of themselves

Humility: ability to assess accurately and acknowledge one's own strengths and weaknesses

Competence: effective deployment of the skills and knowledge needed to do what is required

Fairness: consistent application of appropriate criteria to inform decisions and actions

Wisdom: possession of sound judgement that informs practice

Courage: capacity to act in spite of known fears, risks and uncertainty

Aspiration, not perfection

These lists of qualities and traits are good for aspiration purposes, but should not be seen as a yardstick for self-beating

You should aspire to develop these traits while recognising that you will never actually be able to demonstrate all these qualities all the time

Values in therapy

Therapists must recognise their own values, beliefs, prejudices, biases, etc.

Every single person holds values, beliefs, prejudices, biases, stereotypes, etc.

Existence in a social and cultural world will naturally lead to these tendencies

From a positive perspective, these tendencies can be helpful heuristics to simplify thinking

From a negative perspective, these tendencies can cause us to make assumptions, draw inaccurate conclusions or treat people unfairly

Since we cannot ever counsel from a completely unbiased position, it is important to recognise our own values in order to acknowledge them if and when they affect our work

Tolerance and respect for others is crucial in effective therapy

> By demonstrating these traits as a therapist, you are modelling these positive life habits for your client to develop

However, if you are unable to work with certain clients or problems, recognise this and acknowledge it as an unavoidable limitation in your client base – do not force yourself to work with those who make you uncomfortable (for example, those who have committed certain crimes)

Therapists must demonstrate good self-care

> No need to be perfect, take time for yourself, do not assume responsibility for client, do not lose yourself in the problems of the client, do not feel obliged to self-disclose to your client, always remember that you are just as important as the client

Supervision

Every practising therapist must undergo regular supervision to support his or her therapeutic work

> Both BPS and BACP guidelines suggest 1.5 hours of supervision for every month in contact with clients (although the BPS does suggest that this should increase in line with caseload)

Therapeutic supervision is a specific relationship designed to support therapists

> The supervisor is NOT assuming the role of a line manager – s/he is not there to make sure that the therapist does a good job

> The supervisor is NOT a therapist for the therapist – s/he is not there to give individual personal therapy to the therapist

> The supervisor IS a professional point of support associated directly with the working life of the therapist

Supervision is essential for supporting the following

> Sharing difficult client experiences

> Exploring own emotional and psychological reactions to clients

> Considering different options for working through client problems

> Gaining a different perspective on client issues

> Investigating possible directions for future continuous professional development

Therapeutic notes

Therapists are strongly advised to keep notes about their clients (client notes)

> Notes can provide a clear record of the relationship for improving recall in later sessions and reflecting on development over time

> 'Practitioners are encouraged to keep appropriate records of their work with clients unless there are adequate reasons for not keeping any records. All records should be accurate, respectful of clients and colleagues and protected from unauthorised disclosure' (BACP, 2010b)

However, therapists are not required by law to keep notes and the level of detail produced in the notes is a matter for debate

Some therapists like to keep detailed client notes . . .

Notes can indicate the client life story, significant events reported by the client, significant events in the relationship with the therapist, thoughts and feelings reported by the client, and thoughts and feelings experienced by the therapist

But there are risks associated with producing detailed client notes . . .

Client notes are not completely confidential because certain individuals and organisations can request or demand access

Client notes should always be professional, appropriate and maintain as much confidentiality as possible to minimise risk

Notes should never include personal insults or slights, unsubstantiated suspicions or beliefs about a client, unsupported claims about the activities of the client

Notes should always be written in a factual manner – it is good practice to report the activities, thoughts and feelings of the client verbatim when possible and indicate that they were reported in such a way by the client him/herself

Certain individuals and organisations are legally entitled to access all client notes

Client has a right of access to his or her own notes under the Data Protection Act 1998 and Freedom of Information Act 2000

But the therapist can insist that the client make a formal request for access to notes and follow a specific access procedure

Courts have a right of access to any available evidence so they can request full disclosure of client notes to the defence and prosecution in civil and criminal proceedings

But therapists can request limited disclosure if they feel that some of the records are not relevant to the case

Courts can also request a report or statement from a therapist or even issue a 'subpoena duces tecum' to bring the therapist to court to give evidence using the original notes

Police may request access to client notes to conduct specific investigations

But police have no right to therapeutic records without a warrant issued by a judge – therapeutic records are exempt from police powers of search and seizure

In these cases, it is advisable to maintain confidentiality, ask the client to request access and disclose personally to the police, or request a court order for disclosure

Solicitors may request access to client notes to support a legal claim

But solicitors have no right to therapeutic records without the explicit permission of the client

In these cases, it is advisable to maintain confidentiality, ask the client to request access and disclose personally to the solicitor, or request a court order for disclosure

For further details on appropriate disclosure of notes, please refer to Bond and Jenkins (2007)

Process notes and supervision notes

In addition to client notes, some therapists may keep notes specifically for personal or supervision purposes

Process notes focus on the therapeutic process with a client

Process notes are completely anonymous with no identifiable detail and little explicit content in relation to the client

Instead, process notes focus on the private thoughts and feelings of the therapist in relation to the sessions and the general process of the therapeutic exchanges

In this context, process notes are more about the therapist than the client so they are not subject to the same disclosure rules as client notes

Supervision notes reflect on the experience of supervision

Although these notes may refer to therapy sessions with clients, they will not contain any specific details about the client and will predominantly focus on the development of the therapist

Supervision notes are not subject to the same disclosure rules as client notes

Limits to confidentiality

Clients should have an opportunity to disclose in a safe, non-judgemental, confidential environment

Confidentiality is essential to ensure that the client feels able to discuss his or her life without restraint

In the absence of confidentiality, the client may lie or withhold information and this can make it very difficult to provide effective therapy

However, there are limits to the provision of confidentiality and all clients should be aware of these limits

Confidentiality may be limited to the organisation, rather than the individual

This means that other members of the organisation may have access to the client notes and may discuss the client case with the therapist

This is often done to allow smooth transfer of clients in the event that the therapist has to temporarily or permanently leave the practice

Confidentiality is unlikely to be maintained during supervision

Although most therapists will not provide identifiable details when discussing cases with a supervisor, it is likely that the case will be presented in sufficient detail to allow discussion during the supervision session

Supervisors are, however, also bound by confidentiality guidelines so this information should travel no further

Confidentiality can be breached in response to a court order

As noted in the section on client notes, the court can insist on the therapist revealing details about the client when this is relevant to the trial

Confidentiality can be breached if the client is identified as high risk

Please refer to the previous section explaining the identification of high-risk clients

If a client is identified as high risk through the initial assessment or during subsequent discussions with the therapist, then it is important to disclose appropriately in order to avoid negative ethical or legal consequences

Therapists have a legal obligation to report any client who is at risk of causing harm to self or others and any suspicion of child abuse or terrorist activity irrespective of whether the client is the victim, perpetrator or other

If the client is an immediate risk to self or others (perhaps even the therapist), in an excited state and/or has already hurt him/herself, then the therapist should immediately telephone the emergency services and explain the situation – the emergency services will probably send an ambulance in the event of harm and the police to escort the client to a place of safety (often a local mental health ward)

If the client indicates an immediate intention to harm self or others but is not in danger at that moment, then the therapist should report the disclosure to the head of the therapy service and the police as soon as possible

If the client indicates a future intention to harm self or others, then the therapist should contact the head of the therapy service to discuss the level of risk in order to decide whether to report the disclosure to the police (if in doubt, it is better to report to the police)

If the client indicates knowledge of or involvement in the current or future harm to a vulnerable other (such as a child), then the therapist must immediately report the disclosure to the head of the therapy service, the social services and the police

If the client is not classed as high risk but discloses something with legal or ethical consequences, then the decision to report the disclosure can be less clear

Walfish et al. (2010) surveyed therapists to reveal that many have experienced the client disclosure of an unprosecuted past crime

13% indicated client self-disclosure of murder

33% indicated client self-disclosure of sexual assault

69% indicated client self-disclosure of physical assault

Therapists are not legally bound to report all disclosures of past criminal activity if there does not appear to be a future risk of harm to self or others

Client confidentiality can be maintained in some of these cases in terms of reporting the disclosure, although the therapist may be forced to disclose in court

In these cases, the therapist must consider their own morals and the ethical guidelines of their professional body

If the client discloses a serious past crime (such as murder, assault, robbery, etc.) for which they or another identified individual have not been tried, then the therapist should carefully assess the risk of repeat offending posed by the client

If the client is deemed likely to offend again, then the therapist should report the disclosure

If the client is deemed unlikely to offend again, then the therapist must make his or her own decisions about whether the disclosure is warranted

In all cases of disclosure, it is a good practice for the therapist to outline the intention to disclose prior to disclosure

Therapists should have initially outlined the confidentiality policy to clients at the start of the therapeutic relationship and should reiterate this policy if it appears that the client is going to disclose something important

If the client continues with the disclosure then it can be assumed that they are aware that the information will be passed on, even if they do not appear to be happy about this at the time

Once the disclosure has been made, the therapist should gently explain that the information will need to be reported, outline exactly who will be contacted, and provide guidance on the likely outcome of the report (only to the extent that the therapist is able to advise)

It is important to consider the possible reaction of the client carefully before expressing an indication to disclose

Although this is a preferred method of disclosure, the therapist should not follow this procedure if the client is likely to respond with aggression or violence

In all cases of disclosure or uncertainty about disclosure, it is advisable for the therapist to take the issue to supervision for further consideration (see next section for details about supervision)

Please note that these general guidelines are not comprehensive and could change over time

If a therapist has a concern about the legal limits to confidentiality then s/he must contact his or her professional body to receive the current guidelines

Relationship between therapist and client

Secure

The therapeutic relationship should be secure

Interactions should be warm and friendly

Rapport between client and therapist is essential

Therapy is unlikely to be successful if the client or therapist feels uncomfortable or dislikes the other party

Client should feel safe in disclosing to the therapist

> Client should trust that the therapist would maintain confidentiality and remain non-judgemental irrespective of the nature of disclosure (within the agreed limits)

> Client must be able to be open and honest with therapist in order to explore issues, and therapist should be honest and congruent in return

Working

The therapeutic relationship should be a working relationship

> Sessions should not be little chats, but rather a structured experience of self-exploration working towards an improved understanding of self and a healthier mental outlook

> > Structure and defined boundaries will help to ensure that the relationship stays at a working level rather than altering to a friend level

> > Client should become more independent over time, not more dependent on the therapist and therapy sessions

Therapy in the modern world

Therapeutic variety

Thousands of therapeutic methods in modern psychological interventions

Each method offers a new insight into human nature and a new set of techniques for improving mental wellbeing

> Some of the less typical methods currently gaining popularity include bibliotherapy, cinema therapy and angel therapy

> These are only three of a vast field of possible approaches and these three have been specifically selected as examples to demonstrate how modern therapy draws from self-help, media and spiritual concepts

BIBLIOTHERAPY

Clients are 'prescribed' books to support them through their problems

Recommended books are typically self-help therapy books containing information about the identified disorder and offering guidance or activities designed to encourage self-exploration and enhance coping skills

Book Prescription Wales is a scheme introduced by the National Health Service to support those with mild to moderate emotional problems by prescribing therapy books (NHS, n.d.)

> Mental health professionals write out a prescription for their recommended book and the patient is able to fill the prescription at the local library

> Systematic review of the effectiveness of bibliotherapy in mental health services suggests that it is beneficial for a range of conditions (Fanner & Urquhart, 2008)

CINEMA THERAPY

Wolz (2013) argues that cinema therapy can be a 'powerful catalyst for healing and growth'

Cinema therapy differs from book therapy because the films used during the treatment are not designed specifically to treat emotional problems (like self-help books), but are instead mainstream films produced for entertainment

> These films offer a creative experience to encourage freedom of thought, feeling and expression, rather than specific guidance on how to solve the emotional problem

Clients are 'prescribed' certain films that are associated with their own problem or emotional state

> For example, a client who is struggling to cope with a divorce might be encouraged to watch *Kramer versus Kramer*

Films offer an opportunity to explore an issue from an objective angle

> For example, the client who watches *Kramer versus Kramer* might be able to see the parallels between the plot and her own experiences and then use this parallel as an opportunity to discuss the situation from a more objective perspective (recognising both points of view to advise the characters)

Films also provide a cathartic release of emotion

> For example, the client who feels that she has to stay strong and not show her emotions about her own situation may have an acceptable outlet for her feelings by reacting to the events in the film

ANGEL THERAPY

Angel therapy combines traditional therapeutic methods with non-denominational spiritual healing

Virtue (2010) proposes that everyone has a guardian angel that seeks to guide him/her down his or her natural spiritual path

> Practitioners use the therapeutic relationship to work with the client to contact their own guardian angel to ask for healing, harmonisation and support

Therapy is generally regarded as pseudoscientific (or entirely non-scientific) and typically ignored in the scientific literature

> Norcross et al. (2006) conducted a Delphi poll (consensus of 101 experts) to identify psychological interventions that are unable to consistently generate treatment outcomes beyond base rates, placebos and time expectancies

> Angel therapy was identified alongside crystal healing, rebirthing therapy and prefrontal lobotomy as a 'certainly discredited' psychological treatment

Interested other

Importance of the therapeutic relationship is a concurrent theme across all therapies, irrespective of the unusual nature of the activities within the treatment

Stiles et al. (2008) suggest that all treatment methods are approximately equivalent in terms of outcome and thus it is the relationship between therapist and client that is the key to effective therapy

Common to all of the traditional (and less traditional) methods is the presence of an interested other

Whether the therapist is trying to identify films that parallel the situation of the client or consulting angels on behalf of the client, the other is showing an interest

> Interested other is listening to the life story of the client, appreciating the magnitude of the problems experienced by the client, and seeking to help the client in some way

Technology in therapy (or therapy in technology)

New advances in computer technology and the introduction of the internet have had a massive impact on the field of psychotherapy

> Modern therapy can be conducted in a variety of settings beyond the traditional and therapists have embraced these new opportunities to access a more diverse range of clients

ONLINE THERAPY

Cybertherapy can occur in real time through chat-rooms and Skype or be time delayed through email

Many therapists supplement their traditional relationships with clients by adding the extra dimension of online support

> For example, clients who are unable to attend an appointment because they are out of the country could have a virtual session through a chat program

Some therapists complete all of the treatment through an online platform

> For example, the Association for Counselling and Therapy Online (ACTO) lists over 42 registered therapists offering cybertherapy for depression in the UK

There are many benefits to cybertherapy

> Access problems are reduced because the treatment is less costly (therapist does not have location overheads) and more convenient (therapists can see clients across great distances at any time of the day)

> Distance between client and therapist may promote disinhibition, thus encouraging the reluctant client to be more open

However, there are also a number of significant disadvantages and limitations for this method

> Technical faults during the session can be highly disruptive and may lead to misinterpretations by the client – consider the response if the contact accidentally disconnects immediately after a client has disclosed something extremely personal

> Grohol (2011) noted that people may be reluctant to pay for online therapy since they are used to gaining access to online services for free – it is difficult to imagine

why a client would pay £100 an hour to receive emails from a therapist when they could just access the free support information online instead

Boundaries are more difficult to maintain when the client can email the therapist at any hour or request appointments during holidays, weekends and nights – it can be extremely difficult to retain the boundary if you happen to see an email threatening self-harm at 3am

Herwitz (cited in Hoffman, 2011) argues that cybercounselling creates a 'perverse lower version of intimacy' – clients are able to hide behind the computer and avoid engaging in a genuine therapeutic relationship with the practitioner

It is interesting to note that the concept of distance therapy is not novel, although the application through the internet is new

Many therapists throughout history (such as Freud and Jung) have communicated therapeutically with clients using non-face-to-face means, such as letters or telephone calls

THERAPIST-LESS THERAPY

Movement to an online platform provides a new potential for types of therapy that exclude a physical practitioner

Alongside traditional self-help information online, there are now interactive mobile phone and computer apps designed to provide therapy

Apps guide users through exploratory activities to help raise self-awareness and achieve goals

Cognitive-behaviour therapy is the most common therapy for delivery through a computerised application

Many therapists integrate the use of apps into their practice and many have embraced the new technology as a more interactive form of self-help guide or homework worksheets

However, apps also provide clients with an alternative therapeutic experience excluding the traditional therapist

On a more extreme level, modern advances in chatbots have produced the potential for a fully automated 'counsellorbot'

Artificial semi-intelligence in the form of chatbots is able to mimic (to some extent) the art of human conversation and the most advanced chatbots are very similar to human respondents in the simulated environment

These advances offer the potential for counselling to occur with a non-human therapist

iTherapy (2005) is adopting chatbots to administer initial tests and establish the background story of the client before passing this information over to human counsellors

The Machine called Abel (Genesis Interactive, 2009) offers teenage counselling services using a chatbot that can mimic teenage language in a counselling setting –

the creator argues that 'most teenagers hang out on the internet . . . through support and interest from appropriate social groups we can create an instance of ABEL to have the personality of a teenager, that speaks in their language (the local lingo) and comes across as someone who can relate with what they might be going through . . . at last, the teenagers will have a place to share their emotions – albeit with a machine, but an intelligent one' (Genesis Interactive, 2009)

Counsellorbots could potentially offer the ultimate in unconditional positive regard given the objective non-judgemental programming of the machine, yet perhaps fail to offer genuine empathy in a warm setting

These types of therapy raise new questions about the importance of the therapeutic relationship

Does therapeutic benefit depend on having a genuine interested other present in the relationship?

Or can there be therapeutic advantages to providing an outlet for self-exploration and emotion even in the absence of a receiver?

VIRTUAL REALITY AND AVATAR THERAPY

Modern use of virtual simulations through avatars has provided some novel options for implementing therapeutic interventions

Virtual reality has been used to provide safe graded exposure to fear-inducing stimuli during behaviour therapy (systematic desensitisation)

For example, there are large reductions in anxiety in phobia disorders following virtual reality exposure therapy (Parsons & Rizzo, 2008)

Simulated environments have also been used to provide wider and more diverse access to patient populations

For example, therapy through the online virtual world *Second Life* is feasible for a wide population and effective in reducing social anxiety disorders (Yuen et al., 2013)

Avatar therapy has been used to provide interactive constructs for exploring the various aspects of the self

For example, one novel approach to treating schizophrenic persecutory hallucinations is encouraging patients to create an avatar for the malevolent entity and then allowing the patients to slowly bring the entity under their control (Leff et al., 2013)

SUMMARY

Therapy versus helping: contract, boundaries, direction, advice, criticism, equality, outcome; distinction between advice, guidance and therapy

Client: many reasons for seeking therapy, not always mental illness, safe place to disclose; high-risk clients identified in initial assessment (CORE-OM), high risk = risk of harm to self or others, assessment is subjective, may need to breach confidentiality with certain disclosures; client expectations must be managed at the start of the relationship

Therapist: Wampold lists traits of effective therapists (interpersonal skills, cultural awareness, inspires trust, forms an alliance, confident about therapy, flexible during therapy, self-insight, evidence-based practice and CPD); BACP lists traits to be an effective therapeutic person (empathy, sincerity, integrity, resilience, respect, humility, competence, fairness, wisdom, courage), aspiration not perfection; values, recognise own biases, demonstrate good self-care; attend regular supervision 1.5 hours per month to support work (not line manager or personal therapist); keep appropriate therapeutic notes (client, supervision, process), notes can be accessed by client and legal bodies; confidentiality is essential but limited, info shared with organisation and supervisor, confidentiality can be breached by court order or if client is high risk, legally obliged to disclose risk to children and terrorism – all other cases at the discretion of the therapist

Relationship: secure, honest, open, safe, warm, friendly; working, not 'little chats'; structured, defined, encouraging independence

Therapy in modern world: therapeutic variety, literally thousands of possible methods; bibliotherapy involves self-help book prescriptions (self-help), cinema therapy involves film prescriptions (media), angel therapy involves seeking guidance from guardian angels (spiritual) – regarded as pseudo-scientific; relationship (interested other) is critical in all methods; technology, online therapy through delayed email or real-time chat/Skype (enhances access, but less genuine relationship), therapist-less therapy through apps or counsellorbots (enhances access but eliminates relationship), virtual reality and avatar therapy

BOUNDARIES AND ETHICS IN THE THERAPEUTIC RELATIONSHIP

LEARNING OUTCOMES

After reading this section, you will be able to:

*   discuss the importance of maintaining boundaries in the therapeutic relationship
*   highlight the nature of the therapeutic contract
*   discuss ethical issues in relation to therapy

Boundaries in therapy

Boundaries are defined as the rules that an individual holds about the appropriate and acceptable ways to interact with others

In therapy, boundaries refer to specific lines that should not be crossed by the therapist and/or client

> These lines are put in place to ensure that there is an appropriate amount of emotional, psychological and physical space between individuals

> Boundaries are a relatively new concept and research suggests that therapists did not consider boundaries in this context prior to 1990 (Totton, 2010)

Boundaries are essential in the therapeutic setting as the nature of the relationship between the therapist and the client could lead to misunderstandings

> Clear boundaries will ensure that the client remains aware that the therapist is operating as a professional and this will reduce the likelihood that the client may misinterpret empathy for affection or desire

> Clear boundaries will also reassure the client and the therapist as each individual in the relationship will be confident in their own role and the expectations associated with those roles

Both the BPS and the BACP state that all therapists should seek to establish clear boundaries

> Boundaries will provide a framework for working with clients

> Defining and maintaining boundaries is the responsibility of the practitioner

Boundaries should be established through collaboration between the therapist and client

> Initial sessions should focus on establishing the boundaries of the therapeutic relationship

>> Some boundaries will need to be established by the therapist irrespective of input from the client (such as rules regarding confidentiality), but even those boundaries should be discussed in the initial session

> Mearns and Thorne (2007) note that 'for the counsellor to impose boundaries without a consultative process with the client would be a denial of the essential equality of the relationship which it is hoped to establish'

Some boundaries can be simple to establish, whereas other boundaries may require careful consideration by both the therapist and the client

> Sometimes boundaries can easily be determined when considering extreme behaviour but can be more difficult to establish when considering milder forms of that behaviour

>> For example, present giving is generally regarded as inappropriate and most therapists would refuse an expensive gift like a diamond necklace

>>> But it is difficult to adopt this rule for less extravagant gifts like a home-made cake without hurting the feelings of the client

For example, physical contact is generally regarded as inappropriate and most therapists would refuse to hug or kiss a client in greeting

But it is difficult to adopt this rule for less excessive contact like a touch to the back of the shoulder

Sometimes boundaries can be restricted by the nature of the therapeutic setting

For example, some therapists may work from home or offer home visits and this could result in future difficulties maintaining boundaries

Ryan (2010) noted: 'Working one-to-one from within a client's home generates a different dynamic. This is not a therapeutically neutral space; it is their home, a window on their personal world. Entering the client's home turns the conventional therapist/client relationship upon its head; there is a shift of power. In the therapy room the therapist controls the environment, the timing, and the ambience. In the client's environment the counsellor is in an alien environment, outside of their comfort zone . . . Even though the counsellor is sitting in their client's realm, there has to be separation between client and counsellor; the counsellor is there to counsel, not befriend, and boundaries are essential to keep that therapeutic distance'

Maintaining boundaries

Each therapist is different in their own expectations and requirements for clear boundaries. However, here are some possible suggestions for maintaining clear boundaries in the therapeutic relationship

Establish a therapeutic contract at the start of the relationship

Meet only at agreed times for sessions

Do not allow yourself to be 'on call', even for emergencies

Do not engage in a physical relationship with the client

Avoid self-disclosure if it is not relevant to the therapy

Try to focus the sessions on the therapy rather than simply 'a chat'

Refer to other agencies for problems beyond your own abilities

Therapeutic contract

Encouraging client autonomy

BACP ethical guidelines (2010b) relating to autonomy state that the therapist should 'engage in explicit contracting in advance of any commitment by the client' in order to ensure that both the counsellor and the client give fully informed consent

BPS (2009) noted that practitioners are responsible for making and reviewing 'clear and explicit contracts' that inform clients about confidentiality, record keeping and financial costs of therapy

Therapeutic contract helps to establish clear boundaries relating to the therapeutic relationship, thus encouraging client autonomy

Contracts provide an opportunity for the client to give fully informed consent to the therapeutic process

The contract launches the working alliance between the therapist and the client (Clarkson, 1992). The contract can 'make clients more informed about the process, more collaborative with their helpers, and more proactive in managing their problems' (Egan, 1994)

Advantages of a contract

Clients feel secure about exactly what is expected of them during the process

Clients are aware of all the practical aspects of the sessions such as length, duration, cost, etc.

Clients will feel in control of the therapeutic relationship as they have an active input in the agreement

Types of therapeutic contract (Dale, 2003)

Business contract

Duration of sessions, number of sessions, charges of sessions, cancellation expectations, etc.

Therapeutic contract

Reasons for attending therapy, process of therapy, responsibilities and expectations, limits of confidentiality, etc.

Contracts can vary in terms of style, content, depth, etc.

Some contracts can be very basic

Organisations such as the Samaritans provide drop-in centres with basic provision including little more than the offer of a safe space in which to spend as much or as little time as desired so these contracts are often unwritten verbal agreements only

Some contracts can be very complex

Private practices often use detailed written contracts to reduce the potential risk of litigation in the event of future disagreements with a client

Verbal or written contract

Advantages of verbal contract

Less official and formal so less intimidating to the client

Advantages of written contract

More permanent as a record of agreement to be used in the event of future problems

Recommended, not compulsory

Although contracts are strongly recommended in most practice guidelines (BPS, APA, BACP, etc.), they are not compulsory and some therapists do operate without contracts

> Some therapists do not have an explicit contract, but they do engage in contracting activities in the initial session (discussing limits of confidentiality, agreeing session duration and cost, etc.)

> Risks of operating without any type of contract (informal verbal agreement or formal written agreement) are that the therapist is deemed liable in the event of a disagreement relating to the promised provision

WHAT WOULD YOU DO?

Consider the following ethical dilemmas and try to imagine how you might react as a therapist.

- A man confesses to you that he murdered another man five years ago and has never stood trial for the crime. He says that it was a crime of passion committed under the influence of alcohol. Today, he is an upstanding citizen who strongly regrets his actions and wants to come to terms with what he has done to accept himself. There does not appear to be any risk that he will reoffend. What do you do?

- A female client is booked to see you from 4pm to 5pm on a Friday evening in January. When the session ends, it is dark outside and the weather is terrible. You know that your client will be walking home and that this walk will take her through a dangerous neighbourhood. You are also aware that you will probably be driving past her house on your way home. What do you do?

- Your client has been increasingly friendly over the last few sessions and constantly asks questions about your private life. In this session, the client confesses to having strong feelings towards you and invites you out for a coffee. The client explains that this would not be a breach of ethics because your client intends to terminate the therapy as soon as you agree to a date. What do you do?

- You run a private practice in your own home and you need to lead your clients through your hallway to reach your office. One of your clients is addressing issues of bereavement following the death of her baby. At the start of the third session, you notice that she stops to look at your family photographs in the hallway on her way through your house. During the session, she explains that the photographs make her feel uncomfortable and she asks you to remove them during her sessions. What do you do?

- You have recently been through a difficult divorce due to infidelity by your partner. Your client is currently wrestling with a decision about marrying her childhood sweetheart. She has described her fiancé as flirtatious and she suspects that he may have had an affair in the past. You believe that she would be making a mistake by marrying her fiancé and you are often tempted to give her advice on the basis of your experience. What do you do?

- You have recently suffered the loss of your adult daughter to cancer. You are finding it difficult to sleep and you have lost a lot of weight due to your tendency to forget to eat. You decided to return to work to try to take your mind off your sadness. Your client has recently given birth to a baby girl and she is attending therapy because she is feeling overwhelmed by the new arrival. You are finding it difficult to listen to her discuss her feelings about the new baby without reflecting on your own recent loss. In the last session, you had to leave the room for a few minutes to compose yourself because you began to cry. You are scheduled to see the client again tomorrow and you are dreading the session. What do you do?

Ethical guidelines

Ethical guidelines are designed to protect both client and therapist

Historically, some therapeutic practices have led to serious physical and psychological abuse of vulnerable clients

Recovered memory therapy (hypnosis, medication, dream analysis, etc. to recover repressed trauma) carries a high risk of false memory syndrome

The False Memory Syndrome Foundation reports a large number of cases of child abuse retractors who made accusations as a direct result of false memories (False Memory Syndrome Foundation, n.d.)

In 1992, Beth Rutherford accused her parents of sexually abusing her between the ages of seven and 14 (Loftus, 1997). Beth had 'recovered' memories during therapy of her father repeatedly raping her, her mother helping him by holding her down, being impregnated by her father on two occasions, and being forced to abort her fetus with a coat hanger. However, a medical examination revealed that she had never been pregnant and remained a virgin. Beth successfully sued her therapist for $1million in 1996

Rebirthing therapy carries a high risk of injury or even death

Rebirthing therapy is designed to address attachment disorders by simulating the birthing process to allow the formation of new attachments

Rebirthing therapy has been banned in some US states following the death of a 10-year-old child during the procedure (Josefson, 2001). Candace Newmaker was smothered in pillows and blankets then repeatedly crushed by therapists in an effort to simulate the birthing process in order to help her attach to her new adopted parents. Video evidence shown in court revealed that the child vomited, excreted and cried to be released, but the therapists responded by ignoring her or mocking her for not trying hard enough to be born. Eventually, after 70 minutes of torture, Candace died as a result of asphyxiation. The therapists responsible were convicted of reckless child abuse resulting in death and were sentenced to 16 years in prison

Ethical guidelines issued by professional bodies are designed to reduce the risk of abuse and support the professional practice of therapist members

Formal ethical guidelines support the decision-making process for practising therapists

Ethical issues can often be complex and controversial

Judgements about what is 'wrong' or 'right' can often reflect social conventions or personal opinions

For example, an individual may believe that it is 'wrong' to be unfaithful because it goes against our social convention of marriage

An individual may believe that it is 'wrong' to eat meat because it goes against his own personal beliefs

Therapeutic ethical guidelines can offer a set of rules for all practitioners

These rules allow consistent behaviour across all ethical practitioners

However, many of these 'rules' are flexible to the extent that they are open to the interpretation of the practitioner and this can lead to the same complexities that the rules seek to reduce

Professional therapeutic bodies (BACP, UKCP, BPS, etc.) outline ethical guidelines by which member practitioners must abide

Therapists must adhere to the ethical guidelines issued by their own professional bodies

Every working therapist should be a member (ideally, an accredited member) of a professional body

Each member must follow the ethical guidelines for that professional body

Therapists should avoid membership of professional bodies that do not provide ethical guidelines

Some therapists choose to practise independently of any professional bodies

Membership and accreditation of professional bodies are voluntary (refer to information about protected titles with the HPC in the careers section of this chapter)

It is possible for some individuals to practise without being a member of any professional body; thus they operate without adhering to a formal set of ethical guidelines

While these practitioners may adhere to their own moral and ethical guidelines, therapists who are not members of any professional organisation will find it difficult to obtain adequate insurance and may (or perhaps should) be viewed with mistrust

Some of the key values and principles for three major professional bodies (BACP, UKCP, BPS) are outlined in the next few pages. However, please note that this is just a summary of the main points and it is highly recommended that you consult the references link to read the full guidelines

BACP Ethical Framework for Good Practice in Counselling and Psychotherapy (2010b)

Values of counselling and psychotherapy

> Respect human rights and dignity
>
> Ensure the integrity of practitioner–client relationships
>
> Enhance the quality of professional knowledge and its application
>
> Alleviate personal distress and suffering
>
> Foster a sense of self that is meaningful to the person(s) concerned
>
> Increase personal effectiveness
>
> Enhance the quality of relationships between people
>
> Appreciate the variety of human experience and culture
>
> Strive for the fair and adequate provision of counselling and psychotherapy services

Principles of counselling and psychotherapy

> Fidelity: honouring the trust placed in the practitioner
>
>> Therapists should respect the trust of the client and avoid disclosure of confidential information
>
> Autonomy: respect for the client's right to be self-governing
>
>> Therapists should ensure that advertisements and information about services are accurate, and they should protect the privacy of clients, engage in explicit contracting before gaining fully informed consent, report any conflicts of interest, and refuse to manipulate clients against their will (even for beneficial social ends)
>
> Beneficence: a commitment to promoting the client's wellbeing
>
>> Therapists should act in the best interests of the client (especially those with diminished capacities), provide services on the basis of adequate training or experience, take advantage of supervision to support work with clients, and commit to continuous professional development
>
> Non-maleficence: a commitment to avoiding harm to the client
>
>> Therapists should hold appropriate insurance, refuse to work when unfit due to illness or personal circumstances, seek to minimise harm to clients and assume responsibility to challenge poor practice in others, and avoid any incompetence, malpractice or client exploitation
>
> Justice: the fair and impartial treatment of all clients and the provision of adequate services

Therapists should respect the human rights and dignity of all clients, be committed to equality of opportunity by avoiding discrimination on the basis of prejudice, provide fair access to services for clients with differing needs, remain aware of legal obligations, and remain alert to conflicts between legal and ethical obligations

Self-respect: fostering the practitioner's self-knowledge and care for self

Therapists should use supervision for professional support, seek continuous professional development, obtain appropriate insurance, engage in life-enhancing activities and relationships independent of relationships in counselling, and apply all of these principles to the self as well as clients

UKCP Ethical Principles and Code of Professional Conduct (2009)

General ethical principles

Best interest of clients

Therapist should treat all clients with respect, refuse to exploit or abuse clients, respect the autonomy of clients, not enter into a personal relationship with clients, not harm or collude in the harm of clients or others, and recognise how own behaviour outside of professional life can impact on clients

Diversity and equality

Therapist should actively consider issues of diversity and seek to prevent prejudice from impacting on treatment

Confidentiality

Therapist should respect and protect the confidentiality of clients, ensure consent where possible when information is to be disclosed, and explain to clients prior to the relationship those legal situations in which confidentiality cannot be guaranteed

Conduct

Therapist should recognise the impact of their actions on clients, seek to promote professional conduct at all times, and disclose any criminal convictions, investigations or disciplinary actions to the professional body

Professional knowledge, skills and experience

Therapist should disclose all qualifications to clients and the professional body to avoid any misleading assumptions

Communication

Therapist should explain all pertinent contractual points to the client and notify about ethical issues (including complaints procedure)

Obtaining consent

Therapist should explain the therapeutic approach to the client and gain fully informed consent to participate in therapy and/or any research associated with the therapy

Records

> Therapist should keep appropriate records and store these records in accordance with data protection laws to safeguard client confidentiality

Physical or mental health

> Therapist should not work when unfit to do so due to physical or mental illness or impaired by alcohol, drugs, etc.

Professional integrity

> Therapist should report any breaches of ethical guidelines committed by themselves or colleagues

Advertising

> Therapists should ensure that advertisements for services are fair, accurate and responsible

Indemnity insurance

> Therapists should ensure that they are covered to practise by indemnity insurance

Complaints

> Therapist should ensure that clients are aware of all complaints procedures and should raise ethical concerns to the professional body when observing breaches in the behaviour of colleagues

BPS Code of Ethics and Conduct (2009)

Ethical principles

Respect

> Therapist should respect the dignity and worth of all people, maintain privacy and confidentiality, seek informed consent for any therapeutic intervention, and encourage and support client self-determination

Competence

> Therapist should be aware of professional ethical guidelines, engage in ethical decision making, recognise the limits of their own professional competence, and recognise impairment due to health or personal issues and refrain from practice when unfit to do so

Responsibility

> Therapist should avoid bringing the profession into disrepute through misconduct or allowing harm to clients or others, recognise those conditions under which the therapeutic relationship should be terminated, and seek to protect and debrief all research participants

Integrity

> Therapist should be honest and accurate in dealing with clients and the general public, avoid exploitation and conflicts of interest, maintain personal boundaries, and address ethical misconduct in colleagues

WHAT WOULD YOU DO (AFTER FURTHER REFLECTION)?

Consider the following ethical dilemmas again and how you might react as a therapist based on the ethical guidelines available from professional organisations.

A man confesses to you that he murdered another man five years ago and has never stood trial for the crime. He says that it was a crime of passion committed under the influence of alcohol. Today, he is an upstanding citizen who strongly regrets his actions and wants to come to terms with what he has done to accept himself. There does not appear to be any risk that he will reoffend. What do you do?

> Remember that the therapist should maintain client confidentiality within legal limits and should seek to protect their own clients, clients of colleagues and members of the general public

> Consider the BACP principles of autonomy and justice, UKCP principles of confidentiality and professional integrity, and BPS principles of responsibility and integrity

A female client is booked to see you from 4pm to 5pm on a Friday evening in January. When the session ends, it is dark outside and the weather is terrible. You know that your client will be walking home and that this walk will take her through a dangerous neighbourhood. You are also aware that you will probably be driving past her house on your way home. What do you do?

> Remember that the therapist should not hold multiple relationships with the client and should seek to protect the client

> Consider the BACP principles of autonomy and beneficence, UKCP principles of best interest of clients and conduct, and BPS principles of responsibility and integrity

Your client has been increasingly friendly over the last few sessions and constantly asks questions about your private life. In this session, the client confesses to having strong feelings towards you and invites you out for a coffee. The client explains that this would not be a breach of ethics because your client intends to terminate the therapy as soon as you agree to a date. What do you do?

> Remember that the therapist should not hold multiple relationships with the client and the therapist and client are both entitled to terminate therapy at any time

> Consider the BACP principles of autonomy and non-maleficence, UKCP principles of best interest of clients and conduct, and BPS principles of responsibility and integrity

You run a private practice in your own home and you need to lead your clients through your hallway to reach your office. One of your clients is addressing issues of bereavement following the death of her baby. At the start of the third session, you notice that she stops to look at your family photographs in the hallway on her way through your house. During the session, she explains that the photographs make her feel uncomfortable and she asks you to remove them during her sessions. What do you do?

> Remember that the therapist should seek to protect the client and should also protect their own wellbeing

> Consider the BACP principles of beneficence and self-respect, UKCP principles of best interest of clients and physical or mental health, and BPS principles of respect and integrity

You have recently been through a difficult divorce due to infidelity by your partner. Your client is currently wrestling with a decision about marrying her childhood sweetheart. She has described her fiancé as flirtatious and she suspects that he may have had an affair in the past. You believe that she would be making a mistake by marrying her fiancé and you are often tempted to give her advice on the basis of your experience. What do you do?

> Remember that the therapist should respect the free will of the client and seek to protect the client

> Consider the BACP principles of autonomy and beneficence, UKCP principles of best interest of clients and physical or mental health, and BPS principles of respect and competence

You have recently suffered the loss of your adult daughter to cancer. You are finding it difficult to sleep and you have lost a lot of weight due to your tendency to forget to eat. You decided to return to work to try to take your mind off your sadness. Your client has recently given birth to a baby girl and she is attending therapy because she is feeling overwhelmed by the new arrival. You are finding it difficult to listen to her discuss her feelings about the new baby without reflecting on your own recent loss. In the last session, you had to leave the room for a few minutes to compose yourself because you began to cry. You are scheduled to see the client again tomorrow and you are dreading the session. What do you do?

> Remember that the therapist should seek to protect the client and should protect their own wellbeing

> Consider the BACP principles of beneficence and self-respect, UKCP principles of best interest of clients and physical or mental health, and BPS principles of respect and competence

Can you imagine any other scenarios that could inspire an ethical dilemma? Devise three scenarios that could pose an ethical problem then work with a partner to identify the main principles associated with the scenarios and develop an action plan for working within the situations.

All professional bodies have similar ethical guidelines

Ethical considerations common to most professional bodies (BACP, UKCP, BPS, APA, BABCP, etc.) include the following

Therapist should provide all pertinent information at the start of the relationship (contracting) to obtain fully informed consent

Therapist should maintain client confidentiality (within legal limits)

Therapist should not hold multiple relationships with the client (client cannot be a sexual partner, family member, friend, etc.)

Therapist should not exploit the client in any way (sexual, financial, psychological)

Therapist should respect the free will of the client

Therapist should seek to protect the client, clients of colleagues and members of the general public

Therapist and client are entitled to terminate therapy at any time (given appropriate notice)

Therapist should protect their own wellbeing by withdrawing from work if unfit, using supervision to support practice, and seeking continuous professional development

ETHICAL CONTROVERSY

Ethical guidelines are designed to reduce the risks associated with therapy, but there are still many critics who argue that therapy carries ethical questions irrespective of these regulations. Reflect on the following questions and discuss the ethical issues with a colleague.

Does therapy lead to an unhealthy dependency on the therapist?

Despite all efforts to develop a collaborative relationship, it is inevitable that the client will view the therapist as an 'expert'

As an expert, the therapist wields a great deal of power and this power is very attractive to many clients

Clients who feel better as a result of therapy are reinforced for engaging with the therapeutic process; thus they may begin to believe that therapy is essential for them to be able to cope with everyday difficulties

Will therapy inevitably influence the client in the direction desired by the therapist?

Arguably, it is impossible to interact with another person without influencing the other to some extent

Therapy will inevitably influence the client – indeed, therapy presumably aims to influence the client in the direction of positive change

However, it is difficult to state who should make the decision about which direction is 'positive' and which direction is 'negative'

Therapists often seek to ensure that all decisions relating to change are made by clients, but there will be an inevitable influence of the therapist

This means that the personal beliefs and biases of the therapist will impact on the life choices of any client

Does therapy encourage mental health disorders by providing reinforcing attention for reported symptoms?

Many clients want to be the 'model patient' and seek ways to present exactly as they should

Clients may learn about the diagnosed disorder and the intended treatment then report the correct symptoms to show that they are being a good client – sometimes they may be faking these symptoms and sometimes they may actually experience pseudo-symptoms as a result of the intense desire to please the therapist

For example, 'Lauri' reported her experiences of false memory syndrome as a patient in a multiple personality disorder therapy group (False Memory Syndrome Foundation, n.d.)

Lauri explained that she learnt the traits of multiple personality disorder (now known as dissociative identity disorder) in order to be the 'model patient'

Once she was exhibiting the behaviours associated with this disorder, her therapist explained to her husband, 'Because Lauri now has the behaviour, it follows that she has multiple personality disorder. Thus, some terrible abuse in her childhood must have caused it. So terrible that she's repressed those memories deep in her mind'

During subsequent regression hypnosis, the therapist invited Lauri to create an alter and then used leading questions to encourage this alter to describe childhood abuse

Eventually, Lauri reported a wide range of abuse, including taking part in Satanic rituals, being buried alive, drinking blood and being involved in the murder of a baby

Lauri was rewarded for recovering these memories through attention and sympathy – the therapist described her as his 'best' patient

Is the therapeutic field promoting the overdiagnosis of mental health disorders?

Diagnosis of disorders such as depression and anxiety has increased substantially over recent years to the extent that one in four people will experience a mental health disorder at some point in the next year (Mental Health Foundation, n.d.)

Lutus (2013) is highly critical of psychology and psychotherapy in his report on the absence of science in the field of psychology

Lutus observes that the *Diagnostic and Statistical Manual of Mental Disorders* (DSM) classification of 112 disorders in 1952 rose to 374 disorders by 1994

Lutus argues that the DSM has begun to define many arguably normal emotional states as 'mental health disorders' – for example, he cites sibling rivalry disorder as one diagnosis that should not be classified as a mental health disorder

Lutus claims that this increase in the classification of arguably normal behaviours as 'disorders' will eventually lead to no behaviour being regarded as normal

SUMMARY

Boundaries: rules of appropriate interactions with others, lines between self and other, avoids misunderstandings, advised by professional bodies; established through collaboration between therapist and client, discuss in initial session, agree through consultation with client; maintaining boundaries, no hard rules as they may differ for each individual and situation, suggestions (establish contract at start, meet only at agreed times, do not be on-call, do not have physical relationship, avoid non-relevant self-disclosure), focus on therapy rather than a chat, refer if necessary

Contract: encourages client autonomy; type – business or therapeutic; style – basic or complex, verbal or written; recommended not compulsory; some make explicit contracts, some make implicit contracts, some have no contracts (not recommended)

Ethics: ethical guidelines aim to protect client and therapist; some forms of therapy can be extremely dangerous, recovered memory therapy carries risk of false memory syndrome, rebirthing therapy carries risk of injury or death; ethical issues can be complex and controversial with no clear right or wrong; professional bodies offer some rules, not recommended to operate independently of any professional body; BACP Ethical Framework for Good Practice in Counselling and Psychotherapy (fidelity, autonomy, beneficence, non-maleficence, justice, self-respect); UKCP Ethical Principles and Code of Professional Conduct (best interest of clients, diversity and equality, confidentiality, conduct, professional knowledge, skills and experience, communication, obtaining consent, records, physical or mental health, professional integrity, advertising, indemnity insurance, complaints); BPS Code of Ethics and Conduct (respect, competence, responsibility, integrity);

common guidelines irrespective of which professional body (informed consent, confidentiality, conflicts of interest, exploitation, free will, protect client and others, right to terminate, protect own wellbeing)

APPRECIATING DIVERSITY IN THE THERAPEUTIC RELATIONSHIP

LEARNING OUTCOMES

After reading this section, you will be able to:

- appreciate some of the cultural assumptions in mainstream therapy
- explain multiculturalism in the context of the therapeutic relationship
- self-reflect on your own cultural biases and understanding of cultural diversity
- critique the concept of multicultural therapy
- appreciate the importance of working holistically

Cultural assumptions in mainstream therapy

Modern western-centric therapy

Before we begin to explore our own attitudes to working with clients from different cultural backgrounds, it is worth noting that most therapies are driven by western culture and western values.

Looking at the main theoretical approaches to be explored in later chapters, we can begin to see the 'western-centric' lens through which therapy has been developed

Key figures responsible for developing the main approaches include

humanistic approaches: Rogers, Maslow

psychodynamic approaches: Freud, Jung

behavioural approaches: Watson, Skinner

cognitive approaches: Neisser, Beck

All of these key people are white, western, educated, middle-class, middle-aged men

Some women have made significant contributions to development of theory (for example, Melanie Klein, Karen Horney and Laura Perls), but their contributions have, in some cases, been played down due to the attitudes of men and the values of society in their time

However, these women are still white, western, educated, middle class and middle aged

As therapists, our own values and assumptions, stereotypes and biases are influenced by our society, our culture, our parents and our significant others

> Similarly, all the psychological approaches and therapies discussed in this book will have been developed within the context of the time and place of the founder, who in turn will have been influenced by their upbringing (society, history, context, parents, etc.)

All approaches will have been influenced by the values and assumptions of the society in which the founder was living

> This is one reason why this book includes historical and biographical details of the founding fathers of each approach

> An understanding of these individuals gives an insight into the context for their approach and therapy

> For example, the behavioural approach was developed at a time when behavioural psychology had established research into classical conditioning and assumed that behaviour was learned, could be unlearned and replaced by more effective learning (e.g. the installation and removal of a phobia)

> The humanistic approach has basic assumptions (e.g. individuals striving for actualisation, the importance of the individual, etc.) that are influenced by the values of their time (the 'American Dream', the pursuit of happiness, etc.)

Individualistic versus collectivist cultures

All the therapies that developed from the first three forces of psychology had common values, including

> Belief in the importance of the individual

> Belief that individuals are the drivers of their own destiny

> Belief that personal choice and responsibility should be valued

> Belief that we all have the potential to change

All of these beliefs are common to the individualistic culture in western society

In comparison, collectivist cultures in eastern society may have very different values, including:

> Belief in the importance of the group, family and society

> Belief in the harmony of the individual in connection with the universe

> Belief in the interconnectedness of opposites (dark/light, yin/yang, good/evil)

> Belief in the importance of acting in a way that benefits society rather than the self

Therapies developed in the western world may make assumptions about the 'correct' goals for the client

> For example, these therapies may focus on the importance of the individual client achieving independence and exercising free will

However, these goals might not fit with a culture in which it is expected that a person will contribute to the family and adhere to the family rules of honour

Multiculturalism in the therapeutic relationship

Monocultural to multicultural

In response to the monocultural perspective of traditional counselling theories, there have been developments in approaches to engaging clients from minority groups

> The multicultural approach developed out of the civil rights movements and from equality legislation

> Even in those therapies that emphasise the uniqueness of each individual and strive to understand the world from the client's perspective, the approach itself is grounded in implicit values and assumptions

A basic assumption in the development of a multicultural perspective is that traditional theories of therapy have little understanding of current cultural diversity

> The culture in which a person is brought up influences the development of identity and is the basis for thoughts, feelings and behaviours

> Therefore, culture should be at the centre of the therapeutic relationship rather than only noteworthy when there is an obvious cultural difference between therapist and client

Multiculturalism has been described as the fourth force in therapy, after the behavioural, psychodynamic and humanistic approaches (Pederson, 1991)

> Sometimes the focus of multicultural therapy is described within narrow definitions and assumes that the goals are based around helping individuals assimilate into a new culture

> However, the term 'multiculturalism' embraces a range of diversity and differences

Nelson-Jones (2005) identifies ten areas of difference

> Culture

> Race

> Social class

> Biological sex

> Gender role identity

> Marital status

> Sexual orientation

> Physical disability

> Age

> Religion or philosophy

Multicultural client

Clients from different cultural backgrounds will have different values and assumptions about the therapeutic process

> For example, a client from a non-western society may value collectivism rather than individualism, and so will struggle with the basic goals of striving for self-actualisation, happiness, intimacy, authenticity, independence, etc. that run through many existing western approaches

Clients may present differently on the basis of cultural background

> Some clients may view people of all ages as equal, whereas other clients may be deferential to older people

> Some clients may believe that females should defer to males, whereas other clients may believe that there should be no difference in the treatment of each gender

> Some clients may be comfortable discussing their own feelings, whereas other clients may feel that it is not appropriate to describe their own internal experiences

> Some clients may be able to work openly with the therapist, whereas other clients may not feel comfortable making eye contact or may need to speak with a same-sex therapist

> Some clients may feel that talking negatively about family is a form of betrayal, whereas other clients may enjoy an opportunity to vent feelings of anger and frustration about family members

Clients within the same culture may differ substantially due to subcultures

> Even within any specific culture, there will be many subcultures

>> For example, one client may be a member of a 'drug culture' in which the values and behaviours differ from wider society

>> Those who are deeply religious will have very different values from those who are agnostic

>> Male clients may act, think and feel differently to female clients

> These values are born out of our beliefs and are the principles that drive our behaviours

> We are influenced by the culture and subcultures that we experience

> In this way, everyone is a multicultural individual because it is the combination of our experiences that gives us a unique personal culture

> This has clear implications for the multicultural therapist

Multicultural therapist

The Counselling Psychology Division of the American Psychological Association (APA) identified three areas for competencies (Sue & Sue, 1990)

> Awareness of self (our assumptions, values and biases)

> Awareness of the culturally different client's view of the world

Development of strategies and techniques

In order for therapists to be competent working with issues of diversity in a multicultural society, they need to

Understand their own cultural heritage

Be aware of their own beliefs, values and assumptions

Be sensitive to biases, stereotypes and prejudices

Understand the beliefs, values and cultural differences of others

Develop strategies and techniques for working with others

VALUES AND DIVERSITY

Using the ten areas of diversity noted by Nelson-Jones (2005), make a personal inventory of your understanding and awareness of each area.

Culture
Race
Social class
Biological sex
Gender role identity
Marital status
Sexual orientation
Physical disability
Age
Religion or philosophy

Once you have assessed your own understanding of each area, select an area in which you think that you have limited understanding and do some research into the beliefs, values, customs and practices of a group that differs from your own. For example, if you are an atheist who thinks that he is lacking in understanding of religion, then you could research the beliefs, values, customs and practices of those who actively follow the Catholic religion.

If you are part of a training group, spend some time assuming the role of a person from the chosen group, and role play a short therapy session. In the feedback explore what it felt like as client and therapist in the session.

Self-reflection to recognise bias and prejudice

Importance of self-awareness

There is value in therapists becoming more self-aware

Personal development is integral in training courses and ongoing continuous professional development

Every individual is born and raised in a specific time, society and culture

    Cultures and subcultures in which we are raised will impact on our thoughts, feelings, values, beliefs, etc.

    This can lead to cultural bias and this cultural bias can impact on how we behave towards others

Cultural bias is both inevitable and appropriate

    It is impossible to be culturally neutral

        We all make some assumptions about others

            We are making an assumption if we decide to cross the street rather than walking past a gang of youths late at night

            This could be regarded as stereotyping the youths and our behaviour could be interpreted as discrimination

            However, most people would regard this as an acceptable level of assumption and the resulting behaviour would often be regarded as appropriate

        We all hold some preferences in relation to others

            We are demonstrating a preference if we accept a date with a man who is tall but refuse a date with a man who is short

            This could be regarded as prejudice against shorter men and our behaviour could be interpreted as discrimination

            However, most people would regard this as an acceptable preference and the resulting behaviour would be classed as appropriate

But cultural bias can sometimes lead to inaccurate assumptions and unfair preferences, and the resulting behaviour can be discriminatory and offensive

    Best defence against damaging cultural bias is self-awareness

    It is acceptable to hold some cultural biases, provided that you are aware of these biases and ensure that they do not impact negatively on others

EXPLORING ASSUMPTIONS AND VALUES

Read through the following therapeutic scenarios and consider how you would respond as the therapist. Are any of these particularly challenging to you? If so, why? Are there any in which you want further information? If so, what would you need to know?

1.   An 18-year-old woman comes to you wanting to explore her thoughts and feelings around terminating her pregnancy.

2.   A Chinese student is sent to you for a therapy session as he is struggling with living in a different culture. He appears to be reluctant to discuss how he feels,

agrees with all that you say, and does not make eye contact at all during the session.

3. A 35 year old with heroin addiction talks of the daily round of stealing and scoring.

4. A 72 year old mentions how he regularly drives home from the pub after a few pints and the odd whisky.

5. A 24-year-old woman speaks of how her behaviours are inconsistent with the faith she was brought up in. She is from a Jehovah's Witness family.

6. An elderly lady talks of her husband's terminal cancer, and how they have discussed her role in ending his life.

7. An Indian woman talks about her upcoming arranged marriage.

8. A young man is hesitant to talk, but wants to know your views on transgender issues.

Think of other scenarios which may challenge your beliefs and values, or raise awareness of your lack of understanding of cultural differences.

Finally, what assumptions do you think the author of this section has made in the scenarios?

Criticism of multicultural therapy

Cultural empathy

The Counselling Psychology Division of the American Psychological Association (APA) identifies the following areas for competencies

> Awareness of self (our assumptions, values and biases)
>
> > Good practice to become more aware of ourselves
> >
> > Our beliefs, values, biases and prejudices
>
> Awareness of the culturally different client's view of the world
>
> > Good practice to increase our awareness of cultural differences
> >
> > Others beliefs, values, biases and prejudices
> >
> > Differences in the use of language and non-verbal communication

These competences will help us to build greater cultural empathy

> Genuine understanding of the world of the client from the perspective of his or her own culture

Strategies and techniques

The Counselling Psychology Division of the American Psychological Association (APA) identifies the following area for competencies

Development of strategies and techniques

> Need for this competency has been debated

> Do we really need strategies and techniques to be multicultural?

Patterson (2004) has argued that the basic assumptions for multicultural therapy are flawed

> If everyone is a multicultural individual, then all therapy is multicultural, and there is no need to develop multicultural therapy competencies

>> 'Cultural groups are not pure and discrete, but overlapping. The process of globalization is blurring differences. The only workable product of a multi-cultural society is a society of individuals who must ultimately absorb different cultures into themselves. Thus, no discrete classifications are possible . . . Attempting to develop different theories, methods and techniques for each of these groups would be an insurmountable task . . . This approach is not only impossible, but also irrelevant and harmful in counseling the individual client' (Patterson, 2004)

Patterson (2004) advocates a 'universal system of counseling' and says that the essence of such a system has long been known

> 'It is what is known as client-centred therapy'

Working holistically

Ever-present cultural differences

Cultural (and subcultural) differences and the values that result from these differences are always present in the therapeutic room

> Sometimes this is obvious and explicit

> Sometimes it is subtle and implicit

> But these differences are always present

Therapists need to be aware of these differences

> Self-awareness to understand own cultural bias

> Diversity awareness to understand the cultural biases of others

It may even benefit the therapist to gain some insight into other cultures

> Some knowledge can be helpful and allow a deeper understanding of the world of the client

However, once the therapist is aware of these differences and holds some cultural knowledge, it is important to then put this knowledge on one side so as to be present for the client

> Each client should be viewed as a unique individual rather than the simple output of a cultural context

> The reality is that even the most culturally aware therapist cannot know the subtlety of the multicultural client

Indeed, having knowledge of the cultural background of an individual may lead the therapist to make assumptions about the client

> For example, if the therapist 'knows' that a client from South East Asia will be deferential to authority figures, this may influence the initial behaviour of the therapist regardless of the individual

> Would the therapist be being culturally empathic or stereotyping?

Key to success is to acknowledge cultures and subcultures, yet avoid assumptions on the basis of this knowledge

> Important to recognise potential cultural differences and remain sensitive to potential problems in the therapeutic relationship as a result of these differences

> > For example, it is important to recognise that a female client from Saudi Arabia who follows a Muslim religion may have different values from a male therapist from Scotland who holds an atheist perspective

> But the therapist must not make assumptions about an individual on the basis of knowledge about their culture

> > For example, one must not assume that the female client from Saudi Arabia who follows a Muslim religion is against abortion – it is important to give the client an opportunity to express her own opinions without forming these conclusions on the basis of cultural knowledge

Therapists offer core qualities irrespective of culture

> Therapist must listen to the client's verbal and non-verbal communication

> Therapist must strive to understand the client's world

> If the therapist does not know something, she or he should be honest and ask – this will show interest, equalise any perceived power imbalance and develop the relationship

> Therapist should be aware of difference, but should also look for similarities

> Patterson (2004) noted that 'all clients are alike in one basic essential – they are all human beings'

SUMMARY

Cultural assumptions: modern western-centric therapy, devised by (mainly) white western educated middle-class middle-aged men; therapists influenced by own culture; individualistic (importance of individual, individuals drive own destiny, personal choice valued, all have potential to change) versus collectivist (importance of group, harmony between individual and universe, interconnectedness of opposites, important to act in ways that benefit group) cultures

Multiculturalism: monocultural to multicultural, ten areas of difference (culture, race, social class, biological sex, gender role identity, marital status, sexual orientation, physical disability, age, religion or philosophy); multicultural clients, cultures and subcultures; multicultural therapists, APA's three competencies (self-awareness, diversity awareness, strategies), needs (be aware of own values, understand values of others, understand own cultural heritage, develop strategies for working with others)

Self-reflection: value in being self-aware, cultural bias is inevitable and appropriate, but can lead to inappropriate discrimination if we are not self-aware of own biases

Critique: cultural empathy is important; APA recommends strategies and techniques for multiculturalism but strategies can be impossible and lead to bias; client-centred therapy may be a solution

Working holistically: ever-present cultural differences, need to be aware of differences (self-awareness and diversity awareness), but avoid assumptions on the basis of this knowledge, offer core qualities irrespective of difference, all clients are alike in being human

APPROACHES, THERAPIES AND MODELS

LEARNING OUTCOMES

After reading this section, you will be able to:

* distinguish between an approach, a therapy and a model

* distinguish between purist and non-purist perspectives

* distinguish between effective integration/eclecticism and ineffective syncretism

* define and discuss technical eclecticism, theoretical integration, assimilative integration and common factors

* describe and evaluate Egan's skilled helper model

Defining approaches, therapies and models

Approach

Approach could be described as the umbrella term for all theories and concepts converging on a similar set of principles

> For example, the humanistic approach includes several theories relating to the positive nature of humans, the tendency towards self-actualisation, and the importance of viewing the individual as the expert on the self

Theories and direction of focus may differ between different contributors to the approach, but the key principles are usually similar

For example, in the humanistic approach, Rogers focuses on the concept of congruence between the actual self and the self-concept whereas Maslow focuses on movement up the hierarchy of needs, but both theorists agree on the basic principle of self-actualisation

Four core approaches

Humanistic approach (third force)

Psychodynamic approach (second force)

Behavioural approach (first force)

Cognitive approach (revolution)

Therapy

Therapy could be described as the practical application of an approach to support human growth and development

Several different therapies can operate under a single approach and each therapy may apply the theories within the approach in a slightly different manner

All the therapies under a single approach will share a common philosophy of human nature

For example, person-centred therapy and existential therapy both operate under the humanistic approach

Some therapies can operate under two or more approaches by combining the theories within the approach in a novel manner

These therapies will combine the principles of human nature from two or more different approaches

For example, cognitive-behaviour therapy combines the cognitive approach with the behavioural approach

Some therapies do not operate under any approach, but instead select specific techniques from various different therapies that sit under different approaches dependent on the situation and client

These therapies argue that all the approaches hold some fundamental truths about human nature so they take the most relevant and appropriate parts from each without specifically adhering to all the principles of any

For example, multimodal therapy does not subscribe to the principles of any one approach

Model

Model could be described as a framework for applying a therapy

Models usually involve steps or processes which can be followed by the therapist irrespective of his or her chosen approach and therapy

For example, Egan's skilled helper model (Egan, 2007)

Approach > therapy > model

Approach provides a foundation for therapy

> Approach refers to the general theories about human nature and personality held by the practitioner

> Therapy is the practical application of these theories to improve psychological wellbeing

Therapy can be added to the framework of a model

> Therapy is the practical application of theories to improve psychological wellbeing

> Model is the framework for applying the various therapeutic techniques

Purist versus non-purist perspectives

Purist therapists

Purists exclusively use only one approach and usually remain within the remits of one specific therapy

> For example, a pure person-centred therapist would not agree with any theories or adopt any techniques which conflict with the core principles of the humanistic approach and person-centred therapy

>> Harley Therapy in London adopts a purist approach to both psychodynamic therapy and humanistic therapy with specific therapists rigidly adhering to their own field with no recognisable cross-over in terms of personality concept or therapeutic approach

However, few therapists maintain this strict approach

> Only 4.2% of therapists surveyed by Psychotherapy Networker (2007) identified themselves as purists

> Even those who do regard themselves as 'purists' often deviate towards other therapies to some extent by incorporating additional techniques

> For example, a behavioural therapist may acknowledge the importance of the therapeutic relationship by adhering to the core conditions of the person-centred approach

Non-purist therapists

Non-purists use more than one approach and will often combine elements of different therapies

> For example, a therapist might usually adopt the humanistic approach and use person-centred therapeutic methods, but use cognitive therapy techniques if this is deemed appropriate for the client

This open approach to therapy is regarded as integrative, eclectic or syncretistic

> Dependent on the theoretical motivation underpinning the act of incorporating various therapeutic approaches and techniques

Integration and eclecticism versus syncretism

Integrative therapy

Therapist aims to weld elements of two or more complementary approaches into a single whole

> Ambitious enterprise to bring together elements from different theories to create a new theory (McLeod, 2009)

Many modern practitioners adopt an integrative approach by combining elements of distinct theories to create an entirely new theoretical approach to therapy

> For example, cognitive-behaviour therapy melds the cognitive approach with the behavioural approach to create a new therapeutic method

Eclectic therapy

Therapist aims to bring together a range of therapeutic techniques

> Best or most appropriate ideas and techniques are brought together from a range of different approaches and therapies to suit the needs of the client (McLeod, 2009)

Many modern practitioners select those techniques deemed most appropriate for their individual client on the basis of need without specific subscription to any underlying approach

> For example, multimodal therapy uses a range of techniques from many different therapies without reference to a specific approach

Integration versus eclecticism

'Integration is the process of *bringing together* with the implication of making something whole and new. Eclecticism is a process of *selecting out*, with the implication of taking something apart' (Hollanders, 2000)

'An eclectic counsellor will select what is applicable to the client from a range of theories, methods and practices. Justification is based on the theory that there is no proof that any one theoretical approach works better than all others for a specific problem. Integrative counselling is when several distinct models of counselling and psychotherapy are used together in a converging way rather than in separate pieces' (BACP, 2010c)

Integration involves a combination of different approaches to produce an entirely new therapy on the basis of a new underlying approach

Eclecticism involves a combination of different therapies to produce an entirely new therapy without specific subscription to an underlying approach

'Eclecticism in practice and integration in aspiration' (Wachtel, 1991)

> Many therapists dislike the term 'eclecticism' as it is mistaken for syncretism

> Therapists tend to prefer the term 'integration' even when they are actually practising eclecticism

Both integration and eclecticism should involve careful consideration of client needs and individual circumstances

Provided that the therapist has evaluated the client carefully and has an understanding of the selected approaches or therapies, then integrative and eclectic therapies can be equally successful

Syncretism

Eclecticism involves carefully considered selection of appropriate therapeutic techniques based on a careful evaluation of the client's needs and a deep understanding of the different therapies available

Eclecticism should never be a hotchpotch of different things according to the whims and fancy of the therapist

Lazarus (1992) argued that the arbitrary selection of various random techniques for use in an unreasoned or spontaneous manner is a form of syncretism

Syncretism involves a mix of different approaches and therapies based on what is available to the therapist without an understanding of the underlying theories

Eclecticism versus syncretism

Even though the eclectic therapist might not subscribe to a single underlying approach, s/he is aware of the theoretical underpinnings of each of the approaches that s/he chooses to draw from and is aware of the empirical evidence supporting the therapies that s/he chooses to employ

Eclecticism can be highly effective

All good therapists adopt the eclectic stance (Corsini & Wedding, 2008)

In contrast, the syncretistic therapist would not understand the theoretical underpinnings of different approaches or be aware of the evidence for and against various methods, but would instead choose techniques based simply on a personal whim

Syncretism is at best useless and at worst dangerous

Please refer to Table 1.1 to see some examples of common approaches and therapies in counselling and psychotherapy today

Please note, however, that this list is in no way conclusive or exhaustive

There are many more therapies in the world and many therapists might argue against the categorisation in the table

This list is merely a simplified version of therapy and approach to help you to understand the nature of integration and eclecticism

Types of integration and eclecticism

Four types of eclecticism and integration (Dattilio & Norcross, 2006; Norcross & Beutler, 2008)

Theoretical integration

Assimilative integration

Common factors

Technical eclecticism

Theoretical integration

Theoretical integration will strive to integrate two (or more) core approaches into a novel single approach

> This method has been used to create several new fields of therapy, and many of these new therapies have become even more popular than the preceding pure therapies
>
> In short, theoretical integration involves the integration of two or more approaches
>
> For example, cognitive-behaviour therapy combines the cognitive approach and the behavioural approach

Assimilative integration

Assimilative integration will focus on a single pure approach with the selective incorporation of techniques from some therapies under other approaches

> In short, assimilative integration involves a willingness to selectively incorporate techniques from therapies under other approaches while remaining based within one specific approach
>
> For example, one could argue that transactional analysis is an example of assimilative integration since it appears to have firm roots in the humanistic approach yet it has expanded to incorporate additional theories and techniques

Common factors

Common factors searches for common elements across multiple approaches and therapies in order to pull together the most effective theories into a single new approach and therapy

> In short, common factors involves identifying similarities across different approaches to whittle down to a core approach based on commonalities
>
> For example, family systems therapy is based on a number of common theories across different approaches

Technical eclecticism

Technical eclecticism utilises a variety of techniques from several different therapies without subscribing to any underlying theoretical approach

> This method focuses on applied technique rather than theoretical underpinnings relating to a comprehensive concept of human nature and personality
>
> In short, technical eclecticism involves the selection of techniques based on evidence for the success of the technique without subscription to any underlying theories
>
> For example, multimodal therapy utilises a range of techniques without establishing direct links to any of the pure approaches

Egan's skilled helper model (Figure 1.2)

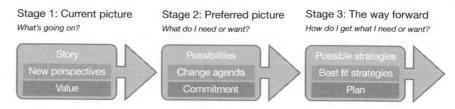

FIGURE 1.2 **Skilled helper model. Adapted from Egan (2007).**

Model

Egan's three-stage model (Egan, 2007) promotes a collaborative relationship between the therapist and the client designed to guide the helper through the process of empowering the client to solve their own problems and develop their own opportunities

Egan argued that previous theoretical models presented in psychology by scientists often failed to inform actual activity in the field by practitioners

> This situation led to a 'lose-lose-lose scenario' with scientists neglecting the real-life problems encountered in therapeutic relationships, practitioners using techniques lacking a scientific basis, and clients failing to reap the benefits of research-informed methods

Egan proposed a problem management and opportunity development perspective in the form of a model founded on the basis of extensive research yet applicable to real-life therapeutic relationships

> Egan stated that the aim of this model is to assist the therapist in helping the client to 'manage their problems in living more effectively and develop unused opportunities more fully'

> This skilled helper model provides a framework for helping by plotting the therapeutic process over three stages in order to highlight the appropriate use of skills during each step of the relationship from problem presentation to solution management

Egan's skilled helper model is arguably the single most enduring and influential helping model in history

> Significant impact on counselling, psychotherapy, psychology, business, nursing, coaching, etc. for over 30 years

Three stages

Therapeutic process is mapped through three stages

> First stage focuses on the current scenario by reviewing the problem situations and unused opportunities

> Second stage focuses on the preferred scenario by developing ideas about the possibilities for the future

Third stage focuses on strategy by determining a plan for realising the goals, solving the problem, taking advantage of the unused opportunities and striving for the preferred scenario

Stages do not follow a clear linear path with precise sequential steps, but rather act as a framework for the techniques and a guide to the process

First stage: current picture – what's going on?

The first stage of the skilled helper model aims to assist clients in exploring, identifying and clarifying their problem situations and unused opportunities

Clients need to be able to tell their story in their own words with the belief that they are being heard, acknowledged and accepted

However, although clients need to feel as though the therapist is listening to their story from their frame of reference, it is also important that the therapist encourages the client to explore their story in more detail with the aim of viewing the situation from a wider perspective and from the perspective of others

Key question: 'what is going on in your world?'

STORY

The first step of the first stage will focus on the client telling their story

This step forms the basis of the therapeutic relationship between the therapist and the client

Deffenbacher (1985) noted that the skilled helper should strive to build rapport with a client by listening in a non-judgemental manner, attending to both thoughts and feelings, and responding with honesty and care

It is essential that the therapist is able to establish this positive connection with the client during the early stages of the therapeutic process in order for the client to feel comfortable and confident enough to tell their story

The client has to trust the therapist in order to be completely honest about their story and this is the first step towards solving their problem

Key questions to encourage story telling will include 'tell me about . . .'

NEW PERSPECTIVES

The second step of the first stage will focus on identifying blind spots

People who are immersed in a problem will often fail to see the situation from a wider perspective and may neglect to account for the perspectives of others within the environment

Clients may experience blindness with regard to certain factors associated with their problem

Therapists should help clients to discover and challenge these blind spots by viewing the problem from a different angle, exploring alternative frames of reference, clarifying the problem details and investigating any unused opportunities

Key questions to address blind spots during this stage may include 'is there any other way of looking at this issue?' and 'how do you think a neutral observer might describe this situation?'

VALUE

The third step of the first stage will focus on the search for leverage

Therapists should help clients to focus on the issues that have a significant impact in their life

Egan (2007) suggests that the principles of leverage should be applied to determine which issue should be addressed: if applicable, priority must be given to crisis management, problems causing extreme pain for the client, problems viewed as particularly important by the client, problems for which the benefits outweigh the costs, problems that are manageable parts of a larger problem, and problems that impact on the general wellbeing of the client

Key questions to help the client prioritise their issues may include 'what is the most important part of all of this for you?' and 'what would you most like to focus on at this moment in time?'

Second stage: preferred picture – what do I need or want?

The second stage of the skilled helper model aims to assist clients in identifying their needs and desires in terms of goals based on an understanding of the current problem situations and unused opportunities

Some people move between problem and action without ever really considering exactly what they want from a solution

Therapist needs to focus on establishing the exact solution desired by the client

Key question: 'what do you want?'

POSSIBILITIES

The first step of the second stage will focus on exploring possibilities for the preferred scenario

Therapists should help clients conceptualise various new future situations as alternatives to the current problematic situation

Clients should be encouraged to be imaginative rather than realistic at this stage and therapists should try to keep these brainstorming activities fun and non-judgemental

Key questions to encourage the client to explore more ideas could include 'what do you really want to happen?' and 'what would your world be like if this problem did not exist and everything was perfect?'

CHANGE AGENDA

The second step of the second stage will focus on developing the range of possibilities into viable goals

Therapists should help clients to identify the realistic possibilities through a reality testing process

It is important that the potential goals are demanding enough to stretch the client, yet realistic enough to give the client an opportunity to succeed

This stage will often incorporate a number of challenging skills, as it requires the client to be honest about their own capabilities and options

Key questions to focus the client on goal setting could include 'which possible future scenario would be best for you?' or 'which future scenario do you think could be achieved?'

There are a number of important elements to consider when setting goals with the client and it may be helpful for the therapist to ask whether the goals are clear and specific, achievable and realistic, and measurable within a set time frame. These questions form the basis of the SMART model for goal setting: specific, measurable, achievable, realistic, time limited

COMMITMENT

The third step of the second stage will focus on establishing a commitment to change

Clients should attempt to conduct a cost/benefit analysis of the goal in order to assess the incentives for change

Key questions to encourage this analysis could include 'what will be better for you if you achieve this goal?' and 'what are the downsides of trying to achieve this goal?'

Third stage: the way forward – how do I get what I need or want?

The third stage of the skilled helper model aims to assist clients in developing action strategies for achieving their goals

Therapist should attempt to work with the client to establish a plan of action

Key question: 'how can you get what you want?'

POSSIBLE STRATEGIES

The first step of the third stage will focus on brainstorming action strategies

Therapists should encourage clients to include all possible strategies without limitations as even silly strategies might lead to realistic possibilities

Key questions to promote free thinking may include 'how could you achieve this goal?' and 'can you think of any wild and wacky ways of achieving this goal?'

BEST FIT STRATEGIES

The second step of the third stage will focus on selecting a set of strategies appropriate to the current situation of the client

Therapists should encourage clients to investigate both internal factors (client needs, values, preferences, etc.) and external factors (resources, support networks, etc.) to ascertain which strategies could be realistic and effective

Clients can be encouraged to focus on appropriate strategies through the use of key questions such as 'which of these ideas is most realistic?' or 'which of these ideas is right for you?'

PLAN

The third step of the third stage will focus on transforming the strategy into a plan of action

Therapists should help clients to formulate a plan of action designed to change the current scenario into the preferred scenario by asking key questions such as 'what will you do first?' and 'what exactly will you do next?'

These plans should be clearly outlined in a step-by-step guide with realistic time frames

SUMMARY

Approach/therapy/model: approach = umbrella term for all theories and concepts converging on a similar set of principles (humanistic, psychodynamic, behavioural, cognitive); therapy = practical application of an approach to improve psychological wellbeing (e.g. person-centred therapy under humanistic approach); model = framework for applying a therapy (e.g. skilled helper model)

Purist versus non-purist: purists exclusively use only one approach and usually remain within the remit of one specific therapy (only 4.2% regard themselves as purist); non-purists use more than one approach and will often combine elements of different therapies (regarded as integrative, eclectic or syncretistic)

Integration/eclecticism/syncretism: integration = combination of different approaches to produce an entirely new therapy on the basis of a new underlying approach; eclecticism = combination of different therapies to produce an entirely new therapy without specific subscription to an underlying approach; syncretism = random selection of techniques without understanding of underlying theory (ineffective)

Types: theoretical integration = integrate two or more approaches into a single novel approach; assimilative integration = focus on one core approach with selective integration of some techniques from therapies under other approaches; common factors = focus on common elements across multiple approaches to pull together the most effective theories into a novel approach; technical eclecticism = utilise techniques from therapies under different approaches without subscribing to any underlying approach

Egan's skilled helper model: problem management model, promotes collaborative relationship with helper guiding client towards solutions, arguably most enduring and influential helping model in history (30 years old); Stage 1 Present scenario, what's going on in your world? Story, new

> perspectives, value; Stage 2 Preferred scenario, what do you want? Possibilities, change agenda, commitment; Stage 3 Strategy for A to B, how do I get what I want? Possible strategies, best fit strategies, plan

REFERENCES AND BIBLIOGRAPHY

American Psychological Association (APA) (2013) Retrieved from www.apa.org

Association for Counselling and Therapy Online (ACTO) (n.d.) Therapists for depression. Retrieved from www.acto-uk.org/depression.htm

Barrott, J. (2008) Culture and diversity in counselling. In: Dryden, W. & Reeves, A. (eds) *Key Issues for Counselling in Action*. London: Sage Publications.

Bond, T. & Jenkins, P. (2007) *Access to Records of Counselling and Psychotherapy*. BACP Information Sheet G1. Lutterworth: BACP.

British Association for Counselling and Psychotherapy (BACP) (2010a) Attitudes to Counselling and Psychotherapy Survey 2010. *Therapy Today*, 21(7), 38.

British Association for Counselling and Psychotherapy (BACP) (2010b) *Ethical Framework for Good Practice in Counselling and Psychotherapy*. Lutterworth: BACP.

British Association for Counselling and Psychotherapy (BACP) (2010c) What does 'orientation' mean? Retrieved from www.bacp.co.uk/accreditation/Accredited%20Course%20Search/course%20modalities.php

British Association for Counselling and Psychotherapy (BACP) (2013) Retrieved from www.bacp.co.uk/

British Psychological Society (BPS) (2009) *Code of Ethics and Conduct*. Leicester: BPS.

British Psychological Society (BPS) (2013) Retrieved from www.bps.org.uk/

Clarkson, P. (1992) *TA Psychotherapy*. London: Routledge.

CORE-OM (n.d.) Clinical Outcomes in Routine Evaluation Outcome Measure (CORE-OM). Retrieved from www.coreims.co.uk/About_Core_System_Outcome_Measure.html

Corsini, R.J. & Wedding, D. (2008) *Current Psychotherapies*, 8th edn. Pacific Grove, CA: Thomson Brooks/Cole.

Dale, H. (2003) *Making the Contract for Counselling and Psychotherapy*. Information Sheet P11. Rugby: BACP.

Dattilio, F.M. & Norcross, C.J. (2006) Psychotherapy integration and the emergence of instinctual territoriality. *Archives of Psychiatry and Psychotherapy*, 8(1), 5–16.

Deffenbacher, J.L. (1985) A cognitive-behavioural response and a modest proposal. *Counselling Psychologist*, 13, 261–269.

Egan, G. (1994) *The Skilled Helper*. Belmont, CA: Brooks/Cole Publishing Company.

Egan, G. (2007) *The Skilled Helper*, 9th edn. Belmont, CA: Brooks/Cole Publishing Company.

False Memory Syndrome Foundation (n.d.) Retractors speak. Retrieved from www.fmsonline.org/retract1.html

Fanner, D. & Urquhart, C. (2008) Bibliotherapy for mental health service users Part 1: a systematic review. *Health Information & Libraries Journal*, 25(4), 237–252.

Genesis Interactive (2009) *The Machine called Abel*. Retrieved from www.genesisweb.co.nz/g6/genesis-interactive/content/30/RnD/Project-ABEL/The-Machine-called-ABEL

Grohol, J. (2011) Telehealth: wait, there's online therapy? *Psych Central*. Retrieved from http://psychcentral.com/blog/archives/2011/07/14/telehealth-wait-theres-online-therapy/

Health Professions Council (HPC) (n.d.) Retrieved from www.hpc-uk.org/

Hoffman, J. (2011) When your therapist is only a click away. Retrieved from www.nytimes.com/ 2011/09/25/fashion/therapists-are-seeing-patients-online.html?_r=2&smid=fb-share&page wanted=all&

Hollanders, H. (2000) Eclecticism/integration: some key issues and research. In: Palmer, S. & Woolfe, R. (eds) *Integrative and Eclectic Counselling and Psychotherapy*. London: Sage.

iTherapy (2005) What is iTherapy? Retrieved from www.itherapy.com/free-therapy-info.html

Josefson, D. (2001) Re-birthing therapy banned after girl died in 70 minute struggle. *BMJ*, 322 (7293), 1014.

Lago, C. (2011) *The Handbook of Transcultural Counselling and Psychotherapy*. Buckingham: Open University Press.

Lago, C. & Thompson, J. (2005) *Race, Culture and Counselling*. Buckingham: Open University Press.

Lazarus, A.A. (1992) Multimodal therapy: technical eclecticism with minimal integration. In: Norcross, J.C. & Goldfried, M.R. (eds) *Handbook of Psychotherapy Integration*. New York: Basic Books.

Leff, J., Williams, G., Huckvale, M., Arbuthnot, M. & Leff, A.P. (2013) Avatar therapy for persecutory auditory hallucinations: what is it and how does it work? *Psychosis*, 1–11.

Loftus, E.F. (1997) Creating false memories. *Scientific American*, 277(3), 70–75.

Lutus, P. (2013) Is psychology a science? Retrieved from www.arachnoid.com/psychology/ index.html

McLeod, J. (2003) *An Introduction to Counselling*. Buckingham: Open University Press.

McLeod, J. (2009) *An Introduction to Counselling*, 4th edn. Buckingham: Open University Press.

Mearns, B. & Thorne, D. (2007) *Person-Centered Counselling in Action*. London: Sage Publications.

Mental Health Foundation (n.d.) Mental health statistics. Retrieved from www.mentalhealth.org.uk/ help-information/mental-health-statistics/

Nelson-Jones, R. (2005) *Practical Counselling and Helping Skills*. London: Sage Publications.

NHS (n.d.) Retrieved from www.nhsdirect.wales.nhs.uk/lifestylewellbeing/bibliotherapyhowitworks

Norcross, J.C. & Beutler, L. (2008) Integrative psychotherapies. In: Corsini, R.J. & Wedding, D. (eds) *Current Psychotherapies*, 8th edn. Pacific Grove, CA: Thomson Brooks/Cole.

Norcross, J.C., Koocher, G.P. & Garofalo, A. (2006) Discredited psychological treatments and tests: a Delphi poll. *Professional Psychology: Research and Practice*, 37(5), 515.

Parsons, T.D. & Rizzo, A.A. (2008) Affective outcomes of virtual reality exposure therapy for anxiety and specific phobias: a meta-analysis. *Journal of Behavior Therapy and Experimental Psychiatry*, 39(3), 250–261.

Patterson, C.H. (2004) Do we need multicultural competencies? *Journal of Mental Health Counseling*, 26(1), 67–73.

Pedersen, P.B. (1991) Multiculturalism as a generic framework. *Journal of Counselling and Development*, 70(1), 6–12.

Psychotherapy Networker (2007) *The most influential therapists of the past quarter-century*. Retrieved from www.psychotherapynetworker.org/component/content/article/81–2007-marchapril/898- ten-most-influential-therapists

Ryan, K. (2010) Flexible boundaries. *Therapy Today*, 21, 10.

Sills, C. (2006) *Contracts in Counselling and Psychotherapy*. London: Sage Publications.

Stiles, W.B., Barkham, M., Mellor-Clark, J. & Connell, J. (2008) Effectiveness of cognitive-behavioural, person-centered, and psychodynamic therapies in UK primary-care routine practice: replication in a larger sample. *Psychological Medicine*, 38, 677–688.

Sue, D.W. & Sue, D. (1990) *Counselling the Culturally Different: Theory and Practice.* New York: Wiley.

Sutton, J. & Stewart, W. (2002) *Learning to Counsel.* Oxford: Spring Hill House.

Totton, N. (2010) Boundaries and boundlessness. *Therapy Today,* 21, 8.

UK Council for Psychotherapy (UKCP) (2009) *Ethical Principles and Code of Professional Conduct.* Retrieved from www.psychotherapy.org.uk/code_of_ethics.html

Virtue, D. (2010) Angel therapy. Retrieved from www.angeltherapy.com/index.php

Wachtel, P. (1991) From eclecticism to synthesis: towards a more seamless psychotherapy integration. *Journal of Psychotherapy Integration,* 1, 43–54.

Walfish, S., Barnett, J.E., Marlere, K. & Zielke, R. (2010) 'Doc, there's something I have to tell you': patient disclosure to their psychotherapist of unprosecuted murder and other violence. *Ethics and Behaviour,* 20(5), 311–323.

Whitbourne, S.K. (2011) 13 Qualities to look for in an effective psychotherapist. *Psychology Today.* Retrieved from www.psychologytoday.com/blog/fulfillment-any-age/201108/13-qualities-look-in-effective-psychotherapist

Wolz, B. (2013) Cinema therapy. Retrieved from www.cinematherapy.com/

World Health Organization (WHO) (2013) Retrieved from www.who.int/en/

Yuen, E.K., Herbert, J.D., Forman, E.M., Goetter, E.M., Comer, R. & Bradley, J.C. (2013) Treatment of social anxiety disorder using online virtual environments in Second Life. *Behavior Therapy,* 44(1), 51–61.

TABLE 1.1 Examples of common approaches and therapies

Approach	Humanistic approach (third force in psychology)	Psychodynamic approach (second force in psychology)	Behavioural approach (first force in psychology)	Cognitive approach (cognitive revolution)
Pure therapies	Person-centred therapy	Psychoanalytic therapy	Behaviour therapy	Cognitive therapy
	Existential therapy	Adlerian therapy	Applied behaviour analysis (behaviour modification)	Rational therapy
Integrated therapies	Gestalt therapy		Rational emotive behaviour therapy	
	Transactional analysis		Cognitive-behaviour therapy	
Eclectic therapies	Multimodal therapy			
	Neurolinguistic programming			

Chapter 2

Humanistic approach and person-centred therapy

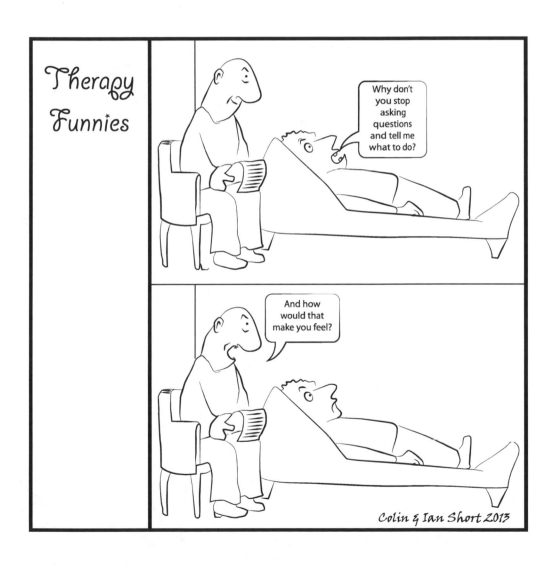

CHAPTER CONTENTS

- Introduction to humanistic approach and person-centred therapy
- Development of the humanistic approach
  - Third force in psychology
  - Major advances in the humanistic approach
  - Key figures in the humanistic approach
- Personal and professional biographies of Carl Rogers and Abraham Maslow
  - Biography of Carl Rogers
  - Significant learnings
  - Biography of Abraham Maslow
  - Significant learnings of Abraham Maslow
- Humanistic theories of human nature and personality
  - Organismic self and self-concept
  - Impact of conditions of worth on the self-concept
  - Tendency towards self-actualisation
  - Hierarchy of needs
  - Characteristics of the fully functioning person
  - Nineteen propositions of personality
- Therapeutic relationship in person-centred therapy
  - Six conditions for constructive personality change
  - Necessary and sufficient?
  - Stages of constructive personality change
  - Relational depth
- Therapeutic techniques in person-centred therapy
  - Absence of techniques
  - Demonstrating congruence
  - Demonstrating unconditional positive regard
  - Demonstrating empathic understanding
- Case study demonstrating person-centred therapy
  - Recorded session: therapy in action
  - Presentation of Phil Thomas: history and symptoms
  - Therapy session: analysis
  - Personal experience of the client

INTRODUCTION TO HUMANISTIC APPROACH AND PERSON-CENTRED THERAPY

This chapter aims to introduce the reader to the humanistic approach to counselling and psychotherapy. Person-centred therapy will be explored as one example of a therapeutic method under the humanistic approach.

LEARNING OUTCOMES

By the end of this chapter, you will be able to:

- describe the development of the third force in psychology: the humanistic approach
- acknowledge the relative impacts of Carl Rogers and Abraham Maslow on the development of the humanistic approach
- discuss the core theories of human nature and personality from the humanistic perspective
- discuss the nature of the therapeutic relationship between therapist and client in person-centred therapy
- outline the main therapeutic techniques utilised in person-centred therapy
- appreciate the application of person-centred therapy in a real-world setting

---

DEVELOPMENT OF THE HUMANISTIC APPROACH

LEARNING OUTCOMES

After reading this section, you will be able to:

- list the three main forces in psychology
- discuss the development of the humanistic approach in a historical context
- acknowledge the main contributors to the development of the humanistic approach

---

Third force in psychology

Three forces in psychology

    Behavioural approach

    Psychodynamic approach

    Humanistic approach

Humanistic psychology is the 'third force'

Reacted against psychodynamic and behavioural approaches dominant in early 20th century

    First force

        Behavioural psychology assumed that human nature was mechanistic and reduced humanity to the link between stimuli and response (see Chapter 4 for further information)

    Second force

        Psychodynamic psychology assumed human nature was deterministic and reduced humanity to basic biological drives (see Chapter 3 for further information)

    Third force

        Humanistic psychology is 'a response to the denigration of the human spirit that has so often been implied in the image of the person drawn by behavioural and social sciences' (Association for Humanistic Psychology, 2001)

Reacted against the medical model

    Medical model and psychiatry focus on illness

        Aim of the medical model is to cure the patient

        This makes the crucial assumption that the individual is sick and that the practitioner is an expert who needs to act on the individual in order to improve his or her mental health

    Humanistic approach focuses on individuals

        Aim of humanism is to offer a safe environment for an individual to re-establish control over his or her own world

Reacted against the values of logical positivism

    Logical positivism focuses on logic and empiricism to understand thoughts, feelings and behaviours

        Logical positivism was developed by the Vienna Circle (Schlick, Godel, Carnap, Hempel, Neurath, etc.)

        Logical positivism attempts to solve the demarcation problem (identify the line between science and pseudoscience) by suggesting that science should build a system of knowledge about the natural world using empiricisms (statements that can be verified as true)

        Logical positivism emphasises rationalism (use of reason, intellect and logic to draw inferences about the world) and empiricism (observational evidence to draw conclusions about the world)

    Humanistic approach focuses on the individual human experience, rather than objective scientific enquiry

        Founding fathers of humanism were heavily influenced by existential phenomenology (Kierkegaard, Husserl, Heidegger, etc.)

Existential phenomenology suggests that the human condition must be considered from the perspective of the individual as a unique whole seeking answers about reality

Existential phenomenology emphasises the subjective nature of meaning and the importance of individual experience

Dedicated to a meaningful human-based perspective

Psychology is predominantly the study of human nature and yet much of the focus appears to be on factors affecting all species

Drive for reward, drive for food, sex drive, etc. are present in almost all species across the world

Humanists in the 1950s began to explore elements of the human that are overlooked in other fields of psychology

Essentially human phenomena such as love, hope, creativity, individuality, the nature of being, self-consciousness, self-awareness, philosophy, language, art and morality

Friedman (1994) argued that the humanistic shift could be described as a move 'from determinism to self-determination, from causality to purpose, from manipulation to self-responsibility, from analysis to synthesis, from diagnosis to dialogue, from solution-oriented models to process, from degradation of human life to celebration of the human spirit'

This approach rejects the objective control of science in favour of an empathic understanding of humanity

Major advances in the humanistic approach

Initial interest in humanistic approach

Rogers suggested that psychology in general and therapy in particular should focus on the individual as a unique human being

Counseling and Psychotherapy published in 1942

Client-Centred Therapy published in 1951

Maslow suggested that psychology should focus on exploring human behaviour in terms of our desire to satisfy needs and argued that theories of motivation should be human centred rather than animal centred

A Theory of Human Motivation published in *Psychological Review* in 1943

Motivation and Personality published in 1954

Formal establishment of humanistic approach

Detroit meetings at the invitation of Maslow and Moustakas took place in 1957 and 1958

Aim of establishing an association focusing on 'the subjective human being' (Rogers, 1962)

Cohen published the first book on humanistic psychology titled *Humanistic Psychology* in 1958

American Association of Humanistic Psychology formed in 1961

> Establishment of this association marked the formal foundation of the humanistic approach

Journal of Humanistic Psychology launched in 1961

> Initially known as The Phoenix

Humanistic Invitational Conference in Connecticut in 1964

> Attendees included psychologists such as Rollo May, Gardner Murphy, Gordon Allport, J.F.T. Bugental, Henry Murray, Charlotte Buhler, Abraham Maslow and Carl Rogers

> Attendees included other humanists such as Jacques Barzun, Rene Dubos and Floyd Matson

> Conference focused on exploring why the first and second forces in psychology (behavioural and psychodynamic approaches) failed to explore the real issues, problems and complexities of the human condition

> Attendees concluded that the 'third force' of humanistic psychology would 'offer a fuller concept and experience of what it means to be human' (Association for Humanistic Psychology, 2001)

American Psychological Association recognised status in 1972

> Humanistic Psychology is Division 32 of the APA and produces its own academic journal, *The Humanistic Psychologist*

Modern humanistic approach

Breadth of the modern humanistic approach

> One of the key principles of the humanistic approach is the idea of individuals being in a constant process of 'becoming'

>> Becoming means to be constantly striving to be more effective and moving towards self-actualisation

> Therefore, it is not surprising that the approach itself is also not static

>> The approach too is in a process of continuous ongoing development

Rogers continued to develop the theories that underpin the humanistic approach, and welcomed others to research and develop their own ideas

> Since producing his theory of personality, and later his ideas on the conditions for therapeutic change and the stages of the process of change, there have been other key theorists who have taken forward the theory and developed this approach further

Key figures in the humanistic approach

Carl Rogers (1902–1987)

Impact on the approach

Introduced person-centred therapy as a therapeutic method of applying the principles of humanism

Emphasised the importance of the therapeutic relationship in moving a client towards self-actualisation

Argued that six conditions were necessary and sufficient for the therapist to encourage positive therapeutic change

It has become common in the person-centred approach to talk about the three 'core' conditions of unconditional positive regard, accurate empathic understanding and congruence (conditions 3, 4 and 5 of the original six), but it is important to recognise that Rogers argued that all six conditions were necessary and sufficient

Focused on the client being 'fully received' (Rogers, 1961) and the idea of 'presence' (Rogers, 1980)

Selected works

Counseling and Psychotherapy published in 1942

Client-centred Therapy: Its Current Practice, Implications and Theory published in 1951

On Becoming a Person: A Therapist's View of Psychotherapy published in 1961

Freedom to Learn published in 1969

A Way of Being published in 1980

Abraham Maslow (1908–1970)

Impact on the approach

Developed a hierarchy of human needs to describe the nature of human motivation

Highlighted the importance of addressing basic needs (such as physiological needs like food and safety needs like security of body) before being able to address higher needs (such as belonging needs like family and esteem needs like confidence) so that the individual can eventually strive towards self-actualisation

Selected works

A Theory of Human Motivation published in *Psychological Review* in 1946

Motivation and Personality published in 1954

Toward a Psychology of Being published in 1968

Rollo May (1909–1994)

Impact on the approach

> Associated existential philosophy with the humanistic movement

> Provided insight into evil and suffering, and encouraged debate about the links between love and sex

Selected works

> The Meaning of Anxiety published in 1950

> Existence published in 1956

> Love and Will published in 1969

James Bugental (1915–2008)

Impact on the approach

> Published a manifesto for the third force in psychology

> Outlined five key postulates for the approach: human beings cannot be reduced to components, have in them a uniquely human context, have an awareness of oneself, have choices and responsibilities, and seek meaning, value and creativity

Selected works

> Humanistic Psychology: A New Breakthrough published in 1963

> The Search for Authenticity published in 1965

Eugene Gendlin (1926–current)

Impact on the approach

> Student and subsequent close colleague of Rogers

> Developed experiential focusing oriented therapy

> Interested in the process of how clients change, and how the therapist can help clients attend to their 'inner experiencing' through the use of empathic responding

Selected works

> Focusing published in 1978

Natalie Rogers (1928–current)

Impact on the approach

> Carl Rogers' daughter

> Developed person-centred expressive art therapy using empathy to help clients explore the personal meanings of their creativity

Selected works

> The Creative Connection: Expressive Arts as Healing published in 1993

Garry Prouty (1937–2009)

Impact on the approach

> Significant contribution in engaging clients who need preparation to engage in the therapeutic process

> Pre-therapy remains very close to the original humanistic concept proposed by Rogers but offers an opportunity to work with those who would ordinarily be excluded from the 'talking cure' (e.g. those unable to communicate)

Selected works

> *Pre-therapy* published in 1976

SUMMARY

Three forces: behavioural, psychodynamic, humanistic; humanistic focused on essentially human traits, reacted against medical model and logical positivism, dedicated to a meaningful human-based perspective

Major advances: initial ideas proposed by Maslow and Rogers in 1940s; Rogers suggested psychology should focus on individuals as unique human beings, Maslow suggested psychology should be human centred and focus on satisfaction of needs; formally established in 1960s, Detroit meetings set up to establish approach in 1950s, American Association of Humanistic Psychology formed in 1961, *Journal of Humanistic Psychology* launched in 1961, Humanistic Invitational Conference held in 1964, APA recognised status in 1972; modern approach is constantly evolving and in a process of 'becoming'

Key figures: Rogers' person-centred therapy, Maslow's hierarchy of needs, May's existential philosophy, Bugental's humanistic manifesto, Gendlin's focusing, Rogers' expressive arts, Prouty's pre-therapy

---

PERSONAL AND PROFESSIONAL BIOGRAPHIES OF CARL ROGERS AND ABRAHAM MASLOW

LEARNING OUTCOMES

After reading this section, you will be able to:

* outline the personal and professional biography of Carl Rogers (1902–1987)

* outline the personal and professional biography of Abraham Maslow (1908–1970)

* appreciate the impact of these key figures on the development of the humanistic approach

Biography of Carl Rogers

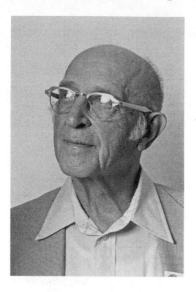

*'I speak as a person, from a
context of personal experience
and personal learnings'*
—Rogers (1961)

Who was Carl Rogers?

Carl Rogers helped to found the humanistic movement

> Possibly the most influential change in modern psychology

Carl Rogers introduced person-centred therapy

> Possibly the most influential therapist in history

In answering the question 'who are you?'. . .

> 'I am a psychologist whose primary interest has been in psychotherapy' (Rogers, 1961)

Early years

Born January 8th 1902 in Chicago

> Fourth of six children – father (Walter Rogers) was a civil engineer and mother (Julia) was a housewife

Successful affluent family

> Strong Christian values: no alcohol or theatre, very little social life, lots of work

> Solitary child who read incessantly and went on only two dates in high school

Educationally advanced from a young age

> He entered school in second grade because he was reading before kindergarten

> His family moved away from the temptations of suburban Chicago to a farm when he was 12 and the advanced methods of agriculture used on the farm instilled in him a love and understanding of science

Education

Agriculture major at Wisconsin College

> He switched major after two years after a powerful religious student conference convinced him to seek a future in the ministry

History major at Wisconsin College

> He visited China for an International World Student Christian Federation Conference
>
>> This experience brought him into contact with German and French enemies and he realised that likable individuals could hold extremely disparate attitudes about politics, religion, etc.
>>
>> He emancipated himself from the religion of his parents and became an 'independent person'
>
> Graduated with a BA in History in 1924

Family

Married Helen Elliot in 1924

> He fell in love with his childhood friend and married her soon after college
>
> This further increased the poor relations with his parents, although they did give reluctant consent to the wedding
>
> He remained married to Helen Elliot until her death in 1979
>
> 'I cannot be very objective about this, but her steady and sustaining love and companionship during all the years since has been a most important and enriching factor in my life' (Rogers, 1961)

Raised two children

> David was born in 1926 and Natalie was born in 1928
>
> '... my son and daughter grew through infancy and childhood, teaching me far more about individuals, their development, and their relationships, than I could ever have learnt professionally' (Rogers, 1961)

Career

Attended the Union Theological Seminary in 1924

> He petitioned the administration to be permitted to establish a credit-free seminar containing no instructor or syllabus in order for students to explore their own ideas
>
> His petition was successful and subsequent discussion in these seminars began to form the philosophy of life evident in the humanistic approach
>
>> He decided that beliefs were so transient that it would be awful to work in a field in which one had to profess a set of beliefs in order to remain in the profession
>>
>> He decided to seek a field of work in which he would have unlimited freedom of thought

Clinical psychology

> Philosophy of Education at Teachers' College of Columbia University
>
>> Clinical work with children under Leta Hollingworth
>>
>> MA in 1928
>>
>> PhD in 1931
>
> Granted a fellowship at the new Institute for Child Guidance
>
>> He was exposed to Freudian therapy through work with David Levy and Lawson Lowrey
>
> Psychologist in the Child Study Department of the Society for the Prevention of Cruelty to Children in New York
>
>> He realised that mental disturbance might not have the sexual basis claimed by psychodynamic theory and that therapeutic work might not require direction and interpretation
>>
>> 'I was moving away from any approach which was coercive or pushing in clinical relationships, not for philosophical reasons, but because such approaches were never more than superficially effective . . . It is the client who knows what hurts, what directions to go, what problems are crucial, what experiences have been deeply buried. It began to occur to me that unless I had a need to demonstrate my own cleverness and learning, I would do better to rely upon the client for the direction of movement in the process' (Rogers, 1961)

Lecturer

> Lecturer on Working with Troubled Children at University of Rochester in 1935
>
>> His work did not fit with the behaviourist approach of experimental psychology or the psychodynamic approach of psychoanalysis
>>
>> He lectured under the Department of Sociology and Department of Education
>>
>> He eventually fitted into the role of psychologist after the formation of the American Association for Applied Psychology
>
> Professor of Clinical Psychology at Ohio State University in 1940
>
>> 'Contrary to expectation, they offered me full professorship. I heartily recommend starting in the academic world at this level. I have often been grateful that I have never had to live through the frequently degrading competitive process of step-by-step promotion in university facilities, where individuals so frequently learn only one lesson – not to stick their necks out' (Rogers, 1961)
>
> Professor of Psychology at University of Chicago in 1945
>
>> He established a therapy centre at the university where he served as Executive Secretary
>>
>> Elected President of the American Psychological Association (APA) in 1946
>>
>> Published *Client-centred Therapy* in 1951 to describe a new approach to therapy and outlined the core conditions for constructive personality change

Award for Distinguished Scientific Contributions by the American Psychological Association (APA) in 1956

Professor at University of Wisconsin in 1957

Joint post in Department of Psychology and Department of Psychiatry

Published *On Becoming a Person* in 1961

Researcher at Western Behavioral Sciences Institute in 1964

Center for the Studies of the Person in 1968

Published *Freedom to Learn* in 1969 outlining applications of the person-centred approach in education

Published *A Way of Being* in 1980

Founded a new centre focusing on therapy and psychoeducation

'We are a face-to-face community of people for whom the Person Centred Approach plays an important role in our personal and professional lives – as a way of Being and of doing. Our commitment is to maintain/build/create an environment where each of us can be heard, where we can be fully ourselves, where we accept and embrace each other as we are. Currently projects offer opportunities for Person Centred personal growth, community leadership development, creative use of conflict, publishing, library and bookstore, organizational development and psychotherapy training' (Center for the Studies of the Person, 2010)

Dedicated later years to applying theories to social conflict

He travelled the world delivering seminars and workshops with the aim of uniting conflicting forces

Protestants and Catholics in Belfast

Blacks and whites in South Africa

He was nominated for a Nobel Peace Prize in 1987

Death

Died February 4th 1987 in San Diego

Cause of death was recorded as heart failure

Significant learnings

'In my relationships with persons I have found that it does not help, in the long run, to act as though I were something that I am not' (Rogers, 1961)

'I have found it of enormous value when I can permit myself to understand another person' (Rogers, 1961)

'The more I am open to the realities in me and in the other person, the less do I find myself wishing to rush in to "fix things"' (Rogers, 1961)

'Evaluation by others is not a guide for me' (Rogers, 1961)

'It has been my experience that persons have a basically positive direction' (Rogers, 1961)

FOUNDING FATHER OF THE HUMANISTIC APPROACH: ROGERS

Consider the life story of Carl Rogers and try to answer the following questions.

1. What was the social and cultural context of the world in which Rogers developed his theories?
2. How might Rogers' life experiences have impacted on his perception of human nature?
3. How can this life story contribute to your understanding of the humanistic approach?

Biography of Abraham Maslow

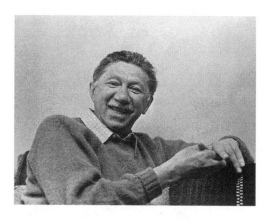

'I was awfully curious to find out why I didn't go insane.'
—Maslow (as cited by Association for Humanistic Psychology, 2011)

Who was Abraham Maslow?

Abraham Maslow helped to found the humanistic movement

Possibly the most influential change in modern psychology

Abraham Maslow introduced the hierarchy of needs

His theories have been applied across many fields, including business, education, therapy, healthcare, social policy, etc.

Early years

Born Abraham Harold Maslow on April 1st 1908 in Brooklyn, New York

Father (Samuel Maslow) was a cooper and mother (Rose Scholofsky) was a housewife

Jewish family

Parents were uneducated first-generation Russian immigrants who were determined that the family should succeed in the US

> He was expected to pursue a career in law, but preferred to read about psychology

Parents expected eldest son to assist with caring for the family

> He was expected to study for many hours then assist father at work and care for six younger siblings

> He had very few friends other than his cousins during his youth because most of his time was spent working

Extensive anti-Semitism within his neighbourhood

Non-Jewish neighbourhood with very few Jewish families

He was a shy and awkward child who suffered abuse from peers, teachers and neighbours

> 'I was a little Jewish boy in the non-Jewish neighborhood. It was a little like being the first Negro enrolled in an all-white school. I was isolated and unhappy. I grew up in libraries and among books, without friends' (Maslow cited in Hall, 1968)

Poor relationship with his parents

He had a poor relationship with his father

> His father was determined that his son would succeed where he had failed, so he constantly pushed him in all academic pursuits

> However, his relationship with his father did improve in later years and they were reconciled before his death

He had a particularly difficult relationship with his mother

> 'What I had reacted to and totally hated and rejected was not only her physical appearance, but also her values and world view, her stinginess, her total selfishness, her lack of love for anyone else in the world – even her own husband and children – her narcissism, her Negro prejudice, her exploitation of everyone, her assumption that anyone was wrong who disagreed with her, her lack of friends, her sloppiness and dirtiness . . .' (Maslow cited in Hoffman, 1988)

His negative feelings towards his mother were extremely strong and he never managed to overcome his hostility, even after extensive therapy as an adult – in fact, it is reported that he did not even attend her burial (Engler, 2008)

Educationally advanced from a young age

Attended Boys High School – top school in Brooklyn

However, he was unconvinced about his own capabilities and often had to be persuaded to exhibit his skills in any way

> Perhaps a result of the negative opinions held (and often expressed) about him by his parents?

Education

City College of New York and Brooklyn Law School

> Withdrew after three semesters against the wishes of his parents

Briefly attended Cornell, but had to withdraw for logistical reasons

Psychology major at University of Wisconsin

> Graduated in Psychology with a BA in 1930, MA in 1931 and doctorate in 1934

Family

Married Bertha Goodman in 1928

> Rebelled against parents by falling in love with his cousin and childhood sweetheart

> Married when he was 20 years old and she was only 19 years old and still in high school

> He describes this marriage as the true start to his life and they remained married until parted by death

Career

Research

> Researched primate dominance behaviour at University of Wisconsin

>> Experimental behavioural research conducted alongside Harlow (attachment theory)

> Researched human sexuality at Columbia in New York in 1935

>> Research conducted alongside Thorndike (theory of learning)

>> Adler introduced him to psychodynamic theory during his time at Columbia and this had a huge impact on his development as a psychologist

Lecturer

> Taught psychology at Brooklyn College in 1937

>> He began to focus on the study of exceptional human beings when he met several intellectuals, including Benedict and Wertheimer

>> He developed many of his initial theories on motivation and the hierarchy of needs during his time in New York

>> Published *A Theory of Human Motivation* in *Psychological Review* in 1946 – paper outlined the hierarchy of needs

> Chair of Psychology at Brandeis in Massachusetts in 1951

>> He worked alongside Goldstein who introduced him to the concept of self-actualisation (Goldstein, 1934)

>> He began promoting humanistic psychology in his role as Psychology Chair and this became the focus of his life's work

>> Published *Motivation and Personality* in 1954 to expand on the hierarchy of needs

>> Published *Toward a Psychology of Being* in 1968

Elected President of the American Psychological Association (APA) in 1968

Resident Fellow of the Laughlin Institute in California in 1969

Semi-retirement, but still updated his more influential books and wrote two more books

Dedicated later years to promoting humanistic psychology

He was responsible for controlling the new 'third force' in psychology and he focused exclusively on this psychological approach

Death

Died June 8th 1970 in California

Cause of death was recorded as a fatal heart attack while jogging in Menlo Park

---

FOUNDING FATHER OF THE HUMANISTIC APPROACH: MASLOW

Consider the life story of Abraham Maslow and try to answer the following questions.

1. What was the social and cultural context of the world in which Maslow developed his theories?
2. How might Maslow's life experiences have impacted on his perception of human nature?
3. How can this life story contribute to your understanding of the humanistic approach?

Significant learnings of Abraham Maslow

'The study of crippled, stunted, immature, and unhealthy specimens can yield only a cripple psychology and a cripple philosophy. The study of self-actualising people must be the basis for a more universal science of psychology' (Maslow, 1954)

'One of the goals of education should be to teach that life is precious. If there were no joy in life, it would not be worth living' (Maslow, 1954)

'If swindling pays, then it will not stop. The definition of the good society is one in which virtue pays' (Maslow, 1965)

'I suppose it is tempting, if the only tool you have is a hammer, to treat everything as if it were a nail' (Maslow, 1966)

'A first-rate soup is more creative than a second-rate painting' (Maslow, 1974)

SUMMARY

Rogers: founded humanistic movement and introduced person-centred therapy; *early years*, born 1902 in Chicago to an affluent Christian family, highly intellectual from a young age; *education*, initially studied agriculture but switched to history to enter ministry, graduated with BA in history; *family*, married childhood sweetheart and raised two children; *career*, moved away from religion and towards education and clinical therapy, took professorship in psychology in several institutes, introduced concept of client-centred therapy, outlined core conditions for constructive personality change, established the Center for the Studies of the Person, applied theories to education and social conflict, nominated for a Nobel Peace Prize; *death*, died of heart failure in 1987

Maslow: founded humanistic movement and developed hierarchy of needs; *early years*, born 1908 in New York to uneducated first-generation immigrants, Jewish family – anti-Semitism in neighbourhood, poor relationship with parents (especially mother), highly intellectual from a young age (possibly due to pressure to succeed from parents); *education*, studied law but withdrew against wishes of parents, studied psychology at University of Wisconsin – BA, MA, doctorate; *family*, married cousin and childhood sweetheart and raised two children; *career*, taught psychology at Brooklyn College, published *A Theory of Human Motivation* in 1946 (hierarchy of needs), Chair of Psychology at Brandeis, President of the APA, Resident Fellow of the Laughlin Institute, dedicated later years to promoting humanistic approach; *death*, died of a heart attack in 1970

HUMANISTIC THEORIES OF HUMAN NATURE AND PERSONALITY

LEARNING OUTCOMES

After reading this section, you will be able to:

*   describe the organismic self and the self-concept
*   discuss the impact of conditions of worth on the self-concept
*   discuss the tendency towards self-actualisation
*   describe the hierarchy of needs
*   describe the characteristics of the fully functioning person
*   outline the 19 propositions of personality

Organismic self and self-concept

Organismic self

Actual self

> Human organism generally provides the individual with trustworthy messages and will naturally strive towards enhancing the self (Mearns & Thorne, 1988)
>
> Children are often completely congruent with their organismic selves
>
> Child falls over = child feels pain = child begins to cry

Self-concept

Self-concept is defined as 'that organisation of qualities that the individual attributes to himself' (Kinch, 1963)

Configurations of self (Mearns et al., 2000)

> Self-concept is not a unified entity
>
> Individual may hold many different concepts of the self
>
>> Most of us hold contrasting views of ourselves
>>
>> We might feel that we can be both spontaneous and cautious or loving and angry
>>
>>> For example, a man with an alcohol addiction may feel as though there are two parts to his self-concept: 'drunk me' and 'sober me'
>>
>> Different configurations of the self may result in different and possibly conflicting thoughts, feelings and behaviours
>>
>>> For example, the man with an alcohol addiction may behave aggressively towards his partner when he is 'drunk me' but behaves in a loving manner when he is 'sober me'
>
> It is important to note that these configurations are different parts of the SAME personality
>
>> This is NOT split personality disorder
>
> Different 'parts' of the self are known as different 'configurations of self'
>
>> 'Configurations of self' is used instead of 'parts of self' so that it is recognised that each 'part' is also made up of many different parts
>>
>>> For example, the man with an alcohol addiction may hold a 'drunk me' configuration that can be further divided into an 'angry me' and an 'impulsive me'
>>
>> 'Configuration is a hypothetical construct denoting a coherent pattern of feelings, thoughts, and preferred behavioural responses symbolised by the person as reflective of a dimension of existence within the Self' (Mearns et al., 2000)
>
> Mearns et al. (2000) note that this notion of 'pluralism' in the self-concept (multiple parts of the self-concept) offers an 'adaptive versatility' because the different parts of the self can be used in different social environments

For example, a teenager might use her 'good daughter me' when at home and her 'rebel me' when with her friends

Perception of self

Social experiences will teach us about the person we 'should' be

Many of the different configurations of the self-concept have been created according to social influence

Children learn how they 'should' act, feel and think through interaction with others in their environment

Child falls over = child feels pain = child begins to cry = child is told that 'big boys don't cry' = child learns that pain should be buried and crying is a sign of weakness

Children eventually internalise these values and these values impact on their perception of the self

Child learns that crying is a sign of weakness = child believes that he is weak for wanting to cry = part of the self-concept of the child involves being a weak person = 'weak me'

OR

Child learns that crying is a sign of weakness = child believes that people who cry are weak = part of the self-concept of the child involves being a strong person who never cries = 'strong me'

Both of these self-concepts are equally damaging

'I am a weak person' can cause low self-esteem

'I never cry' can cause repression and emotional detachment

Perception of self is reinforced by interactions with others over time

Any interaction not fitting with the perception of the self (self-concept) will be ignored or distorted to fit with the self-concept

Self-concept involves being a weak person = individual is complimented for being a strong person = individual believes that the person giving the compliment does not really know him (information is ignored)

Self-concept involves being a strong person who never cries = individual is hurt and wants to cry = feelings of sadness are changed into feelings of anger (information is distorted)

Impact of conditions of worth on the self-concept

Positive regard (Standal, 1954)

Organismic self has a natural desire to receive positive regard from others

Human organisms naturally seek approval and recognition of success from family, friends, colleagues, superiors, etc.

Positive regard is rarely unconditional

Most of the significant people in our lives offer us conditional positive regard

Parents imply that they love us if we are good, spouses imply that they love us if we are faithful, friends imply that they love us if we are nice, etc.

Conditions of worth (Rogers, 1959) (Table 2.1)

Conditions of worth are the evaluations made by significant others about the correct way to act, think and feel in order to receive conditional positive regard

You must do these things in order to be loved, valued, etc.

You must meet these conditions in order to feel worthy

Conditions of worth are often internalised in childhood

Child falls over = child feels pain = child begins to cry = child is told that 'big boys don't cry' by mother = child stops crying = mother tells him that he is a good boy and gives him a hug = child learns that he is only lovable if he does not cry = child learns that crying is a sign of weakness and he will only be valued if he does not cry (condition of worth) = self-concept is influenced by this condition of worth = child believes that he is weak for wanting to cry or that he is a strong person who never cries

Tendency towards self-actualisation

Self-actualisation is the natural drive towards fulfilment

Goldstein (1934) coined the term self-actualisation to describe the driving force that works to move the organism through life towards achieving its true potential

In the absence of blocks and restrictions, all humans will naturally move towards self-actualisation

Each individual has a natural urge towards self-maintenance – we assimilate food, we defend ourselves when threatened, etc.

Child might be unable to find food alone yet all children will naturally know which behaviours to exhibit to seek out this goal (such as crying, suckling, etc.)

Each individual has a natural urge to mature – we start to walk, we start to have sex

Child might experience discomfort or pain when attempting to learn how to walk, and yet all children still strive towards this natural goal

Each individual also has a natural urge towards self-actualisation in a personal sense – we seek self-respect, autonomy, independence, etc.

Child will behave in specific ways designed to enhance their own self-respect and independence

From the perspective of an outside observer, some behaviour might not appear to be optimal for moving towards self-actualisation

However, if we view the world from the frame of reference of the individual and truly understand the private internal world of that individual, then we will see that even this behaviour is an attempt to move towards self-actualisation

Unacceptable behaviours such as stealing might initially appear to be actions moving away from enhancing the self, but we can understand these behaviours as attempts to self-actualise once we appreciate that the individual views financial gain as a means to achieve respect

Actualising tendency refers to the directional movement towards realisation, autonomy, perfection, acceptance, etc.

Note that the important factor here is not the achievement of self-actualisation but rather the constant growth, development and drive towards self-actualisation

All humans have this natural drive towards positivity but they are often confounded in their attempts to grow

Self-actualisation versus enlightenment

Enlightenment (or Nirvana or Knowing) often refers to a state of being

An individual may achieve this state of being through intense meditation or the movement of the self to a higher level of consciousness

Self-actualisation often refers to a process, drive or movement

An individual does not reach self-actualisation any more than one might reach 'running'

To be described as 'self-actualising', an individual must be moving towards his or her true potential

The actualising tendency is a state of movement, rather than a state of being

Congruency between organismic self and self-concept (Rogers, 1951)

In the presence of unconditional positive regard, you will become your 'real self' and experience self-respect, gain positive regard and value yourself as an individual

Your self-concept (perception of self) will be the same as your organismic self (true self)

This is known as congruence

In the presence of conditions of worth, you will develop an 'ideal self' and experience anxiety and gain only conditional positive regard

Your self-concept (perception of self) is not the same as your organismic self (true self)

This is known as incongruence

Self-actualisation is an attempt to reduce the space between the organismic self and the self-concept

Hierarchy of needs

Self-actualisation is a basic human need (Maslow, 1943)

Tendency towards self-actualisation is the highest need for the individual to achieve, but it can only be sought when all other needs are being met

Pyramid of human needs (Maslow, 1954)

Physiological needs

These needs include food, water, sex, homeostasis, sleep, etc.

These are the most basic needs for human life and must be met before the individual can seek to meet any higher needs

If all the basic needs are unsatisfied, then the individual will first strive to meet the physiological needs before focusing on any other needs

For example, a man who is starving will risk life and limb to seek food

Safety needs

These needs include security of self, family and property

Once physiological needs have been met, the individual will seek to meet safety needs

These needs must be met before the individual can focus on attempting to meet the subsequent needs of love, esteem and self-actualisation

For example, an insecure child who lives in fear of physical violence from her mother will seek protection rather than love

Love needs

These needs include intimacy in terms of family, friends and partners

Important to note the distinction between love and sex

Love is a sense of belonging and affection

Sex is a basic physiological need for all animals

Although love can be demonstrated through sexual intimacy, these two needs are mutually exclusive – you can have love without sex and you can have sex without love

However, although this distinction does exist, many people fail to acknowledge the difference and still confuse the expression of sexual desire with the expression of love

Once safety needs have been met, the individual will seek to meet love needs

These needs must be met before the individual can focus on attempting to meet the subsequent needs of esteem and self-actualisation

For example, a woman who feels unloved may show a lack of self-respect by acting in a clingy and needy manner towards her partner

Esteem needs

These needs include self-respect, respect of others, confidence and achievement

Once love needs have been met, the individual will seek to meet esteem needs

These needs must be met before the individual can focus on attempting to meet the highest need of self-actualisation

For example, an artist who believes that his father views him as weak and inferior may focus on succeeding in business, even though this is not a reflection of his true purpose in life

Self-actualisation needs

Self-actualisation is unique to each individual so it cannot be defined as a list of needs

Maslow (1943) explains that 'what a man can be, he must be' and states that self-actualisation involves the individual doing exactly what he is fitted to do: 'A musician must make music, an artist must paint, a poet must write, if he is to be ultimately happy'

Once all other needs have been met, the individual can focus on attempting to meet the highest need of self-actualisation

For example, a successful man who has sufficient resources to live in a secure environment with loving family can work on becoming his true self by doing what he is designed to do and accepting his true purpose in life

Peak experiences

Frankl (1946) suggested that self-actualisation is attainable (although perhaps only for short periods of time)

After achieving self-actualisation, the individual will feel happy with his or her life and enjoy peak experiences

Peak experiences are those events that bring absolute satisfaction and give a meaning or a purpose to a life

For example, a woman might have a peak experience after the birth of her child when she feels intense joy and believes that her life has a purpose

Frankl (1946) argues that this 'will to meaning' is the highest human need

Hierarchical structure (Figure 2.1)

Human needs are positioned in a hierarchy or pyramid

Lower needs must be met before the individual can focus on achieving higher needs

For example, a hungry man (physiological need) can hurt others because he is not seeking their love or respect (love and esteem needs)

A frightened child (safety need) will not be able to focus on learning in school (esteem need)

'Human needs arrange themselves in hierarchies of pre-potency. That is to say, the appearance of one need usually rests on the prior satisfaction of another, more pre-potent need. Man is a perpetually wanting animal. Also no need or drive can be treated as if it

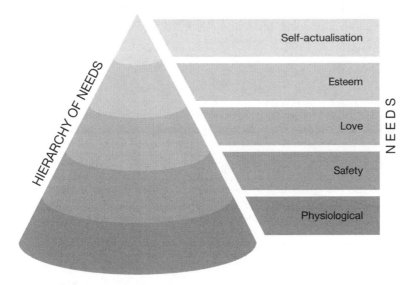

FIGURE 2.1 Maslow's hierarchy of needs. Adapted from Maslow (1943).

were isolated or discrete; every drive is related to the state of satisfaction or dissatisfaction of other drives' (Maslow, 1943)

But is this a simplistic perspective of human needs?

> How can we explain the man who risks his life (safety need) for the woman he loves (love need)?

> How can we explain the woman who does not eat for days (physiological need) because she is so engrossed in her work (esteem need)?

Maslow (1943) argues that we often underestimate the importance of a need until it has not been met at a chronic and extreme level

> Modern western society has adapted to ensure that physiological and safety needs are rarely neglected in the extreme

> 'The average American citizen is experiencing appetite rather than hunger when he says "I am hungry." He is apt to experience sheer life-and-death hunger only by accident and then only a few times through his entire life' (Maslow, 1943)

> Those living in this culture may underestimate the value of these lower needs to the extent that they can afford to risk losing them

Those people who experience true deprivation of a basic need will be dominated by the desire to fulfil that need to the exclusion of all other factors

> 'For our chronically and extremely hungry man, Utopia can be defined very simply as a place where there is plenty of food. Life itself tends to be defined in terms of eating. Anything else will be defined as unimportant. Freedom, love, community feeling, respect, philosophy, may all be waved aside as fripperies which are useless since they fail to fill the stomach. Such a man may fairly be said to live by bread alone' (Maslow, 1943)

Characteristics of the fully functioning person

The good life (Rogers, 1961)

Once basic needs (physiological, safety, love, esteem) are being met, the individual can strive to achieve congruency between the self-concept and the organismic self (self-actualisation)

An individual who is striving towards self-actualisation can be regarded as a fully functioning person

Fully functioning persons are experiencing 'the good life'

> 'The good life is a *process*, not a state of being' (Rogers, 1961)

> 'This process of the good life is not, I am convinced, a life for the faint-hearted. It involves the stretching and growing of becoming more and more of one's potentialities. It involves the courage to be. It means launching oneself fully into the stream of life. Yet the deeply exciting thing about human beings is that when the individual is inwardly free, he chooses as the good life this process of becoming' (Rogers, 1961)

Characteristics of a fully functioning person (Rogers, 1962)

An increasing openness to experience

> An individual who is fully open to experience will allow every single event in life to pass through his or her body and mind without being distorted by the use of defensive mechanisms

>> For example, a man who is open to experience is likely to accept his poor grades in an exam rather than distort them into evidence that he is a failure as a person

> Rogers (1961) argues that one aspect of 'the good life' is a 'movement away from the pole of defensiveness toward the pole of openness to experience'

>> He explains that an individual living the good life would be able to experience internal events so that he can fully accept negative feelings (such as fear, discouragement and pain) and positive feelings (such as courage, tenderness and awe)

Increasingly existential living

> An individual who experiences existential living is able to live fully in each moment

>> For example, many young children do not focus on what has happened previously or on what may happen in the future, but simply enjoy living in the present

> Rogers (1961) argues that each moment in life is new for an individual who is fully open to his new experience without defensiveness

>> He explains that this individual 'becomes a participant in and an observer of the ongoing process of organismic experience, rather than being in control of it' (Rogers, 1961)

An increasing trust in his organism

An individual who places trust in his own self could evaluate each situation and experience based on the available data, rather than relying on prejudice, bias, fear and defensiveness

For example, a woman who is able to interpret each situation based on the stimuli present and trusts her own instincts will be able to make better judgements concerning her career

Rogers (1961) suggests that this individual would have 'access to all of the available data in the situation, on which to base his behavior; the social demands, his own complex and possibly conflicting needs, his memories of similar situations, his perception of the uniqueness of this situation, etc.' (Rogers, 1961)

On the basis of all of this complex information, this individual could then 'permit his total organism, his consciousness participating, to consider each stimulus, need, and demand, its relative intensity and importance, and out of this complex weighing and balancing, discover that course of action which would come closest to satisfying all his needs in the situation' (Rogers, 1961)

Nineteen propositions of personality

Rogers' (1951) theory of personality outlined 19 propositions

1. 'Every individual (organism) exists in a continually changing world of experience of which he is the centre'

    The world around is constantly changing

    From our own perspective, we sit at the centre of this world because we are the main person in our own story

    For each of us, our experiences (what we consciously feel, see, hear, etc.) combine to create an internal private world

    Note that not all stimuli contribute to the private world – many senses are stimulated outside of conscious awareness

    This private world is our experiential field or phenomenal field

    Only you can truly understand your own phenomenal field because you are the only person who has had all of those unique experiences

2. 'The organism reacts to the field as it is experienced and perceived. This perceptual field is, for the individual, "reality"'

    We do not react to an objective actual reality

    Instead, we react to our own perception of reality based on our own phenomenal field

    This is why two people can react in completely different ways to exactly the same stimuli

On a philosophical note, actual reality is nothing more than the agreed acceptance of certain things as real based on overlap between many phenomenal fields

3.   'The organism reacts as an organized whole to this phenomenal field'

It is impossible to adopt a reductionist approach to understanding the reactions of the individual

You always react as an entire entity

We could focus exclusively on the physiological reactions to stimuli only (for example, what happens to the body when you are sexually aroused), but this fails to account for the emotional, cognitive, social and behavioural reactions

Strict physiological or behavioural approaches are insufficient

We need to consider the organism as a whole

4.   'The organism has one basic tendency and striving – to actualize, maintain and enhance the experiencing organism'

Each individual has a natural urge towards self-maintenance – we assimilate food, we defend ourselves when threatened, etc.

Each individual has a natural urge to mature – we start to walk, we start to have sex

These tendencies and strivings exist even in the face of adversity

In the same way, each individual also strives towards self-actualisation in a personal sense – we seek self-respect, autonomy, independence, etc.

Note that the important factor here is not the achievement of self-actualisation, but rather the constant growth, development and drive towards self-actualisation

5.   'Behaviour is basically the goal-directed attempt of the organism to satisfy its needs as experienced, in the field as perceived'

Since our goal is to strive towards self-actualisation, then our behaviour is our way of attempting to move towards this goal

Some behaviour might not appear to be optimal for moving towards self-actualisation

However, if we view the world from the frame of reference and truly understand the private internal world of that individual, then we will see that even this behaviour is an attempt to move towards self-actualisation

Unacceptable behaviours such as stealing might initially appear to be actions moving away from enhancing the self

However, these behaviours can be understood as attempts to self-actualise once we appreciate that the individual views financial gain as a means to achieve respect

6. 'Emotion accompanies and in general facilitates such goal-directed behaviour, the kind of emotion being related to the seeking versus the consummatory aspects of the behaviour, and the intensity of the emotion being related to the perceived significance of the behaviour for the maintenance and enhancement of the organism'

> Significant behaviours are those that you believe will help you survive or move closer to self-actualisation

> Emotional intensity is directly related to the perceived importance of these behaviours

> Those behaviours that may have life or death consequences (for example, jumping out of the way of a racing car) will result in higher emotional intensity than those behaviours that have minimal consequences for the self (for example, cutting your toe nails)

7. 'The best vantage point for understanding behaviour is from the internal frame of reference of the individual himself'

> You are the only person who has had all of your unique experiences from your position in the world – this means that you are an expert about you

>> If someone would like to truly understand you as an individual, s/he would need to view your behaviour while attempting to take into account your own private world

>> They would need to stand in your shoes

> Our attempt at viewing behaviour from the private world or internal frame of reference of the individual is known as empathy

>> Empathy is NOT simply feeling sorry for someone

8. 'A portion of the total perceptual field gradually becomes differentiated as the self'

> 'Self' refers to the individual awareness of being

> Development of the conscious self occurs during childhood as we realise that some parts of the world belong to us (things under our control) and other parts of the world are external to us (things not under our control)

9. 'As a result of interaction with the environment, and particularly as a result of evaluational interaction with others, the structure of the self is formed – an organized, fluid but consistent conceptual pattern of perceptions of characteristics and relationships of the "I" or the "me", together with values attached to these concepts'

> Conscious awareness of self develops during childhood through interaction with the world

> We learn about ourselves as individuals by engaging with objects, environments, experiences, people, etc.

10. 'The values attached to experiences, and the values which are a part of the self structure, in some instances are values experienced directly by the organism, and in some

instances are values introjected or taken over from others, but perceived in distorted fashion, as if they had been experienced directly'

> We will all learn the value of specific experiences – some things have a high value (enjoyable) and other things have a low value (not enjoyable)

> We will learn some of these values through direct experience: for example, I enjoy eating sweet foods

> We will learn some of these values by internalising the values of others: for example, I do not enjoy eating sweets and eating sweets is a bad thing to do

> Internalisation of the values of others happens due to evaluation: for example, my parents tell me that I am a bad girl for eating sweets

> We may then experience a conflict between our evaluation of the self and the evaluation of others: for example, I believe that I am a good girl but my parents tell me that I am a bad girl

> In order to protect our threatened concept of self, we may then internalise the values of others: for example, I do not enjoy eating sweets and eating sweets is a bad thing to do

> This act of internalising the values of others allows us to maintain our concept of self: for example, I can continue to believe that I am a good girl

11. 'As experiences occur in the life of the individual, they are either, a) symbolized, perceived and organized into some relationship to the self, b) ignored because there is no perceived relationship to the self structure, c) denied symbolization or given distorted symbolization because the experience is inconsistent with the structure of the self'

> Some experiences in life will be entirely ignored because they are not related to you as an individual

>> You will experience many things every day that do not have a positive or negative impact on you so they are not noticed – you might pass a tree, postbox and shop on your way to work and never pay attention to them until the moment that you need to post a letter

> Some experiences in life will be noticed because they meet a need (like the postbox) and they are consistent with your perception of yourself and the world

>> You tend to select from your sensory experiences those events that confirm your own view of the world

>> These experiences are then integrated into your concept of the world and yourself to further encourage you to believe that your perception is accurate

> Some experiences in life will be noticed because they meet a need but they will cause conflict because they are inconsistent with your perception of yourself and the world

These experiences are often denied – for example, client with low self-esteem denies the experience of a compliment by saying that he 'doesn't really know me'

These experiences are often distorted – for example, client who has a self-concept of herself as a loving daughter distorts feelings of anger towards her father into a headache

12. 'Most of the ways of behaving which are adopted by the organism are those that are consistent with the concept of self'

Behaviours exhibited by us will be consistent with our perception of ourselves

All behaviours will be driven by desire to satisfy a need, but this behaviour must fit with what we believe about ourselves

For example, a person might have a strong need for food yet he will not steal because this behaviour does not fit with his concept of himself as an honest man

13. 'Behaviour may, in some instances, be brought about by organic experiences and needs which have not been symbolized. Such behaviour may be inconsistent with the structure of the self but in such instances the behaviour is not "owned" by the individual'

Contrary to the above proposition, some behaviour is almost automatic and exists irrespective of whether it matches the self-concept

In these cases, the individual may not admit to the behaviour

For example, a man defending himself against a sudden attack may respond irrespective of his perception of himself as a gentle person and he may then state that he did not know what he was doing and was not responsible for his actions

These behaviours (and the failure to accept ownership of them) can be particularly dangerous when they are the result of an ignored natural urge

For example, a man who constantly represses all sexual urges because they do not fit with his concept of himself as a 'pure man' might eventually commit sexual assault but deny ownership of his criminal behaviour

14. 'Psychological maladjustment exists when the organism denies awareness of significant sensory and visceral experiences, which consequently are not symbolized and organized into the gestalt of the self-structure. When this situation exists, there is a basic or potential psychological tension'

Any refusal to accept organic sensations (natural feelings and perceptions) because they do not match the self-concept will lead to anxiety

For example, a woman might hold a self-concept of herself as a loving mother resulting from the organic sensation of love for her child and internalised conditions of worth from significant others informing her that a mother must be 'loving'

> Any subsequent organic sensations of dislike towards her child will be ignored and the natural behaviour of aggression in response to these feelings will be refused – this will cause psychological tension

> She will seek relief from this tension, but she cannot behave in a way that is not consistent with her self-concept

> However, since her self-concept would justify her to use punishment on a bad child, she will begin to view all of his behaviour as bad so that she can gain relief by exhibiting her aggression

> Her feelings and behaviour will have been distorted to fit with her self-concept

> In the event that she loses control and expresses her dislike of the child, she would then deny ownership of this behaviour and claim 'I was not myself'

15.   'Psychological adjustment exists when the concept of the self is such that all the sensory and visceral experiences of the organism are, or may be, assimilated on a symbolic level into a consistent relationship with the concept of self'

> Contrary to the previous proposition, acceptance of organic sensations and congruence (matching) between the organismic self (true self experiencing organic sensations) and the self-concept (perception of self) will result in relief from psychological tension

> In relation to the previous example, the mother who dislikes her child will be able to cope with these negative emotions if her self-concept allows her to be a mother who experiences both love and dislike

16.   'Any experience which is inconsistent with the organization or the structure of the self may be perceived as a threat, and the more of these perceptions there are, the more rigidly the self structure is organized to maintain itself'

> Any attempt by another person to draw the attention of the individual to things that are inconsistent with the self-concept will fail

> We will naturally defend our own self-concept and we will provide evidence to support our own beliefs about ourselves

> For example, a girl who holds a self-concept of herself as a poor student will defend herself vigorously against the 'attack' of those who claim that she is clever

17.   'Under certain conditions, involving primarily complete absence of threat to the self-structure, experiences which are inconsistent with it may be perceived and examined, and the structure of self revised to assimilate and include such experiences'

If an individual is placed in the unique position of experiencing a complete absence of threats to the self-concept, then they can begin to explore their own sense of self

If others do not judge but simply accept a person without insisting that they are something else other than what they present, that person may feel safe to explore their own organismic self

They might then start to assimilate their organic experiences into their sense of self and true personality change can occur

18. 'When the individual perceives and accepts into one consistent and integrated system all his sensory and visceral experiences, then he is necessarily more understanding of others and is more accepting of others as separate individuals'

> Those who are congruent with the self can often be congruent with others

> If a person denies some aspect of himself or herself then they are constantly defending against 'attack' from those who present conflicting evidence

>> This means that all behaviours exhibited by others can be viewed as threatening

> Once the individual is able to accept all elements of the self, they are less inclined to feel threatened by others

>> This will lead to fewer miscommunications, better interpersonal relations and more acceptance of others

19. 'As the individual perceives and accepts into his self structure more of his organic experiences, he finds that he is replacing his present value system – based extensively on introjections which have been distortedly symbolized – with a continuing organismic valuing process'

> An individual who is able to accept more organic experiences will begin to reject the values of others

> This person will no longer feel the pressures of the conditions of worth because s/he will know that s/he is worthy regardless of behaviour

> In the place of the old value system (shoulds, oughts and musts), a new value system will develop on the basis of genuine organic experience and the natural human desire to move towards growth, honesty and self-actualisation

---

SUMMARY

Organismic self and self-concept: organismic self (actual self) is based on experiences; self-concept (perception of self) is based on interaction with others and is sectioned into configurations of self

Conditions of worth: positive regard is rarely unconditional; values expressed by significant others are internalised to impact on the self-concept – I must do these things in order to receive positive regard (conditional positive regard) and be deemed worthy (conditions of worth)

Self-actualisation: natural drive towards personal fulfilment, can never actually achieve it but we are self-actualising when striving towards it; self-actualisation is different from enlightenment/Nirvana; those striving towards self-actualisation experience congruency between the organismic self and self-concept

Hierarchy of needs: pyramid of basic needs (physiological, safety, love, esteem, self-actualisation); lower needs must be met before seeking higher needs; peak experiences may be regarded above self-actualisation; hierarchy may be regarded as simplistic

Fully functioning person: lives 'the good life' by being congruent and meeting all needs; characteristics include increasing openness to experience, increasing existential living and increasing trust in organism

Nineteen propositions of personality: outlines human nature with links to therapeutic methods (explains organismic self, self-concept, self-actualisation, conditions of worth and core conditions of therapy)

THERAPEUTIC RELATIONSHIP IN PERSON-CENTRED THERAPY

LEARNING OUTCOMES

After reading this section, you will be able to:

- outline the six core conditions required for constructive personality change

- discuss the first condition of two persons in psychological contact

- discuss the second condition of the client being in a vulnerable or anxious state of incongruence

- discuss the third core condition of the therapist being congruent and integrated in the relationship

- discuss the fourth core condition of the therapist experiencing unconditional positive regard for the client

- discuss the fifth core condition of the therapist experiencing an empathic understanding of the client's frame of reference

- discuss the sixth condition of the therapist communicating empathic understanding and unconditional positive regard towards the client

- explain whether the core conditions are both necessary and sufficient
- recognise the seven stages of the client process
- debate the impact of the core conditions on relational depth

Six conditions for constructive personality change

Relationship is key in person-centred therapy

Relationship is the most important part of the therapy

> Techniques, strategies, methods, activities, etc. are not encouraged in this type of therapy

> Instead, the therapist focuses on developing a positive relationship with the client under the assumption that this will give the client the conditions to change in a positive way

Rogers (1957) outlined six therapeutic conditions for constructive personality change in the client. For constructive personality change to occur, it is necessary that these conditions exist and continue over a period of time

1. Two persons are in psychological contact
2. The first, whom we shall term the client, is in a state of incongruence, being vulnerable or anxious
3. The second person, whom we shall term the therapist, is congruent or integrated in the relationship
4. The therapist experiences unconditional positive regard for the client
5. The therapist experiences an empathic understanding of the client's internal frame of reference and endeavours to communicate this experience to the client
6. The communication to the client of the therapist's empathic understanding and unconditional positive regard is to a minimal degree achieved

> No other conditions are necessary

> If these six conditions exist, and continue over a period of time, this is sufficient

> The process of constructive personality change will follow

> Widely misreported to contain only three conditions for change (congruence, unconditional positive regard, empathy), all six conditions are actually described as both necessary and sufficient for constructive personality change

First condition of two persons in psychological contact

TWO PERSONS IN PSYCHOLOGICAL CONTACT

Therapeutic relationship is described as 'psychological contact' because it relates to the contact between two people engaged in the mental – as opposed to physical – relationship typical of therapy

This condition forms the basis for subsequent conditions as it is assumed that there is no potential for a relationship of any kind without initial contact forming between the two individuals

Most forms of therapy involve contact to some extent

Therapy at the student services at a university may involve one-to-one meetings and group meetings

Therapy for a sexual abuse support service may involve telephone discourse

IS CONTACT NECESSARY?

Advancements in modern technology, however, have led to some distortion of the boundaries of human contact

Many forms of therapy can now take place in an anonymous online setting and there is even the potential for a type of therapy to occur without the presence of an actual therapist

Some individuals use online blogs as an attempt to verbalise their own feelings and the return to these blogs at a future point in time allows the writer to reflect on their thoughts

This approach has been common for many years in the form of personal diaries; however, blogging offers one crucial addition to the typical diary in that the writer is actually exposing these thoughts to an anonymous reader

In this respect, the writer is able to share the depths of the self with another individual without forming an actual relationship with the other

CNN reported on the issue of blogging as therapy and cited one widowed blogger as stating 'Right after he died, people kept asking if I was in therapy, and I'd say, "No, but I have a blog"' (Grossman, 2008)

Second condition of incongruence in client

CLIENT IS IN A VULNERABLE OR ANXIOUS STATE OF INCONGRUENCE

Self-concept is incongruent with the organismic self

Individual experiencing a psychological event that is incompatible with their concept of the self may distort or ignore this event

Repeated exposure to experiences that do not fit with the self-concept could lead to vulnerability or anxiety

IS INCONGRUENCE NECESSARY?

Debate as to the extent of malleability and the number of facets of the self-concept

Self-concept is generally both organised and stable, thus giving the personality some degree of consistency (Purkey, 1988)

Self-concept is multifaceted to highlight the different parts or configurations of the individual (Mearns, 1999)

One could find an experience inconsistent with one part yet consistent with another part; for example, a man might feel that he is independent in one sense yet reliant on his partner in another sense. Thus it is difficult to state with certainty that an experience relating to dependency is consistent or inconsistent with the whole self-concept

Third condition of congruence in therapist

THERAPIST IS CONGRUENT AND INTEGRATED IN THE RELATIONSHIP

Congruency is otherwise known as genuineness as it refers to the degree to which one can relate to another individual in a sincere and honest manner

Genuineness is essential for both empathic understanding and unconditional positive regard

> In the absence of congruence, it is very difficult for the therapist to demonstrate the remaining core conditions

MISINTERPRETATIONS OF THIS CONDITION

Success of the therapist depends on his or her achievement of congruence in all areas of life (akin to the attainment of self-actualisation)

> It is not possible for the therapist to be entirely congruent at all times in life. Instead, Rogers (1957) suggests that the therapist need only be congruent and genuine in the moment in the therapeutic setting for the relationship to be successful

Therapy can only be genuine if the therapist discloses all thoughts to the client – Rogers himself disclosed his own feelings of boredom to a client (Landreth, 1984)

> Aim of therapy is not for the therapist to express his or her own feelings

> Instead, therapist should focus on acknowledging and accepting those feelings within him- or herself in order to determine whether the disclosure of such information might be beneficial to the client

IS CONGRUENCE NECESSARY?

Is it possible for a 'fake' therapist to be successful in a therapeutic relationship?

> Patients with dysphoria could not detect a significant difference between congruent and incongruent behaviour in a videotaped therapy session (Hollander & Hokanson, 1988)

>> Conclusion was that there is a lack of interpersonal skills associated with depression, but these findings could also be taken as evidence to suggest that a client suffering from psychological disturbances cannot detect the level of congruency in the therapist

>> However, although these findings suggest that the patient may be unable to consciously detect the genuine therapist, it is not clear whether congruence and incongruence have a therapeutic impact on a subconscious level

Fourth condition of unconditional positive regard from therapist

THERAPIST EXPERIENCES UNCONDITIONAL POSITIVE REGARD FOR THE CLIENT

Rogers (1957) suggests that successful personality change requires the therapist to accept the client with genuine warmth (positive regard) irrespective of the personal traits or behavioural actions of the individual (unconditional)

> This condition highlights the importance of an understanding of oneself to be aware of any potential prejudice in order to maintain a non-judgemental attitude towards the client

Rogers regarded the human condition as inherently worthy, although he did acknowledge that the individual is capable of both positive and negative emotions (Kirschenbaum, 2004)

> For this reason, it is important for the therapist to appreciate that a person is doing the best that they are able to do at that time and any concerns about the behaviour exhibited by a client should be directed towards the actions rather than the character of the individual (Seligman & Reichenberg, 2009)

IS UNCONDITIONAL POSITIVE REGARD NECESSARY?

Is it possible for a therapist to feel genuine unconditional positive regard for a client?

> It is difficult to accept that any individual would be able to experience this level of regard for another, thus the importance of this condition is questioned because this capacity for regard does not appear to exist in reality

> Rogers (1957) acknowledges that the concept of unconditional positive regard operates on a continuum – he even suggests that the concept as an absolute and complete entity could never exist except in theory

>> This is an extremely comforting point as it is tempting to feel that one is a failure as a therapist if one is unable to feel genuine unconditional positive regard for the client at all times

>> It is the attempt to maintain this non-judgemental attitude in the moment that will have the greatest impact on the success of the therapy

Fifth condition of empathic understanding from therapist

THERAPIST EXPERIENCES AN EMPATHIC UNDERSTANDING OF THE CLIENT'S FRAME OF REFERENCE

Rogers (1957) states that the fifth condition for successful therapeutic change is the therapist's ability to experience 'an accurate, empathic understanding of the client's awareness of his own experience'

> Empathic understanding requires the therapist to be able to perceive the world of the client from the client's frame of reference

Therapist should be close enough to the client to appreciate his/her own perspective, yet far enough away from the client to remain objective

In other words, to be able to step in and out of the shoes of the client or to be able to view the world through the eyes of the client (Kirschenbaum & Henderson, 1990)

May (1939) described empathy as 'walking with another person through the deepest chambers of his soul'

Essentially, the therapist should be walking at the side of the client through the journey towards self-actualisation

True empathy is difficult to obtain as it involves an immersion in the world of the client without a loss of the self

Many clients have never had the experience of being truly understood by another person and the expression of empathy by the therapist has resulted in many astonished responses, such as 'yes, that's it . . . I can't believe how well you understand me'

True empathy can enhance rapport, thus opening the lines of communication to a greater extent and allowing the client to engage in deeper self-reflection

Genuine warmth towards the client will be significantly influenced by the experience of empathy in the therapist

Often difficult to feel unconditional positive regard unless one can truly understand the world from the perspective of the client

For example, unconditional positive regard for a man who has abused a child might seem impossible, but a deep understanding of the world from his perspective might aid with this aim

Empathic state appears to be consistently important across all types of therapeutic relationships (both directive and non-directive)

Experts from ten different psychotherapeutic approaches were found to successfully build rapport with clients by being able to understand their feelings, following their line of thought, and never being in doubt about their meaning (Fiedler, 1950)

SYMPATHY VERSUS EMPATHY

Clients with a traumatic background (such as those recovering from rape or sexual abuse) may tempt the therapist to experience sympathy

Compassion for another person may stem from genuine warmth, but sympathy is unlikely to assist the client in exploring a deeper level of his or her own world

Expressions of sympathy ('I really feel for you') will disclose the emotions of the therapist without furthering the self-understanding of the client

True attempts to view the world from the client's frame of reference will help the therapist experience empathy

Expressions of empathy ('I am sensing that you find it really difficult to talk to your partner') can encourage the client to view his or her own feelings from a new perspective

PRIMARY EMPATHY

Primary-level empathy requires the therapist to respond to the feelings and behaviour expressed by the client (Egan, 2007)

> Therapist should actively attend to the client and indicate their understanding of exactly what was expressed by the client

ADVANCED EMPATHY

Advanced empathy requires the therapist to sense the expressions not communicated directly by the client (Egan, 2007)

> Self-disclosure, interpretations and challenges can all be used in advanced empathy
>
> Always need to be aware of the risks associated with advanced empathy – must ensure that the client always remains the expert

IS EMPATHY NECESSARY?

Is positive therapeutic change dependent on empathy?

> Reviews of 75 therapists and 15 research studies revealed no evidence of client change directly related to empathy or warmth in the therapist (Mitchell et al., 1973)

Sixth condition of communication between client and therapist

THERAPIST COMMUNICATES EMPATHIC UNDERSTANDING AND UNCONDITIONAL POSITIVE REGARD TO CLIENT

Effective empathic expressions depend on the level of communication between the client and therapist

> Unconditional positive regard, congruency and empathy are all redundant unless the client is able to detect these states in the therapist

MISINTERPRETATION OF COMMUNICATION

Concept of communication in a person-centred approach is often misunderstood to mean the excessive use of prompts such as 'uhuh' and the question 'how does that make you feel?'

> It is assumed that therapists merely reflect the words of the client and do little else to communicate

In reality, delicate communication of the inner experience of empathy and unconditional positive regard is essential in order to inspire change in the client

IS COMMUNICATION NECESSARY?

As noted for contact, advancements in modern technology have led to some distortion of the boundaries of human communication

> Many forms of therapy can now take place in an anonymous online setting and there is even the potential for a type of therapy to occur without the presence of an actual therapist (for example, iTherapy)

One-way online communication (such as blogs) does not require feedback and yet still appears to serve the purpose of encouraging self-exploration, self-reflection and self-expression

Necessary and sufficient?

Six conditions are reported to be both necessary and sufficient for constructive personality change

> All six conditions are necessary
>
>> There is some debate regarding the necessity of these conditions
>>
>> Please refer to the individual descriptions of each condition for discussion about whether each of these conditions is necessary for successful therapy
>
> These six conditions are sufficient and no other conditions are necessary
>
>> Lots of research debating the sufficiency of these conditions alone and many other approaches utilise specific techniques – difficult to determine whether the conditions alone can inspire therapeutic success
>>
>> Cases have been reported in which the client has reported that the therapist is congruent, accepting and empathic, yet the client did not improve (Lietaer, 2002)
>>
>> Gelso and Carter (1985) argued that 'the conditions . . . are neither necessary nor sufficient, although . . . such conditions are facilitative'
>
> Despite this debate, most therapists agree that the therapeutic relationship is extremely important and almost all therapists will strive to exhibit the core conditions
>
>> Kirschenbaum and Jourdan (2005) note that 'Rogers's core conditions may or may not be necessary or sufficient for effective psychotherapy (the debate is ongoing), but [as] a means to achieve a therapeutic alliance, the value of empathy, unconditional positive regard, and congruence is supported by the latest generation of psychotherapy process–outcome research'

Stages of constructive personality change

Rogers wrote about the six conditions in 1957, but it was not until 1961 that he developed his ideas for 'a process conception of psychotherapy', based upon a 1958 article of the same name

> Rogers identified seven stages in the client's process
>
>> All stages can be viewed from an external frame of reference
>>
>> Stages move from one to seven
>>
>> In stage one, people are unlikely to come to therapy as they lack awareness of self, their views of the world are fixed and rigid, they are out of touch with their feelings, and they take no responsibility for their actions

If people become less rigid in thought processes and begin to get in touch with feelings (through being 'fully received' by another), then they may engage in therapy

Most therapy takes place with clients in stages two to six

If stage six is achieved, then stage seven will inevitably follow and is likely to happen outside the therapeutic relationship

THERAPEUTIC ALTERNATIVES

An individual will choose to seek therapy for many different reasons. Some people seek therapy because they want a safe place to vent frustrations, share feelings, let off steam and generally feel that someone is listening to their problems. Other people seek therapy because they want someone to offer an alternative viewpoint as they explore options with a view to making important decisions. In meeting these needs, it has been said that the modern therapist has taken the place of the religious elder (the more cynical amongst us might argue that the therapist has taken the place of family and friends!). However, modern life does offer many alternatives to therapy and these might be able to meet the needs listed above without involving any kind of therapeutic relationship. Consider trying some of the following activities and compare them with the traditional therapeutic experience to decide whether they are a weaker option, plausible alternative or appropriate addition to therapy.

* Write a diary or a blog describing your experiences and feelings every day for one week
* Express yourself about something that has upset you by talking to a pet
* Vent your frustration by screaming at an inanimate object (you might want to make sure that you do this in private to avoid attracting any unwanted attention)
* Visit a support website to read about issues that are causing you concern (for example, someone who is suffering after the loss of a beloved pet might find helpful information at www.livingwithpetbereavement.com/)
* Google search for a therapy chatbot and explain your current problems in virtual therapy (for example, ELIZA is a web-based person-centred therapist emulator found at www-ai.ijs.si/eliza/eliza.html and FreudBot is a web-based Freudian therapist emulator found at http://psych.athabascau.ca/html/Freudbot/test.html)

Disclaimer: please remember that these suggestions are designed to help you to think about the value of therapy and explore possible alternatives or supplementary options. They are not designed to address any serious personal or mental health issues and you should always contact a professional if you have any concerns in these areas.

Movement from stage one to stage seven involves the following

> Feelings unowned in the past to owned in the present

> Incongruence to congruence

> Experiences changing from remote and fixed to current and fluid

> Communication with self and others from closed to open

> Problems not recognised to accepted as part of the self

> Responsibility put onto others to self-responsibility

People can become less rigid in thought processes and get in touch with feelings through being 'fully received' by another

> Rogers (1961) argued that 'there is implied in this term ['received'] the concept of being understood, empathically, and the concept of acceptance'

> This explains how the six conditions can be used to support the process of therapy

Relational depth

Therapists should strive to achieve relational depth (Mearns & Cooper, 2005)

Relational depth is defined as a 'state of profound contact and engagement between two people, in which each person is fully real with the other, and able to understand and value the other's experiences at a high level' (Mearns & Cooper, 2005)

> Depth in this sense is related to 'honesty' or 'realism'

> A deeper relationship is one that is more honest, genuine, real and true

> This type of relationship is not superficial or artificial, but is instead an honest sharing of an encounter

Relational depth can be experienced within a moment ('a moment of intimacy' or 'a true connection during that conversation') or over a long period of time ('we are extremely connected' or 'we are always very intimate')

Relational depth versus core conditions

Core conditions form the foundation for standard person-centred therapy

> Core conditions indicate what conditions must be met in order for effective therapeutic change to take place (congruence, unconditional positive regard, empathy)

Relational depth goes one step further to explain the quality of the encounter

> Relational depth indicates the level of the intimacy between the therapist and the client

Concept of relational depth has been accused of simply being a new word for standard person-centred therapy

Wilders (2007) argues that the description of relational depth is often nothing more than a description of person-centred therapy (except when the advice given to therapists conflicts with the core conditions – see point below)

It could be argued that relational depth is simply a term to describe what happens when the therapist demonstrates the core conditions

> Rogers used the word 'genuine' to describe the relationship, whereas Mearns and Cooper (2005) refer to the relationship in terms of 'depth'

> 'Mearns and Cooper have failed to understand, or to experience for themselves, that when we, as real and genuine human beings, congruently offer empathy and unconditional positive regard to an other, then the more, not less, likely we are to have intimacy and closeness with our clients' (Wilders, 2007)

Cooper (2007) responds to this criticism by suggesting that relational depth does not need to be viewed as novel or distinct from standard person-centred therapy

> Instead, the intention is that the concept of relational depth will draw attention to the importance of in-depth relating to clients

> Irrespective of whether this is already implied in traditional person-centred therapy, the concept of relational depth aims to bring it to the forefront and make it a critical component of the therapeutic aims

Concept of relational depth has been accused of being in conflict with the core conditions of person-centred therapy

> Purist person-centred therapy is entirely non-directional, yet advice for encouraging relational depth does occasionally indicate that the client may need to be directed or redirected

Wilders (2007) argues that the concept of relational depth lacks an underlying coherent theory because it presents contradictory advice

> Therapists are advised to 'be with' the client, thus suggesting that the therapist should follow rather than lead – this supports the principle of person-centred therapy

> Therapists are invited to 'assume the right to confront or invade or challenge clients if they feel that this "encounter" will help to create a relationship of "depth"'. This conflicts with the principles of person-centred therapy because 'Relational depth at times gives free licence to therapists to offer suggestions, change the direction of the therapy, criticise, or . . . berate clients' (Wilders, 2007)

Cooper (2007) responds to these criticisms by suggesting that it is illogical to assume that the same approach will work with all clients

> Although non-directive methods may be highly effective for some clients, therapy should be flexible enough to incorporate a 'more directive way of engaging' if the therapist feels that this will improve the quality of the encounter (Cooper, 2007)

Value of controversy

Relational depth as a concept has sparked discussion and debate

Perhaps it is not important whether it is a new theory or a contradictory theory or an incomplete theory . . .

Simply reigniting the debate about the nature of the therapeutic relationship had a significant impact on research and development in person-centred therapy

Rogers himself was both flexible and forward thinking, and he would no doubt have embraced the exploration with a view to further improving the therapeutic relationship

---

SUMMARY

Six conditions for constructive personality change: therapeutic relationship is the key component for successful therapy; for constructive personality change to occur, six conditions must exist and continue over a period of time (no other conditions, techniques or methods are necessary)

1. Two persons are in psychological contact

2. The first, whom we shall term the client, is in a state of incongruence, being vulnerable or anxious

3. The second person, whom we shall term the therapist, is congruent or integrated in the relationship

4. The therapist experiences unconditional positive regard for the client

5. The therapist experiences an empathic understanding of the client's internal frame of reference and endeavours to communicate this experience to the client

6. The communication to the client of the therapist's empathic understanding and unconditional positive regard is to a minimal degree achieved

Necessary and sufficient: small debate about whether all conditions are necessary in modern therapy; large debate about whether these conditions are sufficient for successful therapy

Stages: seven stages of the client process; client moves through the stages to become less rigid and more fully functioning

Relational depth: successful application of the core conditions will allow the therapist to work with the client at a deeper level; relational depth describes the intimacy present in a 'genuine' encounter; controversial theory which has sparked debate in the field, questions whether relational depth is just a new word for core conditions, questions whether relational depth conflicts with core conditions, but there is a value in controversy because it provokes discussion

THERAPEUTIC TECHNIQUES IN PERSON-CENTRED THERAPY

> ### LEARNING OUTCOMES
>
> After reading this section, you will be able to:
>
> * appreciate the absence of specific techniques in this approach
> * describe how the therapist uses genuineness, transparency and self-disclosure to demonstrate the core condition of congruence
> * describe how the therapist uses a non-judgemental approach and sensitive cultural awareness to demonstrate the core condition of unconditional positive regard
> * describe how the therapist enters the client's frame of reference by using primary and advanced empathy to demonstrate the core condition of empathic understanding

Absence of techniques

Successful therapy is not dependent on techniques

Successful therapy is dependent purely on the nature of the therapeutic relationship

> Constructive personality change requires only that the client and therapist engage in a positive therapeutic relationship

Person-centred therapy involves simply being with the client

> No use of games, exercises, activities, homework, etc.

Various methods can be taught and utilised to improve skills in communicating the core conditions of congruence, unconditional positive regard and empathy

> But these are simply interpersonal skills, rather than specific therapeutic techniques to be followed according to the instructions
>
> As noted by Thorne (1996), Rogers was horrified to find that the focus on the responses of the therapist became a list of techniques – the whole purpose of person-centred therapy is to be genuine in that moment, rather than to follow a set of protocols according to the book

Therapeutic relationship is more important than therapeutic techniques

Research exploring common factors across multiple types of therapy has often focused on the core conditions of person-centred therapy (Lambert & Barley, 2001)

> Analysis of over 100 empirical and meta-analytic studies of therapeutic interventions reveals that

40% of client improvement is dependent on external events unrelated to the therapy

15% of client improvement is dependent on the placebo effect

15% of client improvement is dependent on the therapeutic techniques used in the sessions

30% of client improvement is dependent on the nature of the therapeutic relationship

These findings are a little disturbing as they suggest that over half (55%) of client outcome is influenced by events that have absolutely nothing to do with what takes place in the therapeutic sessions

These findings also support the suggestion that the relationship itself (and the demonstration of the core conditions) is twice as important as the techniques employed in ensuring a positive outcome for the client

WHO I AM OR WHAT I DO?

Reflect on three people who have had a positive impact on your life; perhaps they inspired you or comforted you or assisted you in some way. Try to think about why you were influenced by these people . . .

Did they show you how to be a better person by demonstrating their own positive traits? Perhaps they were strong in the face of adversity and this taught you to have strength? This would be akin to a therapist demonstrating the core conditions in relation to the self (self-acceptance, etc.) in order to show the client how to move towards self-actualisation.

Did they offer you a warm and safe environment in which to share your feelings? Perhaps they were a shoulder to cry on or inspired you to express yourself? This would be akin to a therapist offering a positive therapeutic relationship in which the client can explore and develop on a personal level.

Did you benefit from something that they did? Perhaps they did something to help you or worked with you to complete a task? This would be akin to a therapist using specific activities and techniques to help a client.

All of the above describe situations in which you may have been significantly influenced by another person – perhaps even to a life-changing extent. However, the person-centred therapist would strive towards the first two situations because these are believed to offer the most lasting benefit to the client. In contrast, the third situation may only assist the client on one specific problem and may foster dependency rather than autonomy. Consider your own experiences to decide whether you agree with this perspective.

An APA task force (Norcross, 2011) explored the association between the therapeutic relationship and the outcomes resulting from therapy

> They concluded that the relationship makes 'substantial and consistent contributions to psychotherapy outcome independent of the specific type of treatment'

> These findings suggest that the relationship, rather than any specific techniques used in the treatment, has the greatest positive impact on the client

Lambert and Barley (2001) state that 'decades of research indicate that the provision of therapy is an interpersonal process in which a main curative component is the nature of the therapeutic relationship . . . clinicians must remember that this is the foundation of our efforts to help others'

Clients themselves often attribute the success of therapy to the core conditions demonstrated by the therapist, rather than any specific activity or task completed in the session

> Qualitative analysis of patients experiencing therapy revealed that those who described the treatment as 'successful' explained that the therapist was 'warm, attentive, interested, understanding, and respectful' (Strupp et al., 1969)

Demonstrating congruence

Genuineness, transparency and self-disclosure can be used to demonstrate congruence.

> Therapist must be congruent and integrated in the relationship (Rogers, 1957)

>> Congruency is the degree to which one can relate to another individual in a sincere and honest manner

>> Essential for both empathic understanding and unconditional positive regard

Genuineness to demonstrate congruence

Congruent therapist will demonstrate non-possessive warmth by conveying friendliness in all verbal and non-verbal communication

Congruent client will try to be genuine in all forms of communication

> Body language, gestures, expressions and tone must all match the sentiment being expressed to demonstrate true genuineness

Transparency to demonstrate congruence

Congruent therapist will not pretend to be an expert

> Therapist does not know more about the client than the client him- or herself

> Therapist may only be knowledgeable in one particular area of psychology or therapy, and this should be made clear to the client

> Therapist should not be afraid to ask for further information, admit that they do not know something or confess that they do not understand

Congruent therapist will be open about all qualifications and feel able to refer or signpost when meeting cases beyond the limits of their ability

It is perfectly acceptable for the therapist to admit to a client that s/he is unable to help with that issue and direct the individual to a more appropriate source of help

Congruent therapist will not attempt to hide things from the client, will seek informed consent and will always be transparent in motives and intentions

All goals should be agreed together

Client should not be secretly manipulated to achieve an aim

If confidentiality has to be broken, client should be honestly told about this in advance if at all possible

The traits discussed above enhance transparency and ensure that the therapist adheres to the British Association for Counselling and Psychotherapy ethical principle of autonomy (BACP, 1992)

Autonomy refers to the practitioner's respect for the client's right to be self-governing

BACP states that practitioners 'should ensure accuracy in any advertising or information given in advance of services offered, seek freely given and adequately informed consent, engage in explicit contracting in advance of any commitment by the client, protect privacy, inform the client in advance of foreseeable conflicts of interest or as soon as possible after such conflicts become apparent, and refuse to manipulate clients against their will, even for beneficial social ends' (BACP, 1992)

Self-disclosure to demonstrate congruence

Congruent therapist will try to be honest with the client about his/her feelings

Therapist should not lie or fake feelings to the client

Disclosure of feelings or personal information by the therapist can help both the client and the therapeutic relationship

Client can be helped if the disclosure normalises his or her own thoughts, feelings and behaviours

For example, client may feel that anxiety about motherhood makes her a 'bad mum', so a therapist who explains that she also found it difficult might help to normalise these feelings

However, it is important for the therapist to avoid trivialising the experience of the client or suggesting that the client is not unique

Client can be helped if the disclosure provides a new insight into a problem

For example, client may feel trapped in his current job so a therapist who explains what he did to find a new job might provide some new ideas for solving the problem

However, it is important for the therapist to avoid giving advice or instructing the client – information signposting should be nothing more than providing new information without any pressure to respond

Therapeutic relationship can be helped if the disclosure enhances genuineness

> 'Spontaneous sharing on the part of both parties is the essence of a genuine relationship' (Carkhuff, 1969)

> However, it is important for the therapist to avoid directing attention away from the client and allowing the discussion to descend into a friendly chat

Congruent therapist will not feel compelled to disclose in all situations

> All disclosures should benefit the client (Patterson, 1985)

> Some information can help the client to gain insight about his or her own actions

>> For example, a therapist who feels bored might wish to share this information because it might give the client insight about the way that s/he presents the self to others

> Disclosures not intended to benefit the client should not be made

>> Therapist can explain that s/he does not wish to disclose this information or could ask the client how the information would help

>> 'Therapy is for the client, not the therapist' (Patterson, 1985)

Demonstrating unconditional positive regard

A non-judgemental approach and sensitive sociocultural awareness can be used to demonstrate unconditional positive regard

Therapist must experience unconditional positive regard for the client (Rogers, 1957)

> Successful personality change requires the therapist to accept the client with genuine warmth (positive regard) irrespective of the personal traits or behavioural actions of the individual (unconditional)

Non-judgemental approach for demonstrating unconditional positive regard

Important to understand oneself to be aware of any potential prejudice in order to maintain a non-judgemental attitude towards the client

> All people are entitled to hold their own views and values, but the therapist should strive to avoid imposing these on the client

> Therapists should strive to avoid passing judgement on others

> Ask yourself whether you would honestly behave differently in their circumstance

>> We often find that we judge others most harshly for those sins that we ourselves commit or wish to commit

> Avoid judgemental expressions

>> Certain words and phrases tend to imply judgement: should, ought, must, got to, don't, etc.

>> If you have an urge to say 'you should . . .', try asking yourself why you think that they should

Sensitive sociocultural awareness for demonstrating unconditional positive regard

Important to recognise cultural differences and accept that others view the world in very different ways

> Different does not mean wrong
>
> Avoid stereotypes and assumptions
>
> Many stereotypes and assumptions about people are held so deeply that it is difficult to realise that they exist
>
> > Consider the concept of love – our understanding of love is often from the perspective of an individualistic culture so it is often difficult to appreciate the concept of arranged marriages and this can lead to assumptions of force
>
> Cultural awareness is dependent on understanding
>
> Acceptance can sometimes mean asking for more information so that you can truly understand the world of the client in order to avoid jumping to conclusions

However, cultural awareness is not dependent on knowledge

> Although it can be helpful if the therapist has some knowledge about the culture of the client, it is not always necessary for the therapist to be a member of that culture or to have a deep and comprehensive knowledge of cultural practices specific to the client
>
> Indeed, cultural knowledge can sometimes lead the therapist to disregard factors relating to the individual in favour of assumptions relating to the background culture
>
> > For example, a therapist who 'knows' that the culture of the client forbids premarital sex may assume that the client was forced to marry after falling pregnant – in reality, however, that client may have intentionally become pregnant in order to be permitted to marry the person that she loved
>
> Dyche and Zayas (2001) argued that we need therapists who are 'knowledgeable about the specifics of particular cultures but who are able to suspend this knowledge when with a client in order to listen openly and without assumptions'

Cultural understanding is sometimes classed as 'cross-cultural empathy' (Dyche & Zayas, 2001)

> Cross-cultural empathy helps the therapist understand the world of the client from a sociocultural perspective
>
> This deeper understanding and appreciation can help the therapist to accept the client unconditionally

Demonstrating empathic understanding

The client's frame of reference can be entered using primary and advanced empathy to demonstrate empathic understanding.

Therapist must experience an empathic understanding of the client's frame of reference (Rogers, 1957)

Successful therapeutic change requires the therapist to experience 'an accurate, empathic understanding of the client's awareness of his own experience' (Rogers, 1957)

> Empathic understanding requires the therapist to be able to perceive the world of the client from the client's frame of reference

Frame of reference for demonstrating empathy

We all view the world from our own internal frame of reference

> We do not see the world as it really exists, but instead we see the world based on our memories, beliefs, values, knowledge, experiences, feelings, etc. in addition to our perceptions and sensations

True understanding of another person can only occur if we attempt to view the world from their frame of reference

> We must accept that this is never truly possible and we must ensure that we never become so immersed in the frame of reference that we cannot withdraw

> But we must still strive to view the world in this way so that the client senses that we are trying to truly understand

Therapists can only enter the client's frame of reference if they listen carefully to the verbal and non-verbal communication from the client, attempt to identify the expressed feelings and underlying behaviours, and respond by showing understanding rather than judgement

Primary-level empathy (Egan, 2007)

> Primary-level empathy requires the therapist to respond to the feelings and behaviour expressed by the client

> Responses will usually involve active attending, paraphrasing content and reflecting feelings

> Active listening and attending require the therapist to listen to the client, respond appropriately (use of minimal encouragers and clarification questions), and be aware of how they are sitting and acting towards the client

> Paraphrasing content and reflecting feelings require the therapist to repeat the content and feelings of the client's expression

>> Paraphrasing will involve repetition of the content

>> Reflecting will involve repetition of the feelings

>> Mirroring will involve the direct repetition of specific words spoken by the client

>> Summarising will involve a brief outline of both the content and feelings indicated in the client's expression, linking thoughts, feelings and behaviours, and identifying themes that have emerged

Advanced-level empathy (Egan, 2007)

> Advanced-level empathy requires the therapist to sense the expressions not communicated directly by the client

Self-disclosure, interpretations and challenges can all be used in advanced empathy

Self-disclosure involves sharing selected information about the therapist in order to enhance insight in the client

> Disclosure might be made to normalise – for example, 'Many people might feel like that in your situation, even I have had similar thoughts when I was grieving for my mum'

> But must beware of the risks of assuming that they are not unique or individual

> Disclosure might be made to indicate how the client presents – for example, 'When you raise your voice like that, I feel a little intimidated'

Interpretation involves detection of emotions on the basis of verbal and non-verbal language

> Interpretation might be made to help the client to see parts of themselves that they have not yet acknowledged or draw their attention to emotions not yet expressed

> For example, 'I notice that you clenched your fist when you said that and I wondered if perhaps you were feeling angry'

Challenges involve drawing the attention of the client towards any apparent contradictions

> Contradictions can exist between two sets of spoken words – for example, 'I notice that you said that you were happy for your sister but last week you mentioned feeling angry towards her, so I was just wondering what might be happening there?'

> Contradictions can exist between spoken words and body language – for example, 'I notice that you said that you were happy for your sister but you seemed to clench your jaw straight afterwards and I was wondering what might be happening there?'

Always need to be aware of the risks associated with advanced empathy

> High risk of focusing on therapist during self-disclosure so must ensure that the client remains the focus

> High risk of therapist appearing 'psychic' during interpretation so must ensure that the client remains the expert

> High risk of therapist appearing threatening during challenges so must ensure that the client remains comfortable sharing

SUMMARY

Absence of techniques: successful therapy is not dependent on techniques, success is dependent purely on the therapeutic relationship; research indicates that the main curative component in therapy is the nature of the therapeutic relationship

Congruence: therapist must be congruent and integrated in the relationship; genuineness; transparency; self-disclosure

Unconditional positive regard: therapist must experience unconditional positive regard for the client; non-judgemental approach; sensitive sociocultural awareness (cross-cultural empathy)

Empathy: therapist must experience an empathic understanding of the client's frame of reference; primary empathy, paraphrasing, reflecting, mirroring, summarising; advanced empathy, self-disclosure, interpretation, challenges, but be aware of the risks of advanced empathy

CASE STUDY DEMONSTRATING PERSON-CENTRED THERAPY

LEARNING OUTCOMES

After reading this section, you will be able to:

Appreciate the application of person-centred therapy from the humanistic approach in a therapeutic setting

Recorded session: therapy in action

This chapter is accompanied by a recorded therapy session which is available for viewing.

This session lasts for one therapy hour (50 minutes) and it is presented as the initial session in a new therapeutic relationship. Prior to this session, the client will have completed an initial assessment questionnaire and the therapist will have read this paperwork to ensure familiarity with the case. This completed assessment and a full transcript of the recorded session are available.

No actors are used in this session. The client was one of the authors and the problem presented was genuine. The therapist is an experienced practitioner in the field. The only 'fake' aspect of this recorded session is that the client did not really seek therapy and this is not really the first session of a series of therapeutic contacts.

After the conclusion of the session, the therapist is invited to answer a few key questions about the session. This question and answer session lasts no longer than ten minutes. The transcript of this session is available.

Presentation of Phil Thomas: history and symptoms

Phil Thomas has been suffering with stress and anxiety over the last few months. He has recently experienced some minor life events and these have had an impact on his mental wellbeing. He feels particularly anxious about his tendency to procrastinate and he believes that this is contributing towards his general feelings of stress. He has previously experienced person-centred therapy and he is generally positive about the possible outcomes for therapy. He would like to gain an understanding of his own behaviour in order to be able to reduce his own procrastination.

Therapy session: analysis

The therapy session can be sectioned as follows.

Introduction

Gentle introduction incorporating humour

Reflection on previous experience with therapy to establish possible expectations and beliefs about therapy

Addressing any questions about the nature of person-centred therapy

Outlining basic contractual details, especially the limits of confidentiality and the nature of sessions (length, number, etc.)

Story

Client is invited and encouraged to share his story – this forms the largest part of the therapy session

Focus on feelings and internal experiences, rather than the specific practicalities of the story

Goals

Establishing goals for therapy is periodically explored throughout the session, rather than forming a conclusion to the session

Goals are explored in terms of the current and ideal locations for the client

Ending

Warning given prior to the end of the session

Reflection on how the session was experienced by the client

Invitation to return for future sessions

Key questions to consider in relation to this therapy session

How could the nature of this client be understood from the humanistic perspective?

* What are the various configurations of the self-concept of this client?
* What possible conditions of worth could be having an impact on this self-concept?
* What might be getting neglected in the hierarchy of needs to prevent self-actualisation?
* Which characteristics of the full functioning person is this client failing to experience?

What is the nature of the therapeutic relationship in this person-centred therapy session?

* Does the client seem incongruent?
* Does the therapist appear congruent in the interaction?

- Does the therapist seem to be experiencing unconditional regard for the client?
- Does the therapist seem to feel empathy for the client's frame of reference?
- How does the therapist communicate congruency, unconditional positive regard and empathy to the client?
- How does the client respond to congruency, unconditional positive regard and empathy from the therapist?
- How deep is the relationship between the client and therapist?

Which person-centred techniques are demonstrated in this therapy session?

- Is the therapist transparent in her actions?
- Is the therapist genuine and how is this displayed to the client?
- Does the therapist self-disclose and what is the effect on the client?
- Is the therapist non-judgemental and how is this understood by the client?
- Does the therapist recognise the sociocultural position of the client?
- Is the therapist entering the frame of reference of the client?
- How does the therapist show primary and advanced level empathy?

Personal experience of the client

I arrived at the session a little apprehensive, hoping that all would go well and that I would be a 'good' client. The opening few minutes of the session gave me time to settle, as the therapist clearly explained confidentiality, and briefly outlined her approach.

In terms of relationship, I felt that Elaine and I developed a good foundation within the session for future work. I felt listened to and understood. I sensed that Elaine had a good degree of empathy, that she made some real connections with how I experienced my issues in the session. This enabled me to explore deeper and come to some new awareness. I also was given the time and space to reflect upon my thoughts and feelings. I can see this more clearly with hindsight, but remember that there were times in the session when I felt discomfort with the nature of therapist responses; that they were reflections, rather than challenges. At the time I remember thinking that there was little happening, and I commented on more than one occasion that I felt stuck and that I didn't know what to do with it (the reflection, the new insight). I think at the time I was hoping that Elaine would step in and rescue me.

I think that says a lot about my process. I guess I need to feel that I am moving in some direction, any direction. From my experience, the person-centred approach doesn't give that kind of external direction (non-directive) and that any direction needed to come from me. I see how that is beneficial, but at the time it was a little uncomfortable.

During the session I became increasingly aware of internal incongruence; that there were 'parts' of me in conflict. Again, in reflection, I see these as 'configurations' and sense that there is an opportunity to have an internal dialogue between these configurations. This new awareness felt challenging, that here is something tangible to get into – an area to explore. I particularly liked Elaine's reflection that she felt sad for the part of me that I wanted to be rid of.

I left the session with a better sense of my issues, some areas were clarified, others areas were newly formed (e.g. internal conflicts). I had a sense that it would need to be a commitment to a process and that there were no short cuts to getting answers and resolutions. It felt like the beginning of a journey and that Elaine had the right qualities to be my guide.

—*Phil Thomas*

REFERENCES AND BIBLIOGRAPHY

Association for Humanistic Psychology (2001) Humanistic psychology overview. Retrieved from www.ahpweb.org/aboutahp/whatis.html

Association for Humanistic Psychology (2011) A brief biography of A H Maslow. Retrieved from www.ahpweb.org/aboutahp/maslow_bio.html

British Association for Counselling and Psychotherapy (BACP) (1992) *Ethical Framework for Good Practice in Counselling and Psychotherapy.* Guidelines available online at www.bacp.co.uk/ethical_framework

Bugental, J.F. (1963) Humanistic psychology: a new breakthrough. *American Psychologist*, 18(9), 563.

Bugental, J.F. (1965) *The Search for Authenticity: An Existential-Analytic Approach to Psychotherapy.* New York: Holt, Rinehart and Winston.

Carkhuff, R.R. (1969) *Helping and Human Relations: Selection and Training.* New York: Holt, Rinehart and Winston.

Center for the Studies of the Person (2010) Welcome to the Center for the Studies of the Person. Retrieved from www.centerfortheperson.org/

Cohen, J. (1956) *Humanistic Psychology.* London: Allen and Unwin Ltd.

Cooper, M. (2007) Relational depth and the person-centred approach. *Person-Centred Quarterly*, May, 14.

Dyche, L. & Zayas, L.H. (2001) Cross-cultural empathy and training the contemporary psychotherapist. *Clinical Social Work Journal*, 29(3), 245–258.

Egan, G. (2007) *The Skilled Helper.* Belmont, CA: Brooks/Cole Publishing Company.

Engler, B. (2008) *Personality Theories.* Boston, MA: Houghton Mifflin.

Fiedler, F.E. (1950) A comparison of therapeutic relationships in psychoanalytic, non-directive and Adlerian therapy. *Journal of Consulting Psychology*, 14, 436–445.

Frankl, V. (1946) *Man's Search for Meaning.* Boston: Beacon Press.

Friedman, S. (1994) The genesis of humanistic psychology. Excerpt from a plenary address. Retrieved from www.ahpweb.org/aboutahp/Freidmanspeech.html

Gelso, C.J. & Carter, J.A. (1985) The relationship in counseling and psychotherapy: components, consequences, and theoretical antecedents. *Counseling Psychologist*, 13(2), 155–243.

Gendlin, E.T. (1978) *Focusing.* New York: Everest House.

Goldstein, K. (1934) *The Organism: A Holistic Approach to Biology Derived from Pathological Data in Man.* New York: Zone Books.

Grossman, A.J. (2008) *Your blog can be group therapy.* CNN Online. Retrieved from http://edition.cnn.com/2008/LIVING/personal/05/07/blog.therapy/index.html

Hall, M.H. (1968) A conversation with Abraham Maslow. *Psychology Today*, 35, 54–57.

Hoffman, E. (1988) *The Right to Be Human: A Biography of Abraham Maslow.* New York: St Martin's Press.

Hollander, G.R. & Hokanson, J.E. (1988) Dysphoria and the perception of incongruent communications. *Cognitive Therapy and Research*, 12(5), 577–589.

iTherapy (2005) What is iTherapy? Retrieved from www.itherapy.com/free-therapy-info.html

Kinch, J.W. (1963) A formalized theory of the self-concept. *American Journal of Sociology*, 68, 481–486.

Kirschenbaum, H. (2004) Carl Rogers' life and work: an assessment on the 100th anniversary of his birth. *Journal of Counselling and Development*, 82, 116–124.

Kirschenbaum, H. & Henderson, V.L. (1990) *The Carl Rogers Reader*. London: Constable.

Kirschenbaum, H. & Jourdan, A. (2005) The current status of Carl Rogers and the person-centred approach. *Psychotherapy*, 42(1), 37–51.

Lambert, M.J. & Barley, D.E. (2001) Research summary on the therapeutic relationship and psychotherapy. *Psychotherapy*, 38(4), 357–361.

Landreth, G. (1984) Encountering Carl Rogers: his views on facilitating groups. *Personnel and Guidance Journal*, 62(6), 323–326.

Lietaer, G. (2002) Remarks at Carl Rogers Symposium. Third World Congress on Psychotherapy, Vienna, Austria.

Maslow, A.H. (1943) A theory of human motivation. *Psychological Review*, 50, 370–396.

Maslow, A.H. (1954) *Motivation and Personality*. New York: Harper and Row.

Maslow, A.H. (1965) *Eupsychian Management: A Journal*. Illinois: Dorcey-Irwin.

Maslow, A.H. (1966) *The Psychology of Science: A Reconnaissance*. New York: Harper and Row.

Maslow, A.H. (1971) *The Farther Reaches of Human Nature*. New York: Viking.

Maslow, A.H. (1974) Creativity in self-actualising people. In: Covin, T.M. (ed.) *Readings in Human Development: A Humanistic Approach*. New York: Irvington Publishers.

May, R. (1939) *The Art of Counselling*. New York: Abingdon Press.

Mearns, D. (1999) Person-centred therapy with configurations of self. *Counselling*, 10(2), 125–130.

Mearns, D. & Cooper, M. (2005) *Working at Relational Depth in Counselling and Psychotherapy*. London: Sage.

Mearns, D. & Thorne, B. (1988) *Person-Centred Counselling in Action*. London: Sage.

Mearns, D., Thorne, B., Lambers, E. & Warner, M. (2000) *Person-Centred Therapy Today: New Frontiers in Theory and Practice*. London: Sage.

Mitchell, K.M, Truax, C.B., Bozarth, J.D. & Krauft, C.C. (1973) *Antecedents to Psychotherapeutic Outcome*. NIMH Grant Report 12306. Arkansas Rehabilitation Research and Training Center, Arkansas Rehabilitation Services, Arkansas.

Norcross, J.C. (2011) Conclusions and Recommendations of the Interdivisional (APA Divisions 12 & 29) Task Force on Evidence-Based Therapy Relationships. Retrieved from www.divisionofpsychotherapy.org/continuing-education/task-force-on-evidence-based-therapy-relationships/conclusions-of-the-task-force/

Patterson, C.H. (1985) *The Therapeutic Relationship*. Monterey, CA: Brooks/Cole.

Prouty, G. (1976) Pre-therapy: a method of treating pre-expressive psychotic and retarded patients. *Psychotherapy: Theory, Research and Practice*, 13(3), 290.

Purkey, W.W. (1988) An overview of self-concept theory for counselors. Retrieved from www.ericdigests.org/pre-9211/self.htm

Rogers, C. (1942) *Counseling and Psychotherapy: Newer Concepts in Practice*. Boston: Houghton Mifflin.

Rogers, C. (1951) *Client-centred Therapy: Its Current Practice, Implications and Theory*. London: Constable.

Rogers, C.R. (1957) The necessary and sufficient conditions of therapeutic personality change. *Journal of Consulting Psychology*, 21(2), 95–103.

Rogers, C. (1959) A theory of therapy, personality and interpersonal relationships as developed in the client-centred framework. In: Koch, S. (ed.) *Psychology: A Study of a Science. Vol. 3: Formulations of the Person and the Social Context*. New York: McGraw-Hill.

Rogers, C. (1961) *On Becoming a Person: A Therapist's View of Psychotherapy.* London: Constable.

Rogers, C. (1962) Toward becoming a fully functioning person. In: Combs, A.W. (ed) *Perceiving, Behaving, and Becoming: A New Focus for Education.* Washington, DC: Association for Supervision and Curriculum Development.

Rogers, C. (1969) *Freedom to Learn: A View of What Education Might Become.* Columbus, OH: Charles Merrill.

Rogers, C. (1980) *A Way of Being.* Boston: Houghton Mifflin.

Rogers, N. (1993) *The Creative Connection: Expressive Arts as Healing.* Palo Alto, CA: Science and Behavior Books.

Seligman, L. & Reichenberg, L.W. (2009) *Theories of Counselling and Psychotherapy.* New Jersey: Pearson Education.

Standal, S. (1954) *The Need for Positive Regard: A Contribution to Client-Centred Theory.* Unpublished PhD thesis, University of Chicago.

Strupp, H.H., Fox, R.E. & Lessler, K. (1969) *Patients View Their Psychotherapy.* Baltimore, MD: Johns Hopkins University Press.

Thorne, B. (1996) Person-centred therapy. In: Dryden, W. (ed.) *Handbook of Individual Therapy.* London: Sage.

Wilders, S. (2007) Relational depth and the person-centred approach. *Person-Centred Quarterly,* February, 1–4.

TABLE 2.1 **My conditions of worth**

Reflect on the following expressions and consider whether you have ever used them yourself or heard them being used by someone you love. Can you identify the unsaid implications of each statement?

Expression	Implication
Example: Real men don't cry	*Example*: If you allow yourself to experience and demonstrate the emotion of sadness then you are unworthy of the respect and love afforded to those who do not exhibit their emotions
Be a good girl/boy	
Don't act like such a big baby	
I wish you were more like your sister/cousin/friend/etc.	
You should know better than that	
You are so clumsy/lazy/stupid/useless	
Hurry up	
I wish you wouldn't do that	
You need to work harder	
I love you when you do that	

Chapter 3
Psychodynamic approach and psychoanalytic therapy

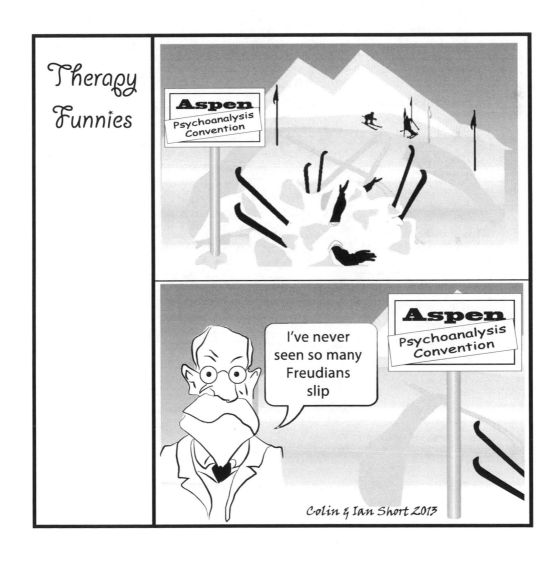

CHAPTER CONTENTS

- Introduction to psychodynamic approach and psychoanalytic therapy
- Development of the psychodynamic approach
  - Second force in psychology
  - Major advances in the psychodynamic approach
  - Key figures in the psychodynamic approach
- Personal and professional biographies of Sigmund Freud and Melanie Klein
  - Biography of Sigmund Freud
  - Significant learnings
  - Biography of Melanie Klein
  - Significant learnings
- Psychodynamic theories of human nature and personality
  - Topographical theory
  - Structural theory
  - Ego defence mechanisms
  - Psychosexual and psychosocial stages of development
  - Patterns of attachment
  - Object relations
- Therapeutic relationship in psychoanalytic therapy
  - Blank screen
  - Transference
  - Counter-transference
  - Use of transference and counter-transference in therapy
- Therapeutic techniques in psychoanalytic therapy
  - Traditional versus modern psychoanalytic therapy
  - Analytic framework
  - Interpretation in therapy
  - Transference analysis
  - Free association analysis
  - Dream analysis
  - Resistance analysis
- Case study demonstrating psychoanalytic therapy
  - Recorded session: therapy in action
  - Presentation of Phil Thomas: history and symptoms
  - Therapy session: analysis
  - Personal experience of the client

INTRODUCTION TO PSYCHODYNAMIC APPROACH AND PSYCHOANALYTIC THERAPY

This chapter aims to introduce the reader to the psychodynamic approach to counselling and psychotherapy. Psychoanalytic therapy will be explored as one example of a therapeutic method under the psychodynamic approach.

LEARNING OUTCOMES

By the end of this chapter, you will be able to:

- describe the development of the second force in psychology: the psychodynamic approach
- acknowledge the relative impacts of Sigmund Freud and Melanie Klein on the development of the psychodynamic approach
- discuss the core theories of human nature and personality from the psychodynamic perspective
- discuss the nature of the therapeutic relationship between therapist and client in psychoanalytic therapy
- outline the main therapeutic techniques utilised in psychoanalytic therapy
- appreciate the application of psychoanalytic therapy in a real-world setting

---

DEVELOPMENT OF THE PSYCHODYNAMIC APPROACH

LEARNING OUTCOMES

After reading this section, you will be able to:

- list the three main forces in psychology
- discuss the development of the psychodynamic approach in a historical context
- acknowledge the main contributors to the development of the psychodynamic approach

---

Second force in psychology

Three forces in psychology

> Behavioural theory
>
> Psychodynamic theory
>
> Humanistic theory

Psychodynamic psychology is the 'second force'

Developed alongside the behavioural approach as the two reacted against one another

First force

Behavioural psychology assumed that human nature was mechanistic and reduced humanity to the link between stimuli and response

Focused exclusively on observable external events (behaviour)

Second force

Psychodynamic psychology assumed human nature was deterministic and reduced humanity to basic biological drives

Focused exclusively on interpreted internal events (unconscious)

Rejection of the scientific method

Behavioural psychology was highly scientific as each principle could be tested in a controlled environment

In contrast, early psychodynamic theory was almost anti-scientific as each principle was based on internal unconscious drives that could only be detected through the subjective process of psychoanalysis

Although Freud considered himself a scientist, early psychodynamic theory did not apply the scientific principles of falsification to the study of the human psyche

This is often a criticism of the psychodynamic approach, but it is important to remember that science is limited by current available methods and it is not accurate to state that something cannot be true simply because it cannot be tested scientifically at that time in history

Modern neuroscience research into psychodynamic theories is now beginning to apply current techniques to exploration of the internal drives described by Freud and some of the findings are consistent with his theories

Neuropsychoanalysis is a new branch of psychology focusing on integrating neuropsychology and psychoanalysis (Solms & Turnbull, 2002)

Major advances in the psychodynamic approach

Initial interest in psychodynamic approach

Brucke presented the argument that every living creature contains dynamic energy governed by the first law of thermodynamics – energy can only be changed from one form to another, but it can never be destroyed

Lectures on Physiology published in 1874

Freud worked under Brucke at the University of Vienna in 1873

Freud was influenced by the lectures on physiology and applied these theories to the human psyche

Freud argued that human personality was a type of psychic energy subject to the same laws of thermodynamics

These early ideas formed the foundation of later psychodynamic theories

Freud and Breuer established the initial idea of repressed traumatic memories impacting on physical symptoms of hysteria during clinical work with hysteria patients

Studies on Hysteria published in 1895

Freud established the idea of dreams revealing repressed memories and unacceptable sexual and aggressive desires

The Interpretation of Dreams published in 1900

Freud began to establish the concept of the psychosexual stages of development as the psychodynamic theories began to form a cohesive approach to understanding human personality

Three Essays on the Theory of Sexuality published in 1905

Formal establishment of psychodynamic approach

Freud failed to get psychoanalysis accepted in the university system as an area of study and this led to the restriction of psychoanalysis training to private institutes (Jarvis, 2004)

Although his basic premises were accepted, the methods were regarded as too non-empirical for experimental psychology based heavily in the behavioural approach

In addition, many academics did not agree with his theories on infantile sexuality

Since his approach was not studied formally by academics, his theories remained free from the academic rigour normally applied to academic study and this led to the 'ossification' of theory (Malan, 1995)

Previous collaboration between Freud and Adler ended in 1911 and collaboration (and friendship) between Freud and Jung ended in 1914 (Bridle & Edelstein, 2000)

Both Adler and Jung struggled to accept the concepts relating to infantile sexuality, although they did agree on the general principles of the psychodynamic approach

Division of the approach at this stage helped to broaden the psychodynamic approach and establish psychoanalysis as the predominant therapeutic method across Europe and the USA

Freud eventually formulated his main theory of personality (structural theory) and this outlined the structure of the mind in terms of the id, ego and superego

The Ego and the Id published in 1923

Structural theory was widely accepted as demonstrating the structure of human personality, but debate continued to rage about the relative importance of each part of the personality on future behaviour

Jung established his own psychodynamic theories based on identifying personality types and archetypes

'Analytical psychology' is the Jungian school of psychodynamic theory

Psychological Types published in 1921

Adler establish his own psychodynamic theories based on a holistic approach to the person

'Individual psychology' is the Adlerian school of psychodynamic theory

Practice and Theory of Individual Psychology published in 1927

Alongside the development of these alternative branches of psychodynamic theory (Adlerian and Jungian), work continued on classic Freudian theory

Melanie Klein developed object relations theory in Britain after applying psychoanalysis to work with young children

The Psycho-Analysis of Children published in 1932

Anna Freud developed the concept of ego defence mechanisms and outlined how these are used in both beneficial and damaging ways

The Ego and the Mechanisms of Defence published in 1936

Both Klein and Freud worked in London using psychoanalysis with young children, and this overlap in activity but difference in perspective brought them into conflict

Eventually, each established her own branch of psychoanalysis, and training in the UK today is predominantly Kleinian whereas training in the US today is predominantly Freudian

Erikson devised an alternative set of developmental stages as a framework for psychoanalysis and this moved the theory away from infantile sexuality to focus on other aspects of human development (thus making it more acceptable to many academics)

Childhood and Society published in 1950 and revised in 1963

Horney presented a less male-oriented view of psychoanalysis, incorporating a new theory of self and a deep understanding of neurosis

Neurosis and Human Growth published in 1950

In the 1950s, the psychodynamic approach was eventually accepted in academia and introduced into the university system

Eysenck (1952) published a review of studies assessing the effectiveness of psycho-analysis

Although these studies have since been criticised, they do demonstrate the acceptance of the theory to the extent that it was regarded as appropriate for empirical evaluation

Bowlby's (1969) attachment theory also provided a framework within which to empirically test psychodynamic principles, particularly those relating to object relations

Modern psychodynamic approach

Today, the psychodynamic approach is accepted in academic circles to some extent

It remains a 'Cinderella paradigm' (Jarvis, 2004) to some extent, as it is still regarded as non-scientific

Modern advances in neuroscience allow some empirical research of the core principles

Psychodynamic approach is split into the following schools of thought

> Modern psychoanalytic therapy focuses on the following

>> Freudian (classic psychoanalysis) – Sigmund Freud, Anna Freud

>> Kleinian (object relations psychoanalysis) – Melanie Klein

>> Independent (mix of Freudian and Kleinian) – Winnicott

> Alternative therapies derived from psychodynamic approach include the following

>> Analytical – Carl Jung

>> Individual – Alfred Adler

Key figures in the psychodynamic approach

Sigmund Freud (1856–1939)

Impact on the approach

> Founding father of psychodynamic theory and psychoanalysis

> Highlighted the effect of the unconscious on the conscious

> Established the structure of personality containing the id, ego and superego

> Presented the psychosexual stages of development, including the Oedipus and Electra conflicts

Selected works

> *The Interpretation of Dreams* published in 1900

> *Three Essays on the Theory of Sexuality* published in 1905

> *The Ego and the Id* published in 1923

Alfred Adler (1870–1937)

Impact on the approach

> Developed 'individual psychology'

> Established a 'holistic' perspective focusing on human behaviour in a social context

> Explained the concept of the 'inferiority complex'

Selected works

> *Practice and Theory of Individual Psychology* published in 1927

Carl Jung (1875–1961)

Impact on the approach

> Developed 'analytical psychology'

> Established the concept of the collective unconscious and 'psychic inheritance'

> Established the concepts of introversion and extraversion

Focused on explaining adult development and the midlife crisis

Discussed roles in terms of archetypes (such as the mother archetype)

Selected works

Psychology of the Unconscious published in 1912

Psychological Types published in 1921

Melanie Klein (1882–1960)

Impact on the approach

Developed 'object relations psychology'

Pioneered work in psychoanalysis for children, with focus on the analysis of play

Established the concept of 'internal objects' to explain how early interactions with parental figures through the paranoid-schizoid and depressive positions impact on later life

Selected works

The Psycho-Analysis of Children published in 1932

Envy and Gratitude published between 1946 and 1963

Narrative of a Child Analysis published in 1961

Karen Horney (1885–1952)

Impact on the approach

Founding mother of feminist psychology

Disagreed with Freudian psychoanalysis and argued that psychological traits (such as gender identity) were not stable factors based in biology, but were instead fluctuating states occurring in response to experience

Established a comprehensive theory of neurosis

Proposed a counterpart to penis envy – 'womb envy' occurs in men who feel envious of the ability to bear children

Selected works

Neurosis and Human Growth published in 1950

Feminine Psychology published in 1967

Anna Freud (1896–1982)

Impact on the approach

Followed in the footsteps of her father to practise psychoanalysis with patients and presented many of her own psychodynamic theories

Pioneered work in psychoanalysis for children and was heavily involved in charity work supporting families and children

Established the concept of defence mechanisms to protect the ego

Selected works

The Ego and the Mechanisms of Defence published in 1936

Donald Winnicott (1896–1971)

Impact on the approach

Introduced the concepts of the 'true self' and the 'false self'

Introduced the 'transitional object' as a means of transferring feelings of security from the mother to another object (such as a security or comfort blanket)

Emphasised the importance of play (in children and adults) for psychological wellbeing

Argued that mothers should trust their own intuition to be 'good enough' for the child

Selected works

Playing and Reality published in 1971

The Ordinary Devoted Mother and Her Baby published in 1949

Transitional Objects and Transitional Phenomena published in 1953

Erik Erikson (1902–1994)

Impact on the approach

Presented the psychosocial stages of development

Coined the phrase 'identity crisis' when working with troubled young adults

Focused on the social aspects of development with specific attention to the ego – different to the classic approach of focusing on the sexual aspects of development with specific attention to the drives of the id

Selected works

Childhood and Society published in 1950

John Bowlby (1907–1990)

Impact on the approach

Developed the concept of attachment theory based on study of maternal deprivation

Highlighted the effect of healthy childhood attachments on adult relationships

Selected works

Attachment and Loss: Attachment (Vol 1) published in 1969

Attachment and Loss: Separation Anxiety and Anger (Vol 2) published in 1973

Attachment and Loss: Sadness and Depression (Vol 3) published in 1980

Final thought . . .

'Anyone who wants to know the human psyche will learn next to nothing from experimental psychology. He would be better advised to abandon exact science, put away his scholar's gown, bid farewell to his study, and wander with human heart through the world. There in the horrors of prisons, lunatic asylums and hospitals, in drab suburban pubs, in brothels and gambling-hells, in the salons of the elegant, the Stock Exchanges, socialist meetings, churches, revivalist gatherings and ecstatic sects, through love and hate, through the experience of passion in every form in his own body, he would reap richer stores of knowledge than text-books a foot thick could give him, and he will know how to doctor the sick with a real knowledge of the human soul' (Jung, 1966)

SUMMARY

Three forces: behavioural, psychodynamic, humanistic; second force developed alongside behavioural but focused on the unconscious rather than the observable, non-scientific originally but recent research has focused on neuropsychoanalysis

Major advances: initial ideas proposed by Freud in late 1800s after exposure to thermodynamics by Brucke; Freud and Breuer introduced concept of repressed memory in 1895; Freud used dreams to reveal repressed memories and unacceptable urges in 1900, psychosexual stages presented by Freud in 1905; formal establishment began after 1920s, acceptance of behavioural approach in academia excluded psychodynamic approach, Adler and Jung diversified the approach and carried the theories across the US and Europe 1910 to 1920, Freud formulated structural theory in 1923, Adler established individual psychology in 1927, Klein introduced object relations in 1932, Freud outlined ego defence mechanisms in 1936, Erikson presented psychosexual stages in 1950, Horney presented a feminist view of psychoanalysis in 1950, accepted as an academic area in 1950s, Eysenck reviewed effectiveness of psychoanalysis in 1952, Bowlby's attachment theory gave a framework for testing psychodynamic theories in 1969; formally established and accepted as an academic area in 1950s; modern approach includes Freudian (classic), Kleinian (object relations), independent (derivatives include analytical (Jung) and individual (Adler))

Key figures: Freud's psychosexual stages and topographical and structural theories, Adler's individual psychology and inferiority complex, Jung's analytical psychology and collective consciousness, Klein's object relations and internal objects, Horney's feminist psychology and theory of neurosis, Freud's ego defence mechanisms, Winnicott's transitional objects, Erikson's psychosocial stages, Bowlby's attachment theory

PERSONAL AND PROFESSIONAL BIOGRAPHIES OF SIGMUND FREUD AND MELANIE KLEIN

LEARNING OUTCOMES

After reading this section, you will be able to:

* outline the personal and professional biography of Sigmund Freud (1856–1939)

* outline the personal and professional biography of Melanie Klein (1882–1960)

* appreciate the impact of these key figures on the development of the psychodynamic approach

Biography of Sigmund Freud

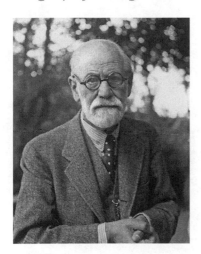

'A certain degree of neurosis is of inestimable value as a drive, especially to a psychologist'
—Attributed to Freud (n.d.)

Who was Sigmund Freud?

Sigmund Freud founded the psychodynamic movement

Possibly the most influential perspective in psychology

Sigmund Freud introduced psychoanalytic therapy

Possibly the most influential therapist in history

Early years

Born May 6th 1856 in the Czech Republic

Named Sigismund Schlomo Freud

Shortened his name to Sigmund at the age of 22

Father (Jacob Freud) was a wool merchant and mother (Amalia Nathansohn) was a housewife

She adored her 'golden Sigi' and revolved the family home around his needs and desires

Her devoted nature established the role for women in his work, and his Oedipus complex was partly based on his own feelings for his parents

Jewish Galician family

In accordance with tradition, both parents favoured him because he was the firstborn son and carried the good omen of having been born with the caul (part of the amniotic sac remaining on the newborn) (Margolis, 1989)

'A man who has been the indisputable favorite of his mother keeps for life the feeling of a conqueror' (Freud, quoted in Jones, 1957)

Family lived in poverty with much of their income going towards the education of their eldest son

Educationally advanced from a young age

Reading Shakespeare at the age of eight

Entered secondary school a year early

Graduated with honours receiving a summa cum laude award (top 5%) in 1873

Education

Law to medicine

Initially intended to study law, but eventually decided on medical school after attending a lecture on the essay 'On Nature' by Goethe

'Anatomy is destiny' (Freud, 1912)

Medical student at Vienna University from 1873

Conducted research on the sexual glands of eels in Trieste then returned to Vienna to work in the laboratory of Ernst Brucke

First scientific paper was published at the age of 20

Attended Meynert's course in psychiatry to learn more about neurology

Awarded a delayed medical degree from the University of Vienna in 1881 after one year of compulsory military service in 1879

Wanted to work in research, but financial difficulties forced him to practise

Career

Initial research in neuroanatomy

Developed a new staining technique using gold chloride to view the microscopic world of the neuron and trace the connections between different parts of the nervous system (Freud, 1884)

First neurologist to trace the course of the spinocerebellar white matter tracts from the lateral portion of the spinal cord to the cerebellum (Amacher, 1965)

Close to being the first to describe the neuron theory of the central nervous system, and his work provided the foundation for later researchers to develop a unified theory of cerebral structure (Galbis-Reig, 2004)

Meynert's psychiatric clinic in 1883

Hermann Nothnagel's medical clinic in 1883

Worked as resident physician at the clinic and was exposed to the use of hypnosis as a treatment for psychiatric disorders

Published *Uber Coca* (an article on cocaine) in 1884

Discovery of cocaine-based anaesthetic

Freud discovered the analgesic properties of cocaine in 1884, but did not conduct formal experiments and instead charged a colleague (Konigstein) to complete the experiments while he visited his fiancée – his colleague never completed the studies

Before leaving, he also described his ideas to another colleague (Carl Koller) who used these theories to test cocaine as an anaesthetic during eye surgery – Koller is now recognised as the person who discovered the anaesthetic properties of cocaine

Modern anaesthetic would not be possible without these early findings about the analgesic properties of cocaine

Personal use of cocaine

Freud frequently used cocaine himself, and the drug may have influenced him when he reflected on childhood (possibly false) memories of sexual desire for his mother and sexual jealousy towards his father

Freud also prescribed cocaine to friend Fleischl von Marxow as a cure for morphine addiction – unsurprisingly, Fleischl became addicted to cocaine and eventually died at only 45 years of age

Freud was criticised significantly in medical circles for this tragedy – Erlenmeyer said that Freud has added a 'third scourge of humanity, cocaine' to morphine and alcohol (Borch-Jacobsen, 2012)

Fellowship to study with Jean-Martin Charcot in Paris in 1885

Charcot was a renowned neurologist who focused on the clinical applications of hypnosis

Observation of patient hysteria and the effects of hypnosis moved Freud from neurology towards psychopathology

Private medical practice in Vienna in 1886

Established a private practice focusing on nervous and brain disorders

Found that symptoms of hysteria could be eased by putting a person in a relaxed position (on the couch) and asking them to talk about whatever passed through their heads – he could then identify the true root of trauma and symptoms would be relieved by this revelation

Found that these procedures could be enhanced by the use of hypnosis and hypnotic suggestion – first use of his technique was in 1887

Published *On Aphasia* in 1891

Reviewed in detail the clinical presentation of aphasia

Argued against the theory that all aphasias are rooted in two or three structures and proposed a unified theory of the mind (Galbis-Reig, 2004)

Still regarded as a classic text containing crucial information about this disorder

Published *Clinical Study of the Unilateral Cerebral Paralyses of Children* in 1891 followed by his last manuscript in the field of neurology, *Infantile Cerebral Paralysis*, in 1897

Questioned the established view that the disorder was due to birth complications (lack of oxygen to the brain during birth) and suggested that the difficult birth was a symptom rather than a cause of the disorder

Argued that the symptoms indicated damage to the brain while the central nervous system was developing in the fetus

Regardless of his work, the birth complication explanation remained until only two decades ago when it was found that the disorder is in most cases due to damage to the brain during fetal development (Galbis-Reig, 2004)

Published *Studies in Hysteria* with Josef Breuer in 1895

Case study of Anna O (real name Bertha Pappenheim)

Anna O suffered a nervous cough, tactile anaesthesia and paralysis but no organic cause could be determined

Talking about traumatic experiences from her life (identifying the root cause of the problem) while under hypnosis appeared to calm her symptoms – this was known as the cathartic method

Formed the basis of the 'talking cure' (term coined by Anna O herself)

Coined the term 'psychoanalysis' in 1896 (Freud Museum)

Psychoanalysis eventually became the fundamental psychotherapeutic method and modern therapy would not have been possible without this initial framework

Began a process of self-analysis in 1897 (Freud Museum)

Abandoned the concept of hysteria and neurosis due to trauma

Began work on the theory of infantile sexuality and the Oedipus complex

Published *The Interpretation of Dreams* in 1900

He felt that this was his favourite book (Freud Museum) and it contained extensive dream analysis

Freud (1900) suggested that 'the interpretation of dreams is the royal road to a knowledge of the unconscious activities of the mind'

Commonly misquoted as 'dreams are the royal road to the unconscious'

Published *The Psychopathology of Everyday Life* in 1901

> Foundation for the concept of the 'Freudian slip'
>
> > Slip of the tongue that can reveal the unconscious drives of the speaker

Published *Fragment of an Analysis of a Case of Hysteria* in 1905

> Case study of 18-year-old Dora (real name Ida Bauer)
>
> Dora suffered depression (suicidal thoughts) and a range of hysterical symptoms, such as a chronic cough and aphonia (loss of voice), with no recognised organic cause
>
> Her father (an intimidating man) brought her to therapy and insisted that she held fantasies about the people in her life
>
> > She babysat for a married couple and reported that the female (Frau K) was having an affair with her own father and the male (Herr K) had propositioned her
> >
> > She explained that her father wanted to exchange her for the married woman – Herr K would permit the affair between his wife and Dora's father to continue provided that he could have Dora in exchange
> >
> > She was diagnosed as repressing her own desire for Frau K and, to a lesser extent, Herr K and her own father
>
> Dora broke away from therapy after 11 weeks and Freud felt that the therapy ended too early to be successful – he later blamed himself for the lack of success as he felt that he had failed to notice key elements of transference during the therapy

Published *Three Essays of the Theory of Sexuality* in 1905

> Outlined the psychosexual stages (oral, anal, phallic, latency, genital) and the Oedipus conflict, but these aspects did not appear in full in the first edition and were instead added at a later date (approximately 1915)

Attended the First International Psychoanalytical Congress in Vienna in 1908

Visited the USA with Jung to give the first lectures on psychoanalysis in America (Clark Lectures) in 1909

> Freud was unimpressed with America – he described it as immature and repressed (Pruner, 1992)
>
> > In conversation with friends, Freud stated that 'America is the most grandiose experiment the world has seen, but, I am afraid, it is not going to be a success' (Pruner, 1992)

Published *Analysis of a Phobia in a Five-year-old Boy* in 1909

> Case study of Little Hans – treated by his father under the guidance of Freud
>
> > Freud acknowledged that the material for this case study was gathered by the father and may have been biased (although he noted that few people other than a parent could encourage a child to express his feelings so openly)

Little Hans had a phobia of horses, possibly relating to an incident in which he witnessed a horse falling in the street

Fear of horses was equated to fear of his father and these feelings of anxiety were explained in terms of the Oedipus conflict

Freud was less convinced by the Oedipus explanation of this case, but the parents were close followers of Freudian theory and the reports of the father did seem to fit with the theory

Published *Notes upon a Case of Obsessional Neurosis* in 1909

Case study of Rat Man (real name possibly Paul Lorenz or Ernst Lanzer)

Rat Man had heard about a military torture involving a bucket of rats tied to the bottom of a prisoner and then heated up so that the rats burrow into the anus to escape the heat

Rat Man suffered obsessive fears that his father and fiancée would be a victim of this torture, and he felt compelled to carry out specific behaviours to cope with his thoughts

Freud suggested that he was repressing homosexual fantasies and displacing aggressive impulses – guilt about his sexual desires and his aggressive feelings towards his father were transferred to fears about the fiancée and father suffering the rat torture

Freud indicated that he made a complete recovery (although there is some controversy about this conclusion)

Delivered introductory lectures on psychoanalysis at University of Vienna in 1915

Published *From the History of an Infantile Neurosis* in 1918 (written in 1914)

Case study of Wolf Man (real name Sergei Pankejeff)

Wolf Man suffered with depression and apathy, and avoided engaging in life (work, family, etc.) to the extent that he was no longer self-sufficient

He reported a terrifying dream from his childhood involving a dozen white wolves sitting in a tree outside his bedroom window – this dream was interpreted to be the result of the trauma of seeing his parents engaged in a primal scene ('coitus a tergo' or sexual intercourse from behind) at a young age

Freud explained that Wolf Man was 'cured' after the initial therapy but returned to work on some transference issues after the war – after this second therapeutic process, Freud reported that Wolf Man was normal and behaved accordingly

Published *Beyond the Pleasure Principle* in 1920

Introduced the concept of the death instinct and suggested that dreams could be forms of wish fulfilment

Published *The Ego and the Id* in 1923

Outlined the structure of the mind (id, ego, superego)

Published *The Future of an Illusion* in 1927

Established himself as an atheist and debunked religion on rational and scientific grounds

Exchanged letters with Einstein on the subject of war in 1932

'Why war?'

Moved to England to escape the Nazi invasion of Vienna in 1938

Continued seeing patients and working on his final books *An Outline of Psychoanalysis* and *Moses and Monotheism*

Family

Married Martha Bernays in 1886

Met in 1882 and were engaged within two months, but then spent four years apart before marrying in 1886

Freud famously wrote over 900 passionate letters to his fiancée and many of these provide an insight into his personality, attitudes and beliefs about masculine and feminine roles

'Woe to you, my Princess, when I come, I will kiss you quite red and feed you till you are plump. And if you are forward you shall see who is the stronger, a gentle little girl who doesn't eat enough or a big wild man who has cocaine in his body' (Freud, quoted in Farber, 1978)

After marriage, she was devoted to her husband and he used his feelings about her role in their relationship to form the basis of many of his theories about female nature

'I know, after all, how sweet you are, how you can turn a house into a paradise, how you will share in my interests, how gay yet painstaking you will be. I will let you rule the house as much as you wish, and you will reward me with your sweet love and by rising above all those weaknesses for which women are so often despised' (Freud, quoted in Farber, 1978)

Raised three sons and three daughters

Anna was born in 1895 and was to eventually work alongside her father and move the therapy forward after his death

Death

Freud was diagnosed with cancer of the jaw in 1923

He suffered more than 30 operations and was eventually fitted with a prosthetic jaw in place of his amputated jaw and palette – this prosthesis allowed him to eat, drink, talk and smoke his beloved cigars

Given his theories about oral fixation, it is interesting to note that Freud remained constantly addicted to the cigars that were responsible for such pain and eventual death

'A cigar is sometimes just a cigar' (attributed to Freud by Wheelis, 1950)

Freud was exiled from Vienna to London following the Nazi invasion in 1938

His Jewish status made his family potential targets

Nazis burnt his books and he was vilified by the regime

'What progress we are making. In the Middle Ages they would have burned me. Now they are content with burning my books' (Freud, quoted in Jones, 1957)

He sought to continue working with patients and writing his final book in the relative safety of London in wartime Britain

Freud eventually died as a result of a lethal injection of morphine at the age of 83

Freud had made an earlier agreement with his doctor and he reminded him of this pledge when he felt that he could no longer work

'My dear Schur, you certainly remember our first talk. You promised me then not to forsake me when my time comes. Now it is nothing but torture and makes no sense any more' (Freud, quoted in Schur, 1972)

Following agreement from his daughter Anna, fatal doses of morphine were administered and he died peacefully in his own study at home on 23rd September 1939

FOUNDING FATHER OF THE PSYCHODYNAMIC APPROACH: FREUD

Consider the life story of Sigmund Freud and try to answer the following questions.

1.   What was the social and cultural context of the world in which Freud developed his theories?
2.   How might Freud's life experiences have impacted on his perception of human nature?
3.   How can this life story contribute to your understanding of the psychodynamic approach?

Significant learnings

'He that has eyes to see and ears to hear may convince himself that no mortal can keep a secret. If his lips are silent, he chatters with his fingertips; betrayal oozes out of him at every pore' (Freud, 1905)

'Psychoanalysis is in essence a cure through love' (letter to Jung, 1906, quoted in Bettelheim, 1984)

'It is always possible to bind together a considerable number of people in love, so long as there are other people left over to receive manifestations of their aggressiveness' (Freud, 1929)

'Homosexuality is assuredly no advantage, but it is nothing to be ashamed of, no vice, no degradation, it cannot be classified as an illness' (letter in response to an American mother's plea to cure her son's homosexuality, 1935, quoted in Grotjahn, 1951)

'The great question that has never been answered, and which I have not yet been able to answer, despite my thirty years of research into the feminine soul, is "What does a woman want?"' (Freud, quoted in Jones, 1957)

Biography of Melanie Klein

'One of the many interesting and surprising experiences of the beginner in child analysis is to find in even very young children a capacity for insight which is often far greater than that of adults'
—Klein (1955)

Who was Melanie Klein?

Melanie Klein revolutionised the psychodynamic approach and psychoanalytic therapy

> Established child psychoanalysis using the play technique
>
> Introduced the concept of object relations
>
> Introduced the psychological positions (paranoid-schizoid, depressive)

Early years

Born 30th March 1882 in Vienna

> Middle-class Jewish family (but religion did not play a role in family life)
>
> Father (Moriz Reizes) was a doctor – his family expected him to be a rabbi but he studied in secret to become a doctor and continued his education throughout his life

Happy childhood, despite the tragedy of loss

> Although Klein felt as though her father favoured her older sister, she always admired his intellectual drive – he died when she was only 18 (Segal, 1980)
>
> Klein had a closer relationship with her mother during childhood
>
>> Although this relationship became more difficult when her mother criticised her through a series of letters in her adult life
>
> Close to her siblings and devastated by the loss of her sister
>
>> Sister Sidonie died at the age of eight – she had taught Klein to read and write in the hope that she could pass on some knowledge before her own death (Segal, 1980)

Education

Passed her entrance exam to study at the gymnasium (responsible for preparing students for university) in 1898

> Initially wanted to become a medical doctor but instead studied humanities (art and history) at Vienna University after getting engaged

Family

Married Arthur Klein in 1903 at the age of 21

Arthur was her second cousin and they met when she was just 17

Married one day after her 21st birthday

> Married while still in mourning for the loss of her beloved older brother – this marked the start of the depression that plagued her life

Marriage ended her dreams of becoming a medical doctor, but she still retained her ambition and drive to help people throughout her life

Raised two sons and one daughter

> Final child Erich was born in 1914 – Klein did not wish to fall pregnant again and her depression increased during her pregnancy (Melanie Klein Trust, 1913)

Travelled frequently across Europe

> Moved to Budapest with her family in 1910

> Separated from her husband and moved with her children to stay with her in-laws in Rosenburg in 1919

> Moved to Berlin in 1920 and her marriage finally ended in 1924

> Moved to London in 1926 after the death of friend and analyst Karl Abraham

> Lived in London for the remainder of her life

Death of her son Hans in 1934

> Accidental death while hiking in Budapest

> Klein was too devastated to attend the funeral (Melanie Klein Trust, 2013)

Estranged from her daughter Melitta in 1942

> Melitta criticised her mother during the Controversial Discussions in 1932, and they remained estranged throughout her life (Donaldson, 2002)

Career

Initially introduced to psychoanalysis through her own depression

> Suffered depression and nervous anxiety reportedly associated with her difficult relationship with her mother followed by her death (Donaldson, 2002)

> As a result of her depression, she began psychoanalysis with Sandor Ferenczi in Budapest in 1914

> Ferenczi encouraged her to analyse her own children (Donaldson, 2002)

>> Klein used this experience to begin establishing a method of child psychoanalysis

>> She developed a 'play technique' for the psychoanalysis of children

>> Play is regarded as symbolic activity indicating underlying drives

Attended the Fifth Psychoanalytic Congress at the Hungarian Academy of Sciences in Budapest in 1918

> Attended a presentation by Freud – a self-confessed pivotal moment in her career (Melanie Klein Trust, 1913)

'I remember vividly how impressed I was and how the wish to devote myself to psychoanalysis was strengthened by this impression' (Klein, quoted in Grosskurth, 1986)

Became a member of the Hungarian Psychoanalytical Society in Budapest in 1919

Presented her first case study of her youngest son, Erich

Became a member of the Berlin Psychoanalytic Society in Berlin in 1923

Karl Abraham supervised her psychoanalysis work and she later received psychoanalysis from him

She incorporated his ideas about the death instinct into her work (Donaldson, 2002)

Published *The Development of a Child* in 1923

Case study of a child named Rita (two and a half years)

Therapy was successful and provided evidence for instinctual drives

Became a member of the British Psychoanalytical Society in London in 1926

Presented papers to the society resulting in critical acclaim

Ernest Jones organised a symposium at the British Psychoanalytical Society focusing on child analysis in 1927

Symposium was a response to a presentation delivered by Anna Freud to the Berlin Psychoanalytic Society earlier in 1927

Freud criticised the Klein approach (Melanie Klein Trust, 1913)

Sigmund Freud regarded the British symposium as a hostile reaction to his theories presented through his daughter (Melanie Klein Trust, 1913)

Sparked the initial divide between Kleinian and Freudian analysis

Published *The Psychoanalysis of Children* in 1932

Argued that children have a primary object relation to the mother

Published *A Contribution to the Psychogenesis of Manic Depressive States* in 1935

Introduced the psychological positions (particularly the depressive position)

Extraordinary Meetings of the British Psychoanalytical Society and Controversial Discussions were held in 1942

These meetings were designed to address the fighting between the members of the society

Anna Freud and Edward Glover argued that Klein was not a qualified psychoanalyst and Melitta Schmideberg (Klein's daughter) criticised the Kleinian method (Melanie Klein Trust, 1913)

Since both Melanie Klein and Anna Freud introduced the concepts of child analysis, discussions are often regarded as a direct battle between these two women

Klein did not, however, participate in the discussions in person until 1944 (Melanie Klein Trust, 1913)

'Kleinian' psychoanalysis established as an alternative to 'Freudian' psychoanalysis

Eventually, the society agreed to form two distinct subschools of psychoanalysis – Kleinian and Freudian

Also a 'middle' group containing those who remained independent and used a mix of techniques

Established the Melanie Klein Trust in 1955

She added her own money to start the running of the trust and invited her closest colleagues to be trustees (Melanie Klein Trust, 1913)

Published *Envy and Gratitude* in 1957

Most controversial of her works introducing the concept of primary envy

Published *Narrative of a Child Analysis* in 1961 (posthumous)

Case study of the analysis of a young boy

Synthesised and evidenced theories relating to object relations and the psychological positions

Death

Diagnosed with anaemia and visited Switzerland to recuperate in the summer of 1960

Unfortunately, her conditioned worsened and she returned to London to be admitted to hospital

Diagnosed with colon cancer after her return from Switzerland

Initially treated with an apparently successful operation but her health became poor again after a fall from her bed

Died on 22nd September 1960

FOUNDING MOTHER OF THE PSYCHODYNAMIC APPROACH: KLEIN

Consider the life story of Melanie Klein and try to answer the following questions.

1. What was the social and cultural context of the world in which Klein developed her theories?
2. How might Klein's life experiences have impacted on her perception of human nature?
3. How can this life story contribute to your understanding of the psychodynamic approach?

Significant learnings

'Feelings of love and gratitude arise directly and spontaneously in the baby in response to the love and care of his mother' (Klein, 1937)

'It was always part of my technique not to use educative or moral influence, but to keep to the psychoanalytic procedure only, which, to put it in a nutshell, consists in understanding the patient's mind and in conveying to him what goes on in it' (Klein, 1955)

'It is an essential part of the interpretive work that it should keep in step with fluctuations between love and hatred, between happiness and satisfaction on the one hand and persecutory anxiety and depression on the other' (Klein, 1955)

SUMMARY

Freud: founded psychodynamic approach and introduced psychoanalysis; *early years*, born 1856 in the Czech Republic, idolised by mother, moved to Vienna after father lost business, educationally advanced from a young age; *education*, originally studied law but moved to medicine after attending lecture On Nature, graduated as a medical doctor, scientific paper published at 20 years, wanted to work in research but forced to practise due to financial constraints; *family*, married after long engagement, wife was devoted and provided a template for female nature, raised six children; *career*, developed new staining technique to view neurons, first neurologist to trace course of spinocerebellar white matter tracts, almost first to describe neuron theory of central nervous system, studied hypnosis as treatment for hysteria, discovered analgesic properties of cocaine (controversy caused by personal use and prescribing as treatment for addiction), studied aphasia to propose unified theory of the mind, investigated cerebral paralysis to propose new explanation (recently found accurate), conducted case studies to establish a novel theory of personality and new approach to treatment of mental disorders (Anna O, Dora, Little Hans, Rat Man, Wolf Man), developed the topographical theory (conscious, preconscious, subconscious) and structural theory (id, ego, superego), outlined psychosexual stages and Oedipus conflict, coined the term 'psychoanalysis' and introduced concepts of Freudian slips and dream analysis; *death*, diagnosed with cancer of the jaw leading to eventual amputation, died following a lethal injection of morphine in 1939

Klein: revolutionised psychodynamic approach and introduced psychoanalysis for children; *early years*, born 1882 in Vienna, happy childhood marred by loss; *education*, passed exam to study at gymnasium, initially wanted to be a medical doctor but instead studied humanities at Vienna University after getting engaged; *family*, married second cousin at a young age, initially wanted to train as a doctor but focused on husband's career, raised two sons (one died at a young age) and one daughter (estranged in later life), onset of depression after death of brother and third unwanted pregnancy; *career*, depression led her to psychoanalysis, analysed her own children to develop a play technique for child psychoanalysis, accepted into various psychoanalysis societies and moved around Europe to eventually settle in London, introduced the concept of object relations and psychological positions through case studies (Rita, young boy), established the Kleinian version of psychoanalysis as an alternative to Freudian after the Controversial Discussions in the British Society, eventually led to three forms of psychoanalysis (Freudian, Kleinian and Independent); *death*, died due to colon cancer in 1960

PSYCHODYNAMIC THEORIES OF HUMAN NATURE AND PERSONALITY

LEARNING OUTCOMES

After reading this section, you will be able to:

- acknowledge the role of unconscious drives in controlling conscious thoughts and behaviour (topographical theory)
- describe the structure of human personality and discuss the interactive roles of the id, ego and superego (structural theory)
- describe and evaluate the ego defence mechanisms
- discuss the psychosexual and psychosocial stages of personality development
- describe the patterns of attachment that recur in childhood and adult relationships
- explain the impact of object relations on psychological development

Topographical theory

Human behaviour is driven by the unconscious (Freud, 1900)

Conscious forms only a small part of the human psyche

   Conscious awareness contains those things of which we are currently aware

      Includes those things that we are thinking about at this moment

      If we consider these psychodynamic theories from a slightly different angle, we could suggest that this is the equivalent of the short-term memory presented in the multistore memory model (Atkinson & Shiffrin, 1968); short-term memory is regarded as the mental desktop of the brain

Preconscious forms a slightly larger part of the human psyche

   Preconscious is not usually within our awareness, but can be accessed if prompted

      Includes all knowledge and information stored in the mind

      If we consider these psychodynamic theories from a slightly different angle, we could suggest that this is the equivalent of the long-term memory presented in the multistore memory model (Atkinson & Shiffrin, 1968); long-term memory is regarded as the mental storage tank of the brain

Unconscious forms the largest part of the human psyche

Unconscious is not within our awareness, but can be explored indirectly through psychoanalysis

Includes all drives, conflicts, desires, etc.

Two major instinctual drives

Life drive (Eros or the libido) to survive and thrive, sparks hunger, thirst, desire, etc.

Death drive (Thanatos or aggression) to self-destruct and return to the inanimate state, sparks aggression, risk taking, inertia, etc.

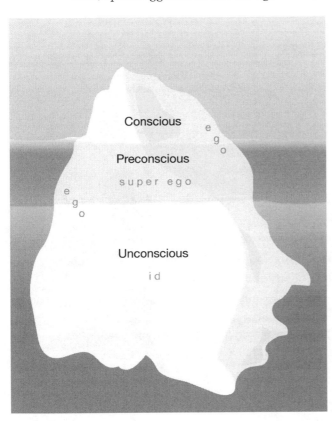

FIGURE 3.1
Topographical and structural theories: iceberg of the mind. Adapted from Freud (1900, 1923).

Structural theory

Personality is composed of three interacting structures (Freud, 1923)

Id

Basic drive for gratification

Located in the unconscious

Governed by instinctual drives

Pleasure principle

Present from birth

Young babies are entirely focused on their own satisfaction without awareness of the wider world

Ego

Understanding of social constraints

Located across the conscious, preconscious and unconscious

Governed by an understanding of the realities of the social world

Reality principle

Develops during the first three years of life

Child becomes aware of the needs and demands of others and responds to the urges of the id with consideration for the real world

Superego

Moral and ethical restraints

Located in the preconscious

Governed by social (particularly parental) constraints

Similar to conscience

Develops during the fifth or sixth year

Child accepts the moral values of caregivers to establish own set of rules for governing behaviour

Ego must be stronger than id and superego

Ego needs to provide satisfaction for the id while avoiding upsetting the superego and remaining within the constraints of the real world

'The poor ego has a still harder time of it; it has to serve three harsh masters, and it has to do its best to reconcile the claims and demands of all three . . . The three tyrants are the external world, the superego, and the id' (Freud, 1923)

'The ego is not master in its own house' (Freud, 1917)

STRUCTURAL THEORY: SIMPSONS OF THE MIND

Imagine *The Simpsons* television cartoon . . .

- Homer is like the Id – childlike, demanding, spoilt, selfish, etc.
- Flanders is like the superego – self-righteous, ethical, judgemental, guilty, etc.
- Marge is like the ego – constantly struggling to appease Homer while impressing Flanders

Weak ego

> Impulsiveness and selfishness would occur if the id became too strong
>
> Judgemental attitudes and guilt would occur if the superego became too strong

Ego defence mechanisms

Intrapsychic conflict leads to anxiety (Freud, 1936)

Conflict between id and superego

> Forbidden impulses are experienced by the id
>
> Condemnation from the superego (and possibly society) would occur if the impulses were expressed openly
>
> Ego will attempt to satisfy the urges of the id while avoiding condemnation from the superego by altering the presentation of the impulse
>
> Ego defence mechanisms are normal and healthy methods to mediate this conflict by denying or distorting reality to protect the fragile balance of the psyche
>
> Ego defence mechanisms operate in the unconscious so we are not aware of their impact on us unless it is interpreted during psychoanalysis

Freud (1936) described various defence mechanisms

> Repression
>
>> Pushing traumatic memories into the unconscious
>>
>> For example, forgetting an incident of sexual abuse in childhood
>
> Regression
>
>> Reverting to a prior stage of development (usually in childhood)
>>
>> For example, throwing a temper tantrum when your computer loses an important document
>
> Denial
>
>> Claiming that an anxiety-provoking stimulus does not exist
>>
>> For example, refusing to accept that a loved one has died
>
> Projection
>
>> Ascribing own desires and emotions to other people
>>
>> For example, accusing your partner of cheating on you instead of accepting own desire to have an affair
>
> Displacement
>
>> 'Kick the cat' syndrome
>>
>> Redirecting emotions from the source to a less threatening target
>>
>> For example, kicking the cat when you are angry with your computer

Sublimation

    Expressing unacceptable impulses in an acceptable manner

    For example, establishing a career in boxing to express aggressive urges

Reaction formation

    Adopting a belief that is completely opposite to true feelings

    For example, insisting that you would be very happy to get a third-class degree to hide the real desire to get a first-class degree

Compensation

    Developing specific traits to make up for deficiencies in other areas

    For example, buying a big car to make up for a small physique

IN MY DEFENCE . . .

For each of the following cases, explain how the ego defence mechanism might yield a positive and/or negative outcome.

A man in his late twenties has a criminal record for assault and burglary committed in his teenage years. He has not committed any crimes in recent years after starting a family with his childhood sweetheart and he has been employed as a labourer on a building site. However, he has just been told that he will be made redundant at the end of the week. He is angry with his boss and he is embarrassed about telling his partner the news.

A woman in her thirties has just lost her father. She has spent the last three years caring for him during the late stages of terminal cancer. Now that he has passed away, she is left with the task of distributing his property according to his last will and testament. She is devastated by the loss and overwhelmed by the responsibility of fulfilling his final wishes.

A teenage boy has had three dreams about being kissed by another boy in his class. He feels ashamed by these dreams when he wakes up and he thinks that his father would be angry if he knew about them.

A young girl was removed from her parents after a neighbour told the police that he had seen her father touching her in an inappropriate way. She is taken to live with foster parents, but the memory of the abuse prevents her from being able to form a close relationship with her new family.

An elderly man has been experiencing severe pains in his stomach and he has lost a significant amount of weight. His older brother died of colon cancer when he was 60 and he seemed to have similar symptoms before his death. However, the elderly man feels uncomfortable discussing his body with the doctor and does not want to worry his family.

Rationalisation

> Formulating a logical and sensible, but false, reason to explain behaviour

> For example, claiming that you failed your exam because you had a cold rather than accepting that it was because you did not revise

Intellectualisation

> Focusing excessively on intellectual details rather than dealing with the associated emotions

> For example, obsessing about the details of the funeral rather than focusing on feelings of grief after the death of a loved one

Psychosexual and psychosocial stages of development

Freud (1905) described the psychosexual stages from birth to adulthood

Oral stage – 0–1year

> Focus of gratification is the mouth and oral exploration of the world

> Child demonstrates a tendency to insert things into the mouth and a desire to suck on objects (typified by sucking at the breast of the mother)

> Weaning is a key event during this stage

>> Child learns the importance of delayed gratification (does not always instantly get to suck on objects), independence of the self (not always able to control environment) and behavioural control (some behaviours lead to gratification, such as crying)

> Too much or too little gratification at this stage of development can lead to an oral fixation

>> Orally aggressive individuals may chew gum and other objects

>> Orally passive individuals may engage in smoking, overeating, etc.

>> Both individuals will be passive, immature and gullible

Anal stage – 1–3 years

> Focus of gratification is the bottom and elimination from the bowel and bladder

> Child demonstrates a tendency to touch the bottom, eliminate bodily waste at inappropriate times, and play with faeces

> Toilet training is a key event during this stage

>> Child learns how to resolve the basic conflict between the id and ego – id will want instant gratification in response to the urge to eliminate bodily waste but the ego has begun to encourage delayed gratification and parental demands will support this desire

Too much or too little gratification at this stage of development can lead to an anal fixation

> Child who seeks to retain bodily waste to spite the ego (and parents) and enjoy the sensation of pressure on the bowel and bladder will become anal-retentive (excessively organised and neat)

> Child who seeks to expel bodily waste at inappropriate times to spite the ego (and parents) and enjoy the sensation of expulsion will become anal-expulsive (excessively disorganised and reckless)

Phallic stage – 3–6 years

Focus of gratification is the genitals and sexual stimulation

Child demonstrates a gradual understanding of the difference between males and females, a desire to explore their own and other bodies, and a tendency to play with their genitals

Oedipus and Electra complex are key events during this stage

Oedipus complex

> Applicable to boys

> As the boy begins to develop a sexual identity (I am a boy) and experience some sexual feelings (touching feels good), he will direct these feelings towards the main person in his life

> Sexual desire is focused on the mother (I want to marry mummy)

> Jealousy is directed towards the father who is viewed as more advanced (daddy is bigger than me) and already in possession of the mother (mummy loves daddy)

> Id wants to kill father, but ego is aware that father would probably win a battle and could castrate the boy

> Boy bonds with father to minimise this risk and possess the mother vicariously – male sexual role develops as boy identifies with father

Electra complex

> Applicable to girls, although Freud did argue against the use of this term

> As the girl begins to develop a sexual identity (I am a girl) and experience some sexual feelings (touching feels good), she will direct these feelings towards the main person in her life

> Sexual desire is initially focused on the mother but realisation of the absence of a penis means that this desire (can never possess mother) is redirected towards the father

> Girl experiences both envy and desire for her father (penis envy) and resentment towards her mother (mother is assumed to have castrated her)

> Girl bonds with mother to possess the father vicariously – female sexual role develops as girl identifies with mother

Too much or too little gratification at this stage of development can lead to a phallic fixation

> Unresolved Oedipus or Electra complex will involve the development of inappropriate sexual roles due to a failure to identify with the appropriate person

> Phallic character traits will involve recklessness, pride, narcissism and vanity

Latency stage – 6–12 years

Gratification is not sought during this stage because sexual feelings lie dormant

Child will use this time to pursue other, non-sexual interests prior to puberty

Genital stage – 12+ years

Focus of gratification is sexual interest in members of the opposite sex

Child will begin to develop sexual relationships with members of the opposite sex

Inability to focus on this stage of development due to fixation in one of the earlier stages can lead to frigidity, impotence and failure to develop satisfactory adult relationships

Erikson (1963) described psychosocial stages from birth to death

Infancy: trust versus mistrust – 0–1 year

Child begins to develop the ability to trust others based on relationships with caregivers, particularly during feeding

Successful completion of this stage leads to confidence and security

Unsuccessful completion of this stage leads to anxiety and insecurity

Early childhood: autonomy versus doubt – 1–3 years

Child begins to develop control over physical body through toilet training

Successful completion of this stage leads to independence and autonomy

Unsuccessful completion of this stage leads to shame and doubt

Preschool: initiative versus guilt – 3–6 years

Child begins to develop control over the surrounding environment through exploration

Successful completion of this stage leads to a sense of purpose

Unsuccessful completion of this stage leads to guilt

School: industry versus inferiority – 6–12 years

Child begins to develop coping skills for new social situations through school

Successful completion of this stage leads to competence

Unsuccessful completion of this stage leads to inferiority

Adolescence: identity versus role confusion – 12–18 years

Teen begins to develop a sense of self and personal identity through relationships beyond the immediate family

Successful completion of this stage leads to a strong sense of self

Unsuccessful completion of this stage leads to role confusion and a weak sense of self

Young adult: intimacy versus isolation – 18–35 years

Adult begins to develop intimate relationships with others

Successful completion of this stage leads to strong relationships

Unsuccessful completion of this stage leads to loneliness and isolation

Middle age: generativity versus stagnation – 35–60 years

Adult begins to develop a need to create things that will last after their death

Successful completion of this stage leads to accomplishment and usefulness

Unsuccessful completion of this stage leads to shallow involvement in life

Later life: integrity versus despair – 60+ years

Adult begins to develop self-reflection and the ability to reflect on life

Successful completion of this stage leads to wisdom and self-fulfilment

Unsuccessful completion of this stage leads to regret, despair and bitterness

Patterns of attachment

Attachment is a 'lasting psychological connectedness between human beings' (Bowlby, 1969).

Attachment is more than simple provision

Responses of rhesus monkey infants differ between carers who provide food versus carers who provide comfort (Harlow & Zimmerman, 1958)

Infants reared in isolation suffered physical and behavioural problems – unable to adjust to normal social life as adults

Infants reared with dummy mothers preferred to spend time with the dummy covered in soft towelling rather than the wire dummy holding the bottle – when frightened, infants would cling to the 'soft mother' rather than the 'providing mother'

Finding suggests that a connection with a warm figure to which the infant can cling is essential in the critical attachment period of the monkey

In humans, the absence of a warm attachment figure in the first two years leads to psychological problems in later life

In a monograph for the World Health Organization, Bowlby stated that 'the infant and young child should experience a warm, intimate, and continuous relationship with his mother in which both find satisfaction and enjoyment' (Bowlby, 1951)

Widespread changes in institutional childcare have resulted from these theories – for example, introduction of parental visits for hospitalised children and foster parent placements for orphaned infants

Early relationships between primary caregivers (parent) and care receivers (child) establish attachments

Attachment is an evolutionarily advantageous strategy for the vulnerable child to stay safely within close proximity of a figure who offers care and protection

Child develops a range of behaviours designed to maintain close proximity to the caregiver, such as crying, clinging, etc.

In the first year of life the child forms an attachment with those who provide care (Bowlby, 1969)

0–3 months = indiscriminate responses to any caregiver

3–7 months = initial preference for most common caregivers

7–9 months = special preference for main caregiver (attachment) with clear distress when the mother is absent (separation anxiety) and fear of unknown replacement caregivers (stranger fear)

9–12 months = as the child matures, s/he will use the caregiver as a 'secure base' from which to explore the world; child negotiates with the caregiver to stretch the boundaries of proximity while retaining feelings of security

Patterns of attachment emerge from these early experiences with caregivers

Ainsworth (1967) identified four distinct individual differences in infant attachment patterns through the 'strange situation' experimental paradigm

Infant and parent play in an unfamiliar space

Parent leaves the infant alone for a short while and infant responses are observed

Parent returns to the infant and infant responses are observed

Secure attachment

Child is able to cope with minor separation to explore the immediate environment comfortably

Child protests the departure of the caregiver and is comforted by the return of the caregiver

Child has a clear preference for the primary caregiver, but will accept comfort from strangers to some extent

Caregiver has formed a secure parental bond with the child

Avoidant attachment

Child is unaffected by separation

Child does not protest the departure of the caregiver and shows no response to the return of the caregiver

Child treats strangers in the same way as the primary caregiver

Caregiver encourages independence and offers minimal response to a distressed child

Anxious attachment

Child is unable to cope with any type of separation and refuses to explore the immediate environment

Child is extremely distressed by the departure of the caregiver and refuses to be comforted by the return of the caregiver

Child has a clear preference for the primary caregiver and will not accept any comfort from strangers

Caregiver is inconsistent in responses to the child, and may display neglectful or abusive behaviours on occasions

Research suggests that only 65% of children have a secure attachment pattern and the remaining 35% display avoidant or anxious attachment patterns (Prior & Glaser, 2006)

Patterns of attachment formed in childhood are repeated in adulthood relationships (Hazan & Shaver, 1987)

Romantic relationships (in particular) tend to mimic the patterns established in childhood

Secure attachment

Adult is secure in the relationship

Adult feels confident about depending on others and being depended upon, without losing a sense of independence

Avoidant attachment

Adult will avoid close relationships

Adult is fiercely independent and does not like depending on a partner and being depended upon

Adult may be cold, distant or act out to push people away

Anxious attachment

Adult will feel very anxious about the relationship

Adult will lack independence and rely completely on a partner

Adult may feel angry or distressed in response to any suggestion that a partner is not similarly dependent

Hazan and Shaver (1987) found similar distributions of attachment patterns in adults as those identified in infants

60% reported a secure attachment in their relationships

'I find it relatively easy to get close to others and am comfortable depending on them and having them depend on me. I don't worry about being abandoned or about someone getting too close to me'

20% reported an avoidant attachment in their relationships

> 'I am somewhat uncomfortable being close to others; I find it difficult to trust them completely, difficult to allow myself to depend on them. I am nervous when anyone gets too close, and often, others want me to be more intimate than I feel comfortable being'

20% reported an anxious attachment in their relationships

> 'I find that others are reluctant to get as close as I would like. I often worry that my partner doesn't really love me or won't want to stay with me. I want to get very close to my partner, and this sometimes scares people away'

Some research suggests that patterns of attachment recur through life, but the evidence to date is far from conclusive (Fraley, 2010)

> Minor correlations between attachment styles to parents, partners and friends

> One unpublished study identifies very little link between attachment pattern at the age of one and attachment pattern in later romantic relationships

> Fraley (2010) noted that the 'existence of long-term stability of individual differences should be considered an empirical question rather than an *assumption* of the theory'

Object relations

Klein (1923) argued that adult relationships are based on interactions with significant others in infancy

> Childhood relationships set a pattern of relating that is repeated in our connections with others as an adult

>> Self relates to objects – object relations

Self and objects

Self is the subject (me, myself and I)

> Self exists at the centre of my universe and relates to objects around it

Objects are people or events that have a psychological impact on the self

> Objects can be anything that is not categorised as the self

Objects can be whole or part

> Whole objects are entire people

>> For example, the mother

> Part-objects are only part of a person

>> For example, the breast of the mother

> Infants tend to understand the world in terms of part-objects as they are focused on only those small parts of the world that satisfy needs

Whole objects develop when the child begins to understand the world from a wider perspective and appreciate that people are complete individuals

Objects can be external or internal

External objects are real things in the outside world

For example, my actual mother

Internal objects are internalised representations of things held in the subconscious

For example, my internal image of my mother

Internal objects are created through experience with external objects

Our subconscious creates internal objects following contact with external objects

For example, an internal representation of 'mother' is created in response to contact with the external actual mother in infancy

Once created, internal objects provide a template for interacting with future external objects

Future external objects can be associated with current internal objects so that our responses are predetermined

For example, an internal representation of 'mother' can be applied to people who exhibit mothering traits in the future

Objects can be 'good' or 'bad'

Good objects are those that fulfil the needs of the self

For example, the good breast is one that will feed the hungry child

Bad objects are those that fail to fulfil the needs of the self

For example, the bad breast is one that is absent or lacking milk when the child is hungry

Polarised views of 'good' and 'bad' minimise ambivalence in infancy

It is confusing for an infant to understand that every person has both positive and negative personality traits and that every person is capable of both kind and cruel actions

It is simpler for the infant to split each object into good and bad versions

For example, 'good' mother is kind and affectionate whereas 'bad' mother is unkind and withdrawn

Mother–infant dyad

Klein (1932) noted that the mother is a critical figure for the infant

Mother is the first external object for whom an internal object is created

Relationship with the external and internal mother-object will have a life-long impact on the individual

More specifically, the breast of the mother is the very first significant part-object in the world of the infant

Good breast will give milk and bad breast will deny milk when the child is hungry

This early relationship with the breast forms the basis of the psychological positions during childhood

Psychological positions

Klein (1935, 1937, 1957, 1961) argued that infants pass through two psychological positions during childhood

Paranoid-schizoid position – birth to six months

Depressive position – six months to one year

Paranoid-schizoid position

Characterised by anxiety, part-objects, splitting, projection and introjection

Vulnerable infant suffers a lot of anxiety

Infant experiences frustration whenever he does not have his needs immediately fulfilled

For example, hunger leads to anguish, frustration and fear of death (death instinct)

Anxiety leads to intense hatred towards the cause

For example, hatred of the breast because it is not satisfying his needs immediately

Infant deals with his anxiety by using defences

Negative (anxiety) and positive (satisfaction) feelings are projected into the world onto part-objects

Part-objects are split into either 'good' or 'bad' and this distinction is based on whether they satisfy or deny

Good and bad part-objects are then introjected and this internal part-object will impact on future thoughts, feelings and behaviours

For example, feelings of frustration and hatred towards the breast that fails to provide milk are projected onto the breast so that it is regarded as 'bad' and this 'bad breast' may impact on feelings about other providers in later life

Depressive position

Characterised by integration, reparation and loss

Infant begins to integrate the different part-objects into whole-objects

For example, the breast that feeds, hand that strokes and voice that soothes are all part of the same mother-object

Infant begins to integrate good and bad into holistic objects

For example, the 'good' mother who gives food and the 'bad' mother who denies food are the same person

This new understanding of the object (whole, good and bad) leads to regret about the previous hatred towards bad part-objects and fear that this hatred may have harmed the object

For example, the child who hated the bad breast now understands that it forms part of the whole mother, and this leads to regret for his previous hatred and fear that his aggression may have driven her away

Infant will experience guilt and a desire to repair the damage done by prior hatred and aggression

For example, this reparation deepens the bond of love between mother and child

Infant will also experience a sense of grief due to the loss of the completely 'good' object

For example, the child grieves the loss of the totally good mother now that she has been replaced by a mother who is a mix of good and bad elements

Positions in adulthood

Paranoid-schizoid and depressive positions can be retained to some extent in adulthood if these stages are not completed successfully in childhood

Those regressing to the paranoid-schizoid position may experience hatred leading to aggression

Those regressing to the depressive position may experience guilt and grief leading to depression

Transitional objects (Winnicott, 1953)

Transitional objects are the first 'not-me' possessions

Physical items that can be held, hugged, etc.

For example, blanket, stuffed toy, etc.

Transitional objects offer comfort to an infant because they are linked to the feelings attached to the mother-object

Infant experiences feelings of loss as the realisation of being an independent entity begins to highlight the mother as a separate entity – infant experiences the 'loss' of the mother during this transitional stage

At this point, feelings associated with the mother (warmth, security, etc.) are transferred over to an available object to provide a substitute in her absence

Transitional phenomena serve the same purpose as transitional objects, but these are thoughts or behaviours instead of objects

Transitional phenomena are often repetitive actions (such as rocking) or recurrent thought patterns (such as fantasies)

In adulthood, transitional objects can be used to provide comfort during times of difficulty

Many adults use objects that remind them of home when travelling as these transitional objects provide a feeling of security at insecure locations

Hotel chain Travelodge revealed that 35% of adults in Britain admit to sleeping with a teddy bear to alleviate stress and 25% of male respondents admit to taking the bear with them when travelling on business (Ahmed, 2010)

SUMMARY

Topographical theory: conscious, preconscious, unconscious (life/Eros and death/Thanatos instincts)

Structural theory: id, ego, superego; problems of a weak ego

Ego defence mechanisms: intrapsychic conflict between id and superego leads to anxiety, ego develops defence mechanisms to cope with anxiety; repression, regression, denial, projection, displacement, sublimation, reaction formation, compensation, rationalisation, intellectualisation

Psychosexual stages: oral, anal, phallic (Oedipus and Electra conflicts), latent, genital

Psychosocial stages: infancy, early childhood, preschool, school, adolescence, young adult, middle age, later life

Patterns of attachment: lasting psychological connectedness, more than provision, Harlow's monkeys; attachment forms between 3 and 9 months, three patterns shown in 'strange situation' (secure, avoidant, anxious); patterns repeated in adult relationships (though evidence is inconclusive), 60% secure, 20% avoidant, 20% anxious

Object relations: objects are people or events that relate to the self, whole or part-objects, internal objects created through experience with external objects, good or bad objects; mother is the first internal object; psychological positions include paranoid-schizoid and depressive; transitional objects and phenomena provide a security object in the absence of the mother

---

THERAPEUTIC RELATIONSHIP IN PSYCHOANALYTIC THERAPY

LEARNING OUTCOMES

After reading this section, you will be able to:

- describe and evaluate the 'blank screen' anonymity of the therapist
- discuss the theoretical assumptions underlying transference
- discuss the theoretical assumptions underlying counter-transference
- explain how transference and counter-transference are used in psychoanalytic therapy

Blank screen

Therapist remains an anonymous blank screen

Therapist does not present the inner self

> No self-disclosures, no personal information, neutral responses

Client can project own needs, desires and values onto the therapist

> Client is unable to form feelings about the therapist based on the actions or revelations of the therapist
>
> Any apparent feelings towards the therapist must, therefore, give an indication of the inner world of the client
>
> Feelings towards the therapist may be a projection of feelings towards other significant people in the life of the client
>
> > For example, reacting with anger to a therapist who has done nothing to provoke this response might indicate that the client has projected these feelings from someone in their own past to the therapist
> >
> > This is known as transference

Transference

Twin concepts of transference and counter-transference

Freud noted that female patients would often indicate amorous intentions towards the therapist during psychoanalysis

> For example, Freud was saved from one potentially embarrassing situation by the sudden intrusion of a housemaid just as a female patient had announced her affections by throwing her arms about his neck. Freud resisted the urge to attribute this behaviour to his own sexual desirability and focused instead on the nature and cause of the phenomenon

Observation revealed that the behaviour would often be exhibited at a point when the patient had begun to explore a previously repressed childhood trauma, typically relating to the Oedipus or Electra complex (Freud, 1905)

> Freud argued that the patient would fail to recall the actual trauma, but instead would reproduce the feelings associated with those involved in the trauma and refer these feelings to the therapist through a 'mistaken mental connexion' (Racker, 1982)
>
> These feelings were displaced from important figures in childhood, such as siblings and parents, to be repeated in reactance to the therapist as a strategy for resisting further disclosure of childhood events
>
> In short, Freud proposed that feelings of love, hate, desire and fear were *transferred* from the original object to the therapist (Racker, 1982)

Definition of transference

Transference as a psychological concept refers to the redirection of feelings about one individual to another individual

'Transfer of feelings originally experienced in an early relationship to other important people in a person's present environment' (Luborsky et al., 2008)

Transference relationship can be classed as the cornerstone of psychoanalysis

In a therapeutic setting, transference will occur when the client redirects feelings about a significant person in their life towards the therapist

Transference refers to the transfer of unconscious feelings about a significant figure from childhood (such as the father) to a current figure (such as the therapist)

For example, a client is reminded of her father when she interacts with the therapist so her feelings of love and rebellion towards the father in the past may be transferred to the therapist

This may, however, be a simplified perspective of transference

An alternative definition for transference would be 'an unconscious pattern of relating developed from early "object" relationships' made real in the current situation (Leiper & Maltby, 2004)

Clients will transfer emotions from their own internal world created through experience in the past onto some aspect of the current external world

This definition suggests that the client is trapped in an unconscious cycle of re-enacting old relationship patterns throughout their life and it is argued that the resulting experience of frustration can lead to significant psychological disturbance

Pattern of relationships

Transference reflects a constant pattern of old relationships repeatedly emerging in current life (Luborsky et al., 2008)

Understanding the nature of transference in the therapeutic setting can provide the therapist with vital clues about the way that the client relates to others in the world beyond therapy

For example, the client who transfers feelings of love and rebellion from her father to the therapist may have a tendency to demonstrate this behaviour in all areas of her life: trapped within this relationship, she may constantly seek to repeat her father/daughter interactions by transferring feelings about the father of her past into her current relationships. This could lead to a search for father figures in personal relationships followed by inevitable rebellion against this authority, resulting in the destruction of the relationship

This hypothetical case provides evidence of how transference can be both beneficial to the client in the short term by providing her with a framework for relating to authority figures, yet damaging in the long term by trapping her in a cycle of rebellion against the desired authority figure

Positive and negative transference

Transference can result in both negative and positive feelings

> Anger and hostility may be examples of negative transference

> Love and desire may be examples of positive transference

Client could exhibit both negative and positive transference at the same time

> Similar to the manner in which one might experience both positive and negative feelings towards a parent

> For example, a client could experience feelings of love and seek to obtain the approval of the therapist whilst simultaneously experiencing feelings of anger and exhibit resentment towards the therapist

Transference or genuine emotion?

Important to be cautious about labelling all emotional responses to the therapist as evidence of transference

> Freud is reported to have said that 'a cigar is sometimes just a cigar' (Wheelis, 1950)

> It is likely that most behaviour may be based on genuine here-and-now emotions, rather than the displacement of emotions from the past

> Rogers (1951) noted that many attitudes of the client are 'of a reality, rather than a transference, nature'

>> For example, initial apprehension may give way to annoyance before eventually settling on a warm rapport (Rogers, 1951)

> Some clients will feel a natural liking or dislike on the basis of the behaviour exhibited by the therapist

> Some clients may feel sexually attracted to the therapist as a result of immediate desire rather than the misplaced attribution of past feelings

>> Indeed, it would be entirely normal for any individual to develop feelings for another person located in close proximity for a prolonged period of time

> Although these emotions may be inappropriate and should be dealt with accordingly by addressing boundaries or ending the therapeutic relationship, the existence of such emotions is not always evidence of transference

>> It is important to be able to distinguish between the transference of feelings and genuine here-and-now feelings in order to explore the revelations inherent in the former

Detecting transference

> Key features of transference (Leiper & Maltby, 2004)

>> Transference is typified by inappropriate and irrational emotions based in fantasy

>> Basis of these emotions will be protected by the distortion of reality to conform to the fixed pattern of response

Emotions will often be repeated indiscriminately across different settings

For example, a client who is transferring her early feelings of love for her father to her therapist might develop fantastical delusions of their supposed love affair, maintain these beliefs despite evidence to the contrary, and have a history of engaging in similar relationships and/or fantasies

This kind of transference can be dangerous for the therapist because he may find it extremely difficult to prove that they have not embarked on such a relationship

Counter-transference

Counter-transference = transference for therapists

Transference in the client during therapy is generally recognised as a natural response to human interaction

It is inevitable that s/he will base relations with the therapist on past relationships to some extent

But transference is not restricted to the client

Therapist may also experience similar emotional carryover effects

Therapists are human beings who cannot be entirely objective in their responses to clients as they will be subject to various biases, prejudices and desires

In a therapeutic setting, counter-transference may be exhibited on those occasions when the therapist reacts to the client in a manner that is not appropriate to that particular therapeutic relationship at that moment in time

Definitions of counter-transference

The term 'counter-transference' has been applied to a large number of psychological concepts in the therapeutic setting (Little, 2003)

Counter-transference refers to a specific unconscious attitude towards the client in response to transference from the client (objective transference – responding to transference from client)

Counter-transference refers to repressed elements of previous events leading to the displacement of past feelings from the source to the client (subjective transference – similar to transference in the client but acting in the opposite direction)

Counter-transference (objective)

Therapist responds to the transference exhibited by the client by acting in the role of the transferred figure

For example, a therapist treating a client who demonstrates transference by rebelling against the therapy in the same way that she rebelled against her own father might be experiencing counter-transference if he responds to the rebellious behaviour of the client by adopting the role of a critical father (responding to transference)

IDENTIFYING TRANSFERENCE

Read the following short transcript of a (rather inappropriate) therapy session and try to pick out examples of possible transference and counter-transference.

Therapist: Hello Suzy, what would you like to talk about today?

Client: I'm not sure. I just feel so lonely. I have just split up with my girlfriend and I feel so depressed.

Therapist: Could you tell me a little about this relationship?

Client: Well, at first, it was really good. We met at the gym when she showed me how to use the treadmill. She's a bit older than me and she was always teaching me stuff – she'd been to uni and had a good job. I've never really done anything like that – been working on the checkout at my supermarket since I was 15. She used to take me places. Like, we went down to London after we had been seeing each other for about a month. She wasn't really into clubbing like my other mates, but she took me shopping. She bought me a completely new outfit and a really expensive handbag. And I just felt really safe with her, you know? Even though London can be a bit rough, I knew that she'd take care of me.

Therapist: So when did things start to go wrong in your relationship?

Client: About six months ago. We were really close and then she just drifted away. Like, she used to wash my hair on the weekend and she used to cuddle me in bed, but she suddenly didn't want to do that any more. She said that she was too tired but it seemed like something more. I tried to talk to her about it but she said that I was just being demanding. I guess I was a bit demanding – it made me really angry that she wasn't, you know, with me any more, looking after me . . . I shouted at her a lot, sometimes I would smash up her stuff just so that she would pay me a bit more attention. But she just spent less and less time with me. Eventually, I stopped talking to her altogether. We were still living together but we didn't really communicate. When she tried to talk to me, I just didn't say anything back because I didn't want another argument. And then, last Sunday, I got home and she was gone. Packed her stuff and gone to her mum's. (Client begins to cry) I really miss her and it's all my fault. Do you think that I did something bad?

Therapist: No, not at all.

Client: But am I a bad person? I just don't know how to cope on my own.

Therapist: I don't think that you are a bad person. Relationships can be difficult and sometimes they do not work out. The important thing is to take care of yourself while you are going through this emotional distress.

Client: But I don't know how to do that!

Therapist: Well, my daughter has recently separated from her husband and she found it really helpful to join a local sports club. It got her out and about meeting new people.

Client: Do you think that I should do that?

Therapist: Yes, I do. . .

Counter-transference (subjective)

> Therapist exhibits his own transference by redirecting feelings about a significant person in their life towards the client

> For example, a therapist treating a client who demonstrates transference by rebelling against the therapy in the same way that she rebelled against her own father might be experiencing counter-transference if he behaves in a fatherly manner because he is reminded of his own past relationship with his daughter (transference acting in the opposite direction)

Use of transference and counter-transference in therapy

Person-centred therapy

Person-centred models of therapy highlight the importance of being able to recognise transference in the client and counter-transference in the therapist in order to prevent this phenomenon from impacting negatively on the therapeutic relationship

> Rogers (1951) suggested that the client-centred therapist should strive to understand and accept client transference in the same way that one would strive to understand and accept any other client attitude

Similarly, counter-transference should be addressed through a process of self-reflection aimed at understanding the attitude within oneself as a therapist in order to ensure that this attitude does not have an impact on the client

> Therapist should monitor and deal with any indication of counter-transference at the earliest stage through self-reflection, supervision, and continuous professional development

Minimising impact of transference and counter-transference

> Can be accomplished by ensuring that the relationship between the therapist and the client remains professional at all times

>> Establishing fixed session times

>> Limiting personal interaction beyond the sessions

>> Refusing gifts or gratuities

>> Maintaining a degree of professional distance

It must be recognised, however, that it is practically impossible to completely eliminate transference in the therapeutic relationship

> Even Rogers has been accused of fostering transference and counter-transference in his renowned exchange with Gloria: the client wishes that Rogers were her father and he responds by stating 'you look like a pretty nice daughter to me' (Thorne, 1992)

>> This aspect of the session has achieved some notoriety as it has been described as an indication that Rogers is unable to cope with transference; however, Thorne (1992) argues that this response from Rogers was essential in order to cement the relationship and further encourage the client to open up in future discourse

Transference and counter-transference are accepted within the relationship provided that the therapist remains aware of these forces and seeks to reduce the potential impact of these attitudes on the therapeutic process

Psychoanalytic therapy

In contrast to person-centred approaches to therapy, the psychodynamic approach actively uses transference and counter-transference to enhance understanding of the client

While transference is regarded as a dangerous phenomenon in most schools of psychotherapy, the interpretation of transference is essential in psychoanalytic therapy in order to explore the repressed experiences of childhood (Little, 2003)

Both Freud and Jung argued that transference was critical to the analytical process and that the exploration of transference was essential for the success of therapy. Indeed, Jung reportedly stated to Freud that transference was the 'alpha and omega of the analytical method' to which Freud remarked that Jung had 'grasped the main thing' (Jung, 1946)

Transference is allowed to develop in the psychodynamic relationship

Transference provides the therapist with crucial information about the childhood traumas of the client

For example, client who rebels against the therapist might be demonstrating transference of feelings from her father and this can provide crucial information about the nature of this past relationship

Transference provides the client with an opportunity to resolve past traumas by acting on the feelings within a safe environment, thereby potentially breaking the cycle of behaviour in the external world

Working through these transferences allows the client to become aware of these patterns of behaviour, address any unresolved conflicts, and seek to eliminate infantile regression by improving the relationship with the therapist

For example, a client may be able to resolve her anger issues in relation to her father by addressing her transferred feelings about her therapist – at the very least, the client will recognise this pattern of behaviour in her real-world relationships and possibly be able to break the cycle

---

SUMMARY

Blank slate: anonymous therapist does not reveal inner self so client can project own needs and values onto the therapist

Transference: redirection of feelings about one individual to another individual, demonstrates a pattern of relationships based on past experience; can involve positive and negative feelings; difficult to determine between transference and genuine emotion, can be detected by the distortion of reality contrary to evidence

Counter-transference: transference experienced by the therapist; objective involves responding to transference from client, subjective involves transference in the opposite direction

Use of transference and counter-transference: person-centred therapy focuses on acknowledging transference so that it does not interfere with the therapeutic relationship; psychoanalytic therapy focuses on detecting transference to reveal information about past traumas and possibly resolve issues from the past

THERAPEUTIC TECHNIQUES IN PSYCHOANALYTIC THERAPY

LEARNING OUTCOMES

After reading this section, you will be able to:

- appreciate the differences between traditional psychoanalysis and modern psychodynamic therapy
- explain the value of the analytic framework
- explain the value and risks of interpretation in therapy
- discuss the use of transference analysis in therapy
- discuss the use of free association analysis in therapy
- discuss the use of dream analysis in therapy
- discuss the use of resistance analysis in therapy

Traditional versus modern psychoanalytic therapy

Traditional psychoanalytic therapy

Typically referred to as 'psychoanalysis'

Therapist is the expert analysing a patient to treat neurosis

Modern psychoanalytic therapy

Not often referred to as psychoanalysis, but instead described as 'psychodynamic therapy' or a more specific term (Kleinian, Freudian, brief psychodynamic, etc.)

Therapist is working collaboratively with the client to solve problems

TRADITIONAL VERSUS MODERN PSYCHOANALYTIC THERAPY

Traditional	Modern
Patient lies down on the couch and therapist is positioned on a chair out of sight	Client sits in a chair opposite the therapist (also in a chair)
Therapist strives to restructure personality of patient and focuses on fantasy material	Therapist focuses on practical concerns and strives to address specific objectives
Therapist will see patient several times every week and treatment lasts many years	Therapist will see the client once a week with treatment as short as 1–20 sessions
Therapist will remain silent as much as possible	Therapist will speak frequently and be active in the treatment process
Therapist offers no self-disclosure	Therapist might offer some self-disclosure
Therapist offers few expressions of reassurance, support or empathy	Therapist will try to uphold the core conditions of person-centred therapy (empathy, unconditional positive regard, congruence), provided it does not conflict with the goals of therapy (for example, transference analysis)

Analytic framework

Rules of the therapeutic relationship

Analytical framework refers to the basic rules of the therapeutic relationship

> Sessions of a particular length at a particular time each week

> Fees for sessions are non-negotiable

> Structure of each session follows a pattern of reflecting on last session, discussing current state, reflecting current session, confirming next session, and paying fees

Analytic framework should be fixed and structured

> Mirroring the preferred relationship between parent and child

Value of maintaining the analytic framework

> Therapist should strive to maintain the framework

>> Do not agree to meet outside of scheduled sessions

>> Do not offer discounts or free sessions

>> Do not interact on a personal basis

> Strict adherence to the framework has many benefits

>> Relationship remains professional (rather than a chat)

>> Relationship mimics preferred parent–child relationships, thus encouraging revealing examples of transference

Relationship helps client to understand the value of structure

Importance of beginnings and endings

Beginnings can tell us a lot

Explore the feelings that emerge in an initial meeting

Endings can help the client more than anything else

Letting go of the important therapeutic relationship can be a positive step for those with attachment, bereavement and control issues

Breaches to the framework

Always work with breaches to the framework

It is always easier to work with a genuine emotion in the here and now rather than exploring a past emotion

Whatever happens, work with it

Client failure to adhere to the rules of the therapeutic relationship can indicate something crucial

Client might repeatedly invite the therapist out for a drink or bring small gifts to the session

Client may be demonstrating a dependency that exhibits in all personal relationships and this can be explored in the here and now of the session

Client responses to necessary breaches in the framework made by the therapist can indicate something crucial

The therapist who has to cancel a session (breaching the agreed rule of weekly meetings) may find that the client cancels the next session or seems withdrawn

Client may be angry about the missed session so exploring this might give access to inner state in the here and now

Concept of 'holding'

Winnicott (1949) identified the concept of 'holding' as the actions of a 'good enough' mother

An ordinary (good enough) mother will offer loving care for her child by creating a safe and secure environment (holding)

Holding environment is created literally by holding the infant and metaphorically by protecting, feeding, bathing, touching and stroking the infant

Infant feels secure in the holding environment and the feeling of being 'held' allows the child to explore the wider world without fear

Winnicott (1986) argued that psychotherapy should seek to parallel this early relationship between mother and child

Therapist should strive to 'hold' (metaphorically, not literally!) the client by providing a safe and understanding environment in which the client can begin to explore

Within the safety of the therapeutic setting, the client is able to explore the true self while the therapist holds and constrains the emotional output within the session

Analytic framework provides this 'holding' environment for the client

Interpretation in therapy

Therapist explains meanings

Meaning of. . .

  Transference

  Free associations

  Dreams

  Resistance

See following sections for more details on interpretation in each of these areas

Client is able to assimilate the information revealed through the interpretations

  Ego can accept this information because it is presented in a safe therapeutic environment

    Winnicott suggested that 'a correct and well-timed interpretation in an analytic treatment gives a sense of being held physically that is more real . . . than if a real holding or nursing had taken place' (Casement, 1990)

  Revelations must be carefully timed

    Interpretation should be unknown by the client, but the client should be very close to discovering the information for themselves

    Client will not accept interpretations if they are revealed too early (ego defence mechanisms)

Risks of interpretation

False memory syndrome

  Memory for something that did not happen

    Often something traumatic, such as abuse

  People can mistakenly attribute an imagined event (mental imagery, thoughts, dreams, etc.) to a real event

    Participants who are asked to imagine some actions and actually carry out some actions (such as combing hair or picking up an object) tend to recall actually carrying out actions that had been imagined (Goff & Roediger, 1998)

  Misleading questions or descriptions by others can influence memories for real events (Loftus, 1979)

Recovered false memories

  Suggestions, interpretations and questions can all implant false memories in the client (especially when also using hypnotherapy) (Loftus, 1979)

Client can assimilate inaccurate interpretations

> If the therapist interprets client behaviour as evidence of repressed trauma and identifies the trauma as abuse, the client could begin to formulate false memories of this abuse
>
>> It may appear as though the client is recovering repressed memories, when in reality they are creating new memories

False memories can be exceptionally realistic

> Many people have been prosecuted for crimes they did not commit, families have been torn apart, relationships have been destroyed . . .

Katrina Fairlie made accusations of child sexual abuse against her father in 2003 (Fairlie, 2010)

> Ms Fairlie had been taken into hospital with stomach pains and was referred to a psychiatrist when a physical cause could not be obtained (later evidence suggests that the hospital failed to detect her inflated gall bladder due to chronic cholecystitis)
>
> Extensive recovered memory therapy revealed a catalogue of abuse including protracted sexual abuse of her and other children at the hands of her father and 17 other men (even recalled observing her father beat a six-year-old girl to death with an iron bar)
>
> Accusations destroyed the family and the career of her father (MP)
>
> Subsequent investigation revealed absolutely no evidence to support these claims and Ms Fairlie later retracted all her accusations
>
> Ms Fairlie claimed that her recovered memory was actually a false memory implanted by the therapist and she successfully sued the NHS for £20,000
>
> Positive outcome for this case (Mr Fairlie did not face criminal proceedings as a result of the false accusations) but many other cases are less positive

Recommendations for therapists

> Brandon Report (Brandon et al., 1997) is a set of training, practice and research recommendations produced by the UK Royal College of Psychiatrists
>
>> Advise psychiatrists to avoid any recovered memory therapy techniques, as there is minimal evidence to suggest that these memories are accurate and not false
>>
>> 'Evidence does not support the view that memory enhancement techniques actually enhance memory. There is evidence to support the view that these are powerful and dangerous methods of persuasion . . . there is sufficient evidence of distortion and/or elaboration of memories to assert that entirely new and false memories can be created, not only experimentally but also in clinical practice . . . The evidence suggests that this is true of . . . drug abreaction, hypnosis, age regression, dream interpretation, imagistic work, "feelings work", art therapy, survivors' groups. Therapist and/or patient expectations, reinforced by guided reading, particular techniques and survivors' group participation may

distort any existing memory or implant a wholly new one . . . Given the prevalence of childhood sexual abuse, even if only a small proportion are repressed and only some of them are subsequently recovered, there should be a significant number of corroborated cases. In fact there are none . . . There is no reliable means of distinguishing a true memory from an illusory one other than by external confirmation . . . There is no means of determining the factual truth or falsity of a recovered memory other than through external evidence . . . The damage to families if the accusations are untrue is immense. Patients who are mistakenly diagnosed as having been abused frequently end as mental health casualties. Where apparent improvement is based upon a false belief, there seems a serious possibility of further mental distress' (Brandon et al., 1997)

Transference analysis

Transference

Transference relationship can be classed as the cornerstone of psychoanalysis

> In a therapeutic setting, transference will occur when the client redirects feelings about a significant person in their life towards the therapist

>> Transference refers to the transfer of unconscious feelings about a significant figure from childhood (such as the father) to a current figure (such as the therapist)

> For example, client is reminded of her father when she interacts with the therapist so her feelings of love and rebellion towards the father of the past may be transferred to the therapist

Analysis of transference

Transference is encouraged and supported in psychoanalytic therapy

> While transference is regarded as a dangerous phenomenon in most schools of psychotherapy, the interpretation of transference is essential in psychoanalytic therapy in order to explore the repressed experiences of childhood (Little, 2003)

Transference is allowed to develop in the psychodynamic relationship as it can . . .

> Provide the therapist with crucial information about the childhood traumas of the client

>> For example, a client who rebels against the therapist might be demonstrating transference of feelings from her father and this can provide crucial information about the nature of this past relationship

> Provide the client with an opportunity to resolve past traumas by acting on the feelings within a safe environment, thereby potentially breaking the cycle of behaviour in the external world

>> Working through these transferences allows the client to become aware of these patterns of behaviour, address any unresolved conflicts, and seek to eliminate infantile regression by improving the relationship with the therapist

For example, the client may be able to resolve her anger issues in relation to her father by addressing her transferred feelings about her therapist – at the very least, the client will recognise this pattern of behaviour in her real-world relationships and possibly be able to break the cycle

Free association analysis

Freedom of speech

Throughout therapy, clients are encouraged to say whatever enters their heads without any attempt at self-censorship

> No matter how silly, illogical, stupid, shocking or trivial it may appear

> Freedom of speech means that the client is able to share fully with the therapist

> Freedom of speech results in revealing Freudian slips and blocks

Freudian slip

> Free expression without self-censorship will sometimes lead to slips of the tongue

> These slips can reveal deeper emotions being repressed by the client

> Freudian slips provide a glimpse into the conflicts located in the unconscious

Blocks

> Things not said by the client can indicate areas of repressed trauma

> Since the client has free rein to say anything, refusal to discuss certain topics or problems expressing certain emotions could reveal a significant repression

> Blocks provide a glimpse into the conflicts located in the unconscious

Listening with the third ear

Interpretation of the apparently mundane thoughts verbalised by a client can lead to revelations

> Listening to the unconscious by interpreting the hidden meanings beneath speech is known as 'listening with the third ear' (Reik, 1948)

>> Therapist will search for surface and hidden meanings in the speech

>> Therapist will interpret Freudian slips and blocks

Free association activities

Therapist says a series of words and the client says the first thing that enters their head in response to the expressions

> For example, Tree, Horse, Table, Love, Work, Book, Father, Shelf, News

> Often a key word relating to an important part of the client history is integrated into the series of words (for example, 'father')

Client does not have time to self-censor so responses can be very revealing

For example, a client who is repressing his anger towards his father might respond to the word 'father' with the word 'hate' and this would reveal the repressed emotion

Free association activities are stereotypically associated with psychoanalysis

However, they are very rarely used in modern psychotherapy

Instead, therapists listen out for any natural free association during speech

Dream analysis

Royal road

Freud (1900) suggested that 'the interpretation of dreams is the royal road to a knowledge of the unconscious activities of the mind'

Defences are lowered during sleep so the ego is less likely to successfully hide repressed trauma

Dream analysis can reveal hidden conflicts, fears, feelings and needs

Latent and manifest

Although defences are lowered, the ego is still working to protect the sleeper

Unacceptable trauma and emotion will often be altered to a more acceptable form

Repressed conflicts, fears, feelings and needs are able to break through from the unconscious, but they are presented in a disguised, symbolised way

Manifest content of dreams

Content of the dream as it appears to the dreamer

Latent content of dreams

Hidden content in the form of symbols

Can be interpreted through psychoanalysis

Manifest content can reveal latent content

Therapist seeks to interpret dreams

Dreams are interpreted by considering the manifest content, suggesting possible meanings for different parts of the dream, observing reactions from client, exploring resistances, discussing the dream experience, etc.

Interpretation is unique to each client

Books on dream meanings cannot possibly be accurate because each meaning is unique to that individual and can only be accessed through extensive analysis

For example, a dream about searching for a lost ring could be interpreted in the following way

Feelings about father have been displaced to a neutral object (ring)

Abstract feelings of loss are represented in a visual form (searching)

Unacceptable emotions of anger and grief are symbolised by a dream event (searching for ring)

INTERPRETIVE DANGERS

Consider the following dreams and use your imagination to write two possible interpretations of the possible latent content of these dreams.

The dreamer is a 30-year-old woman who has suffered with depression since losing her job three months ago. She has previously described a happy childhood raised by a single mother.

> 'I was walking through a forest and it was beginning to get dark. I felt quite anxious that I might get lost and that I might never find my way out of the trees again. I was worried about how my mum might react if she never saw me again. It was not windy but all of the branches on the trees seemed to be moving and the leaves started to fall on me. I felt so helpless. I was weighted down with the leaves and I thought that I was never going to be free again. And then I heard a wolf howling in the distance and I knew that night had fallen. I was terrified and I struggled to escape the leaves before the wolf found me. I woke up tangled in my bedding and shaking with fear.'

The dreamer is a 30-year-old woman who has suffered with depression since losing her job three months ago. She has previously described an unhappy childhood raised by a single father with a drug addiction.

> 'I was walking through a forest and it was beginning to get dark. I felt quite anxious that I might get lost and that I might never find my way out of the trees again. I was worried about how my mum might react if she never saw me again. It was not windy but all of the branches on the trees seemed to be moving and the leaves started to fall on me. I felt so helpless. I was weighted down with the leaves and I thought that I was never going to be free again. And then I heard a wolf howling in the distance and I knew that night had fallen. I was terrified and I struggled to escape the leaves before the wolf found me. I woke up tangled in my bedding and shaking with fear.'

As you have probably noticed, these dreams are identical. But did you feel as though the manifest content might represent different latent content for each dreamer? Perhaps the first case seemed to indicate the woman's feelings of loss about her job and perhaps the second case seemed to indicate repressed trauma of abuse?

These examples highlight the individual nature of dream interpretation. They also demonstrate how easy it can be for the therapist to draw unsubstantiated conclusions based on the client history. It could be the case that a family friend abused the first client but the therapist is unaware of the existence of this person. It could be the case that the second client has moved on from the trauma of her childhood but feels overwhelmed by her recent unemployment. It is always difficult to draw any final interpretive conclusions so it is important to collaborate fully with the client throughout the process.

Resistance analysis

Defence mechanism

Resistance operates as an effective defence mechanism

> Some memories, thoughts and emotions are too traumatic to be experienced so resistance occurs to prevent these threatening experiences from entering consciousness

> Similar to the repression ego defence mechanism (Freud, 1936)

Resistance can hinder the therapeutic process

> Extreme pain or anxiety is avoided by resisting the process of therapy

> Since the aim of therapy is often to reveal these repressed traumas in order to work through them constructively, resistance is commonly employed unconsciously by the client to avoid facing these difficult revelations

Client may use a range of methods to resist the therapeutic process

> Refusing to discuss certain topics

> Using humour or sarcasm to hide true feelings

> Being flippant about important subjects

> Changing the subject away from the difficult area

Analysis of resistance

Analysis of the resistance can reveal repressed trauma

> For example, client who refuses to discuss school and cracks jokes about being a 'loner' when asked about friends may be demonstrating resistance and further analysis could reveal the trauma of childhood bullying

If resistance is overcome, repressed trauma can be addressed

> For example, client could begin to explore their feelings and experience a cathartic release of emotion in relation to this event – insight might also help them in understanding why they respond in certain ways and help them modify their behaviour to avoid getting caught in unhelpful cycles

BUT therapist should not suggest that all resistance is negative

> Remember that resistance is actually an effective defence mechanism to protect the fragility of our conscious emotional state – it is only negative when it hinders the therapeutic process

---

SUMMARY

Traditional psychoanalytic therapy: psychoanalysis; client on couch, therapist out of sight, focus on personality and fantasy, many sessions, silent therapist with no self-disclosure or empathy

Modern psychodynamic therapy: both on chairs, focus on practical concerns, possibly brief, interactive, core conditions

Analytic framework: rules of the relationship, should be fixed and structured to mirror parental relationship, beginnings and endings are crucial; breaches give an insight into the client; concept of 'holding' as the actions of a 'good enough' mother, therapy should parallel mother–child relationship by 'holding' the client

Interpretation: therapist explains meaning of expressions by client, revelations must be carefully timed; risk of false memory syndrome, Katrina Fairlie case, Brandon Report advises against memory recovery techniques

Transference analysis: transfer feelings from past significant others to therapist; encouraged in therapy, can reveal information about past relationships, can provide opportunity to resolve past trauma by acting on repressed emotions

Free association analysis: freedom of speech in therapy, no self-censorship; Freudian slips and blocks reveal deeper emotions; interpretation involves listening with the third ear; free association activity is rarely done in modern therapy, therapist listens to all speech content instead

Dream analysis: royal road to knowledge of unconscious; manifest (actual) and latent (hidden) content interpreted during psychoanalysis

Resistance analysis: defence mechanism, helpful for protecting self, can hinder therapy by hiding trauma; analysis of resistance can reveal repressed trauma and emotions; repressed trauma can then be addressed (but not all resistance is negative)

CASE STUDY DEMONSTRATING PSYCHOANALYTIC THERAPY

LEARNING OUTCOMES

After reading this section, you will be able to:

* appreciate the application of psychoanalytic therapy from the psychodynamic approach in a therapeutic setting

Recorded session: therapy in action

This chapter is accompanied by a recorded therapy session which is available for viewing.

This session lasts for one therapy hour (50 minutes) and it is presented as the initial session in a new therapeutic relationship. Prior to this session, the client will have completed an initial assessment questionnaire and the therapist will have read this paperwork to ensure familiarity with the case. This completed assessment and a full transcript of the recorded session are available.

No actors are used in this session. The client was one of the authors and the problem presented was genuine. The therapist is an experienced practitioner in the field. The only 'fake' aspect of this recorded session is that the client did not really seek therapy and this is not really the first session of a series of therapeutic contacts.

After the conclusion of the session, the therapist is invited to answer a few key questions about the session. This question and answer session lasts no longer than 10 minutes. The transcript of this session is available.

Presentation of Phil Thomas: history and symptoms

Phil Thomas has been suffering with stress and anxiety over the last few months. He has recently experienced some minor life events and these have had an impact on his mental wellbeing. He feels particularly anxious about his tendency to procrastinate and he believes that this is contributing towards his general feelings of stress. He has previously experienced therapy (though this was person-centred, not psychoanalytic) and he is generally positive about the possible outcomes for therapy. He would like to gain an understanding of his own behaviour in order to be able to reduce his own procrastination.

Therapy session: analysis

The therapy session can be sectioned as follows.

Introduction

Gentle introduction

Reflection on previous experience with therapy to establish possible expectations and beliefs about therapy

Addressing any questions about the nature of psychoanalytic therapy

Outlining basic contractual details, especially the limits of confidentiality and the nature of sessions (length, number, etc.)

Story

Client is invited and encouraged to share his story – this forms the largest part of the therapy sessions

Focus on feelings and internal experiences, rather than the specific practicalities of the story

Goals

Establishing goals for therapy is periodically explored throughout the session, rather than forming a conclusion to the session

Goals are explored in terms of the current and ideal locations for the client

Ending

> Warning given prior to the end of the session
>
> Reflection on how the session was experienced by the client
>
> Invitation to return for future sessions

Key questions to consider in relation to this therapy session

How could the nature of this client be understood from the psychodynamic perspective?

- Are there any unconscious drives likely to be controlling thoughts and behaviours?
- Is it evident that the id, ego and superego are in conflict?
- Are any ego defence mechanisms being exhibited?
- Does the client appear to be stuck at any psychosexual or psychosocial stage?

What is the nature of the therapeutic relationship in this psychoanalytic therapy session?

- Is the therapist a 'blank screen'?
- Is there any evidence of transference or counter-transference?

Which psychoanalytic techniques are demonstrated in this therapy session?

- Is the therapist using traditional psychoanalysis or modern psychodynamic therapy?
- Does the therapist direct or interpret the behaviour, thoughts and feelings of the client?
- Does the therapist analyse transference, resistance, defence mechanisms, free association or dreams?

Personal experience of the client

My apprehension at being a filmed client was very present for me at the start of the session. However, this subsided quickly as Tina gave an outline of what she would be hoping to focus on, and the 'permission' for me to free associate, to talk about whatever emerged as the session progressed. She was clear about being interested in relationships – in my early relationships, current relationships (including the therapist–client relationship), and my relationship with aspects of self.

As the session progressed, and I felt more comfortable and less anxious, some connections were made. Firstly how my not wanting to let people down might be something we needed to be aware of in the therapeutic relationship. I particularly liked the way she commented about things to 'notice', for example my feeling stuck early in the session, and losing my train of thought later. This felt very freeing, that I could talk about anything without it being pursued in this first session. I wasn't aware of being guarded or defensive in the session. The question asking whether I could connect thoughts and feelings to any earlier experiences was interesting, and again I felt comfortable enough to talk about my first day at secondary school, something that came to mind ('free association').

The session felt as though it had a direction, even though at times I seemed to be moving from one line of thought to another. I sensed that Tina was tracking content and making sense of my thoughts, acknowledging them, noticing them, and redirecting me as appropriate. I always felt in control of the session despite this 'directing'. For example, about 20 minutes in, after my comments about my first day at school, she refocused me on what had happened about six weeks ago (the start of my current anxiety). This brought up a potentially important point about feeling valued.

I also liked the way Tina used the image that I offered (the cloak of invisibility) and gave me a new interpretation. From that I came to what I think was the most significant part of the session for me, the discrepancy between learning from mistakes, but wanting to do anything creative perfectly. This would be an area for future sessions.

I am aware of the possibility of transference in the session, but overall I felt a close connection to Tina. The relationship felt comfortable but challenging. I felt supported, listened to and understood. I really enjoyed Tina being so engaged in the process, in offering possible interpretations, in 'noticing', in guiding and gently directing. It gave me much to take away and reflect upon. I know that I would welcome the opportunity to work with Tina in future.

Phil Thomas

REFERENCES AND BIBLIOGRAPHY

Adler, A. (1927) *The Practice and Theory of Individual Psychology*. New York: Harcourt, Brace, Jovanovich.

Ahmed, S. (2010) Over a third of British adults still sleep with a teddy bear. Retrieved from www.travelodge.co.uk/press_releases/press_release.php?id=393

Ainsworth, M.D. (1967) *Infancy in Uganda*. Baltimore, MD: Johns Hopkins.

Amacher, P. (1965) Freud's neurological education and its influence on psychoanalytic theory. *Psychological Issues*, 4, monograph 16.

Atkinson, R.C. & Shiffrin, R.M. (1968) Human memory: a proposed system and its control processes. In: Spence, K.W. & Spence, J.T. (eds) *The Psychology of Learning and Motivation, Vol 2*. New York: Academic Press.

Bettelheim, B. (1984) *Freud and Man's Soul*. New York: Random House.

Borch-Jacobsen, M. (2012) Freud's patients, a serial. Ernst Fleischl von Marxow. *Psychology Today*. Retrieved from www.psychologytoday.com

Bowlby, J. (1951) *Maternal Care and Mental Health*. Geneva: World Health Organization.

Bowlby, J. (1969) *Attachment and Loss: Vol 1: Attachment*. International Psychoanalytical Library. London: Hogarth Press and Institute of Psychoanalysis.

Bowlby, J. (1969) *Attachment and Loss: Vol 2: Separation Anxiety and Anger*. International Psychoanalytical Library. London: Hogarth Press and Institute of Psychoanalysis.

Bowlby, J. (1969) *Attachment and Loss: Vol 3: Sadness and Depression*. International Psychoanalytical Library. London: Hogarth Press and Institute of Psychoanalysis.

Brandon, S., Boakes, J., Glaser, D., Green, R., MacKeith, J. & Whewell, P. (1997) Reported recovered memories of child sexual abuse: recommendations for good practice and implications for training, continuing professional development and research. *Psychiatric Bulletin*, 21, 663–665.

Bridle, S. & Edelstein, A. (2000) Was ist 'das Ich'? *EnlightNext Magazine* 17, 126–129, 176–177.

Casement, P. (1990) *Further Learning from the Patient: The Analytic Space and Process*. London: Routledge.

Donaldson, G. (2002) Melanie Klein. *Feminist Psychologist*, 29, 3.

Erikson, E.H. (1963) *Childhood and Society*. New York: Norton.

Eysenck, H.J. (1952) The effects of psychotherapy: an evaluation. *Journal of Consulting Psychology*, 16, 319–324.

Fairlie, J. (2010) *Unbreakable Bonds: 'They know about you Dad'*. London: Austin and Macauley Publishers.

Farber, A. (1978) Freud's love letters: intimations of psychoanalytic theory. *Psychoanalytic Review*, 65, 166–189.

Fraley, C. (2010) A brief overview of adult attachment theory and research. Retrieved from http://internal.psychology.illinois.edu/~rcfraley/attachment.htm

Freud, A. (1936) *The Ego and the Mechanisms of Defence* (trans. G. Baynes). New York: Hogarth Press.

Freud, S. (1884) Uber coca (on cocaine). Reprinted in Byck, R. (ed) *Cocaine Papers*. New York: Stonehill Publishing.

Freud, S. (1891) On aphasia. Reprinted in *On Aphasia: A Critical Study* (trans. E. Stengel). Oxford: International Universities Press.

Freud, S. (1900) The interpretation of dreams. Reprinted in *The Standard Edition of the Complete Psychological Works of Sigmund Freud, Volume IV (1900) and Volume V (1900–1901): The Interpretation of Dreams* (trans. J. Strachey). London: Hogarth Press and Institute of Psychoanalysis.

Freud, S. (1901) The psychopathology of everyday life. Reprinted in *The Standard Edition of the Complete Psychological Works of Sigmund Freud, Volume VI (1901): The Psychopathology of Everyday Life* (trans. J. Strachey). London: Hogarth Press and Institute of Psychoanalysis.

Freud, S. (1905) Three essays on the theory of sexuality. Reprinted in *The Standard Edition of the Complete Psychological Works of Sigmund Freud, Volume VII (1901–1905): A Case of Hysteria, Three Essays on Sexuality and Other Works* (trans. J. Strachey). London: Hogarth Press and Institute of Psychoanalysis.

Freud, S. (1905) Fragment of an analysis of a case of hysteria. Reprinted in *The Standard Edition of the Complete Psychological Works of Sigmund Freud, Volume VII (1901–1905): A Case of Hysteria, Three Essays on Sexuality and Other Works* (trans. J. Strachey). London: Hogarth Press and Institute of Psychoanalysis.

Freud, S. (1909) Notes upon a case of obsessional neurosis. Reprinted in *The Standard Edition of the Complete Psychological Works of Sigmund Freud, Volume X (1909): Two Case Histories ('Little Hans' and the 'Rat Man')* (trans. J. Strachey). London: Hogarth Press and Institute of Psychoanalysis.

Freud, S. (1909) Analysis of a phobia in a five-year-old boy. Reprinted in *The Standard Edition of the Complete Psychological Works of Sigmund Freud, Volume X (1909): Two Case Histories ('Little Hans' and the 'Rat Man')* (trans. J. Strachey). London: Hogarth Press and Institute of Psychoanalysis.

Freud, S. (1912) On the universal tendency to debasement in the sphere of love. Reprinted in *The Standard Edition of the Complete Psychological Works of Sigmund Freud, Volume XI (1910): Five Lectures on Psychoanalysis: Leonardo da Vinci and Other Works* (trans. J. Strachey). London: Hogarth Press and Institute of Psychoanalysis.

Freud, S. (1917) A difficulty in the path of psychoanalysis. Reprinted in *The Standard Edition of the Complete Psychological Works of Sigmund Freud, Volume XVII (1917–1919): An Infantile Neurosis and Other Works* (trans. J. Strachey). London: Hogarth Press and Institute of Psycho-analysis.

Freud, S. (1918) From the history of an infantile neurosis. Reprinted in *The Standard Edition of the Complete Psychological Works of Sigmund Freud, Volume XVII (1917–1919): An Infantile Neurosis and Other Works* (trans. J. Strachey). London: Hogarth Press and Institute of Psychoanalysis.

Freud, S. (1920) Beyond the pleasure principle. Reprinted in *The Standard Edition of the Complete Psychological Works of Sigmund Freud, Volume XVIII (1920–1922): Beyond the Pleasure Principle* (trans. J. Strachey). London: Hogarth Press and Institute of Psychoanalysis.

Freud, S. (1923) The ego and the id. Reprinted in *The Standard Edition of the Complete Psychological Works of Sigmund Freud, Volume XIX (1923–1925): The Ego and the Id and Other Works* (trans. J. Strachey). London: Hogarth Press and Institute of Psychoanalysis.

Freud, S. (1927) Future of an illusion. Reprinted in *The Standard Edition of the Complete Psychological Works of Sigmund Freud, Volume XXI (1927–1931): The Future of an Illusion, Civilization and its Discontents, and Other Works* (trans. J. Strachey). London: Hogarth Press and Institute of Psychoanalysis.

Freud, S. (1929) Civilization and its discontents. Reprinted in *The Standard Edition of the Complete Psychological Works of Sigmund Freud, Volume XXI (1927–1931): The Future of an Illusion, Civilization and its Discontents, and Other Works* (trans. J. Strachey). London: Hogarth Press and Institute of Psychoanalysis.

Freud, A. (1936) *The Ego and the Mechanisms of Defence* (trans. G. Baynes). New York: Hogarth Press.

Freud, S. (1939) Moses and monotheism. Reprinted in *The Standard Edition of the Complete Psychological Works of Sigmund Freud, Volume XXIII (1937–1939): Moses and Monotheism, An Outline of Psychoanalysis, and Other Works* (trans. J. Strachey). London: Hogarth Press and Institute of Psychoanalysis.

Freud, S. (1940) An outline of psychoanalysis. Reprinted in *The Standard Edition of the Complete Psychological Works of Sigmund Freud, Volume XXIII (1937–1939): Moses and Monotheism, An Outline of Psychoanalysis, and Other Works* (trans. J. Strachey). London: Hogarth Press and Institute of Psychoanalysis.

Freud, S. & Breuer, J. (1895) Studies on hysteria. Reprinted in *The Standard Edition of the Complete Psychological Works of Sigmund Freud, Volume II (1893–1895): Studies on Hysteria* (trans. J. Strachey). London: Hogarth Press and Institute of Psychoanalysis.

Galbis-Reig, D. (2004) Sigmund Freud, MD: forgotten contributions to neurology, neuropathology, and anesthesia. *Internet Journal of Neurology*, 3, 1.

Goff, L.M. & Roediger, H.L. (1998) Imagination inflation for action events: repeated imaginings lead to illusory recollections. *Memory and Cognition*, 26, 20–33.

Grosskurth, P. (1986) *Melanie Klein: Her World and Her Work*. New York: Knopf.

Grotjahn, M. (1951) Historical notes: a letter from Sigmund Freud. *International Journal of Psychoanalysis*, 32, 331.

Harlow, H.F. & Zimmermann, R.R. (1958) The development of affective responsiveness in infant monkeys. *Proceedings of the American Philosophical Society*, 102, 501–509.

Hazan, C. & Shaver, P. (1987) Romantic love conceptualised as an attachment process. *Journal of Personality and Social Psychology*, 52(3), 511–524.

Horney, K. (1950) *Neurosis and Human Growth: The Struggle Towards Self-Realization*. New York: Norcross.

Horney, K. (1967) *Feminine Psychology*. New York: Norton.

Jarvis, M. (2004) *Psychodynamic Psychology: Classical Theory and Contemporary Research*. London: Thomson Learning.

Jones, E. (1953) *The Life and Work of Sigmund Freud: Vol. 1 The Young Freud 1856–1900*. New York: Hogarth Press.

Jones, E. (1955) *The Life and Work of Sigmund Freud: Vol. 2 The Years of Maturity 1901–1919*. New York: Hogarth Press.

Jones, E. (1957) *The Life and Work of Sigmund Freud: Vol. 3 The Last Phase 1919–1939*. New York: Hogarth Press.

Jung, C.G. (1912) *Psychology of the Unconscious* (trans. B. Hinkle). London: Kegan Paul Trench Trubner.

Jung, C.G. (1921) *Psychological Types* (trans. G. Baynes). Princeton, NJ: Princeton University Press.

Jung, C.G. (1946) The psychology of the transference. Reprinted in *Collected Works*, 16. Princeton: Princeton University Press.

Jung, C.G. (1966) *Two Essays on Analytical Psychology*. London: Routledge and Kegan Paul.

Klein, M. (1923) The development of a child. Reprinted in *The Writings of Melanie Klein Vol. 1*. London: Hogarth Press.

Klein, M. (1932) The psychoanalysis of children. Reprinted in *The Writings of Melanie Klein Vol. 2*. London: Hogarth Press.

Klein, M. (1935) A contribution to the psychogenesis of manic-depressive states. Reprinted in *The Writings of Melanie Klein Vol. 1*. London: Hogarth Press.

Klein, M. (1937) Love, guilt, and reparation. Reprinted in *The Writings of Melanie Klein Vol. 1*. London: Hogarth Press.

Klein, M. (1955) The psychoanalytic play technique. *American Journal of Orthopsychiatry*, 25, 223–237.

Klein, M. (1957) Envy and gratitude. Reprinted in *The Writings of Melanie Klein Vol. 2*. London: Hogarth Press.

Klein, M. (1961) Narrative of a child analysis. Reprinted in *The Writings of Melanie Klein Vol. 2*. London: Hogarth Press.

Leiper, R. & Maltby, M. (2004) *The Psychodynamic Approach to Therapeutic Change*. London: Sage Publications.

Little, M. (2003) Counter-transference and the patient's response to it. *Influential Papers from the 1950s*, 35.

Loftus, E.F. (1979) *Eyewitness Testimony*. Cambridge, MA: Harvard University Press.

Luborsky, E.B., O'Reilly-Landry, M. & Arlow, J.A. (2008) Psychoanalysis. In: Corsini, R.J. & Wedding, D. (eds) *Current Psychotherapies*. Belmont, CA: Brooks/Cole.

Malan, D. (1995) *Individual Psychotherapy and The Science of Psychodynamics*. London: Butterworth-Heinemann.

Margolis, D.P. (1989) Freud and his mother. *Modern Psychoanalysis*, 14, 37–56.

Masson, J.M. (1985) *The Complete Letters of Sigmund Freud to Wilhelm Fliess, 1887–1904*, v–492. Cambridge, MA, and London: Belknap Press.

Melanie Klein Trust (1913) Melanie Klein. Retrieved from www.melanie-klein-trust.org.uk/

Prior, V. & Glaser, D. (2006) *Understanding Attachment and Attachment Disorders: Theory, Evidence and Practice*. Child and Adolescent Mental Health. London: Jessica Kingsley Publishers.

Pruner, H.W. (1992) *Sigmund Freud: His Life and Mind*. New Jersey: Transaction Publishers.

Racker, H. (1982) *Transference and Counter-transference*. London: Karnac Books.

Reik, T. (1948) *Listening with the Third Ear: The Inner Experiences of a Psychoanalyst*. New York: Grove Press.

Rogers, C. (1951) *Client-centred Therapy: Its Current Practice, Implications and Theory*. London: Constable.

Schur, M. (1972) *Freud: Living and Dying*. Michigan: International Universities Press.

Segal, H. (1980) *Melanie Klein*. New York: Viking Press.

Solms, M. & Turnbull, O. (2002) *Brain and the Inner World*. New York: Other Press.

Thorne, B. (1992) *Carl Rogers*. London: Sage Publications.

Wheelis, A. (1950) The place of action in personality change. *Psychiatry: Journal for the Study of Interpersonal Processes*, 13, 135–148.

Winnicott, D.W. (1949) *The Ordinary Devoted Mother and Her Baby*. Nine Broadcast Talks.

Winnicott, D.W. (1953) Transitional objects and transitional phenomena. *International Journal of Psychoanalysis*, 34, 89–97.

Winnicott, D.W. (1971) *Playing and Reality*. London: Tavistock Publications.

Winnicott, D.W. (1986) *Holding and Interpretation: Fragment of an Analysis*. London: Hogarth Press and Institute of Psychoanalysis.

Chapter 4
Behavioural approach and behaviour therapy

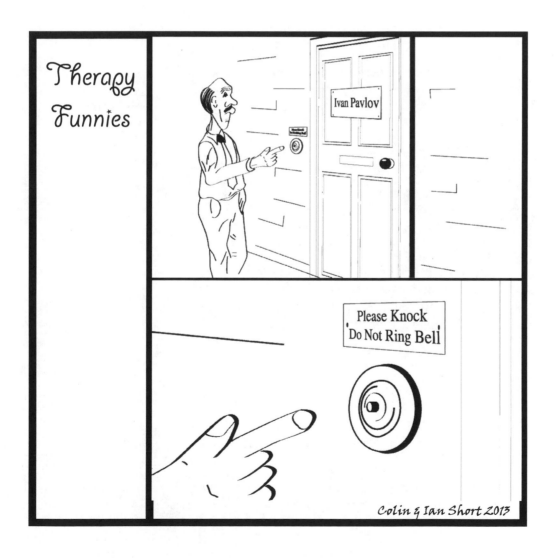

INTRODUCTION TO BEHAVIOURAL APPROACH AND BEHAVIOUR THERAPY

This chapter aims to introduce the reader to the behavioural approach to counselling and psychotherapy. Behaviour therapy will be explored as one example of a therapeutic method under the behavioural approach.

LEARNING OUTCOMES

By the end of this chapter, you will be able to:

- describe the development of the first force in psychology: the behavioural approach

- acknowledge the relative impact of Ivan Pavlov, John Broadus Watson and Burrhus Frederic Skinner on the development of the behavioural approach

- discuss the core theories of human nature and personality from the behavioural perspective

- discuss the nature of the therapeutic relationship between therapist and client in behaviour therapy

- outline the main therapeutic techniques utilised in behaviour therapy

- appreciate the application of behaviour therapy in a real-world setting

---

DEVELOPMENT OF THE BEHAVIOURAL APPROACH

LEARNING OUTCOMES

After reading this section, you will be able to:

- list the three main forces in psychology

- discuss the development of the behavioural approach in a historical context

- acknowledge the main contributors to the development of the behavioural approach

---

First force in psychology

Three forces in psychology

> Behavioural theory

> Psychodynamic theory

> Humanistic theory

Behavioural psychology is the 'first force'

Psychology was initially defined as the study of the human mind and linked to work in medicine and philosophy

> However, animal research in the early 1900s produced results that could be generalised to human behaviour (Thorndike, 1898; Pavlov, 1928)

> This led to psychology being redefined as the study of human behaviour

Tabula rasa

    Behavioural approach focuses exclusively on observable and measurable behaviour

    Emphasises the importance of nurture

        Humans are born as a *tabula rasa* or blank slate on which experience writes the patterns of their future behaviour

Major advances in the behavioural approach

Initial interest in the behavioural approach

Thorndike identified the Law of Effect in 1898

    Proposed that behaviour can be predicted and controlled according to consequences

    'Animal intelligence: an experimental study of the associative processes in animals' published in 1898

Pavlov presented at the International Medical Congress in Madrid in 1903

    Reported physiological research revealing a system of conditioning to explain human behaviour

    Introduced the idea that psychological processes can be studied scientifically

    Lectures on Conditioned Reflexes: Twenty-Five Years of Objective Study of the Higher Nervous Activity Behavior of Animals published in 1928

Formal establishment of behavioural approach

Watson published the Behaviorist Manifesto in 1913

    Foundation of the behavioural approach

    'Psychology as the behaviorist views it' published in 1913

Skinner introduced the concept of behaviour shaping through operant conditioning in 1938

    Established the principles for the experimental study of human behaviour

    The Behavior of Organisms published in 1938

Radical behaviourism was popular from 1940s to 1950s

    Objective study of behaviour with no focus on cognition, emotion, etc.

    All human processes are described as 'behaviour'

        Internal states and mental existence are disregarded as hypothetical constructs that do not exist

        Instead, internal processes are redefined as covert behaviours

        Emotions are regarded as physiological reactions to external events

        Thought is regarded as internal speech

Modern behavioural approach

Popularity of behaviourism decreased in the 1960s to 1980s

> Cognitive revolution redirected psychological research away from the study of behaviour to focus on theoretical models about the nature of the mind

Radical behaviourism softened into behaviour analysis

> Behaviourism that refused to accept the existence of cognitive states was rejected in favour of a less extreme version which focused on analysing behaviour as an external (measurable) evidence of cognitive states

> Staats (1996) argued that radical behaviourism failed as an approach in psychology because it did not incorporate other known phenomena, such as cognition

>> Psychological behaviourism should aim to unify all elements of psychology (biology, environment, cognition, emotion, etc.) into a single grand theory

Behaviour analysis adopts an interdisciplinary approach

> Theories include elements from other approaches such as cognitive, humanistic, etc.

> UK Society for Behaviour Analysis describes it as the science of learning

>> Experimental branch is the experimental analysis of behaviour and this aims to conduct research on how humans learn new behaviours

>> Applied branch is applied behaviour analysis (ABA) and this aims to promote behaviour change by analysing behaviours and developing interventions to modify these behaviours in a positive direction for individuals and society

Key figures in the behavioural approach

Ivan Pavlov (1849–1936)

Impact on the approach

> Classical conditioning

> Found that repeatedly pairing a neutral stimulus with an evocative stimulus eventually leads to a reflexive response to the neutral stimulus

>> For example, pairing saliva-inducing food with a neutral bell eventually causes a dog to salivate in response to the bell only

Selected works

> *Conditioned Reflexes: An Investigation of the Physiological Activity of the Cerebral Cortex* published in 1927

> *Lectures on Conditioned Reflexes: Twenty-Five Years of Objective Study of the Higher Nervous Activity Behavior of Animals* published in 1928

Edward Lee Thorndike (1874–1949)

Impact on the approach

> Established a theory of association through work on animal behaviour

Measured the time taken for cats to escape from a puzzle box by pressing a lever

Found that responses would initially be made accidentally (stepping on the lever) but were repeated when the consequence was desirable (escaping from the box)

Identified a learning curve in which behaviours are more readily completed if they have previously resulted in a satisfactory outcome

Law of Effect

Selected works

'Animal intelligence: an experimental study of the associative processes in animals' published in 1898

John Broadus Watson (1878–1958)

Impact on the approach

Behaviourism

Established the Behaviorist Manifesto in 1913

Produced the oft misquoted 'give me a dozen healthy infants'

Introduced the concept of adult behaviour resulting from childhood stimulus–response associations

Fear conditioning of Little Albert

Selected works

'Psychology as the behaviorist views it' published in 1913

Behavior: An Introduction to Comparative Psychology published in 1914

Conditioned Emotional Reactions published with Rayner in 1920

Behaviorism published initially in 1925 and revised in 1930

Burrhus Frederic Skinner (1904–1990)

Impact on the approach

Operant conditioning

Discovered that behaviour did not appear solely dependent on preceding or co-existing stimulus (classical conditioning), but was also dependent on the consequences of behaviour

Reinforcement and punishment occurring after the behaviour had an impact on the future occurrence of the behaviour

For example, rats rewarded with food when they press a lever are more likely to press the lever again in the future

Selected works

The Behavior of Organisms published in 1938

Arthur Staats (1924–current)

Impact on the approach

Transformed radical behaviourism into a human-oriented form of behaviourism known as psychological behaviourism – a unified approach aiming to integrate multiple psychological perspectives (biology, learning, cognition, emotion, etc.)

Introduced the concept of and coined the term 'time out' – temporarily removing a child from the situation as a method of punishing him/her for inappropriate behaviour, thus reducing the likelihood of the behaviour being repeated in the future

Selected works

Learning, Language, and Cognition published in 1968

Behavior and Personality: Psychological Behaviorism published in 1996

SUMMARY

Three forces: behavioural, psychodynamic, humanistic; first force in psychology, study of behaviour, *tabula rasa*, humans born as blank slates on which experience writes patterns for future behaviours

Major advances: initial ideas based on animal research by Thorndike who identified the Law of Effect in 1895 and Pavlov who presented classical conditioning at a conference in 1903; formally established through the Behaviorist Manifesto by Watson in 1913; Skinner introduced behaviour shaping through operant conditioning in 1938; radical behaviourism popular 1940s to 1960s (objective study of behaviour with no focus on cognition – all human processes are behaviours); modern approach is less radical, softened into behaviour analysis which adopts an interdisciplinary approach

Key figures: Pavlov's classical conditioning, Thorndike's Law of Effect, Watson's Behaviorist Manifesto, Skinner's operant conditioning, Staats' psychological behaviourism and time out

---

PERSONAL AND PROFESSIONAL BIOGRAPHIES OF IVAN PAVLOV, JOHN BROADUS WATSON AND BURRHUS FREDERIC SKINNER

LEARNING OUTCOMES

After reading this section, you will be able to:

* outline the personal and professional biography of Ivan Pavlov (1849–1936)
* outline the personal and professional biography of John Broadus Watson (1878–1958)

- outline the personal and professional biography of Burrhus Frederic Skinner (1904–1990)

- appreciate the impact of these key figures on the development of behavioural therapy

Biography of Ivan Pavlov

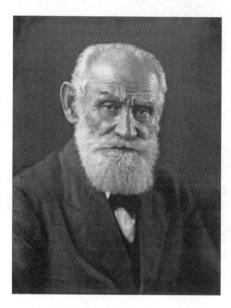

'Perfect as the wing of a bird may be, it will never enable the bird to fly if unsupported by the air. Facts are the air of science. Without them a man of science can never rise.'
—Attributed to Pavlov (n.d.)

Who was Ivan Pavlov?

Ivan Pavlov established the concept of classical conditioning and this formed the foundation for the behavioural approach

> Watson and Skinner also made critical contributions to this approach
>> Watson introduced the concept of behaviourism
>> Skinner established operant conditioning

Early years

Born on 14th September 1849 in Ryazan in Russia

> Father (Peter Pavlov) was the village priest and mother (Varvara Uspenskaya) was a housewife

> Eldest of 11 children – six siblings died before adulthood

Highly religious family

> Active childhood with positive relationships with his parents and siblings (Asratyan, 1953)

Encouraged to pursue a religious career in the footsteps of his father

A serious injury following a fall placed him in the care of his grandfather and he did not attend formal schooling until the age of 11 (Asratyan, 1953)

> Grandfather encouraged his educational development and he was educationally advanced from a young age

> Able to read at the age of seven

Education

Originally intended on a religious career

> Attended the Ryazan Theological Seminary to study for the priesthood

> Transferred to the University of St Petersburg in 1870

>> Moved from theology to science after reading work by Charles Darwin

Graduated with a degree in natural sciences from the University of St Petersburg in 1875, then a medical qualification from the Military Medical Academy in 1879

> Presented his doctoral thesis on the basic principles of the nervous system in 1883

Family

Married Seraphima (Sara) Karchevskaya in 1881

> Early married life was marred by financial difficulties and a miscarriage

> Sara became depressed after the death of her next child, Wirchik, during childhood

> Remained married until the end of his life – Sara survived her husband by 11 years

Raised four sons and one daughter

> Son Wirchik died in early childhood

Career

Academic at the Military Medical Academy from 1880 to 1925

> Laboratory assistant and postgraduate student then lecturer to professor to chair in pharmacology and physiology

Organised and directed the Department of Physiology at the Institute of Experimental Medicine between 1890 and 1900 (Babkin, 1949)

> Studied physiology of digestion in dogs

> Demonstrated the role of the nervous system in controlling digestion – physiology maintains this position today (Babkin, 1949)

Explored the concept of 'psychic secretion' in 1895 (Nobel Lectures, 1967)

> Psychic secretion refers to salivation at the distant sight of food, rather than the taste of food

>> Rejected the subjective interpretation of this phenomenon and developed a scientific approach to the study of the brain and nervous system

Discovered that psychic secretion could also occur in the absence of visual food stimuli if the food has previously been paired with an auditory stimulus

> Reflexive (automatic) responses can be conditioned by associating the natural stimuli (e.g. food) with a novel stimulus (e.g. bell) – conditioned reflexes

Concluded that even psychic activity (thought processes) is reflexive (based on prior conditioning)

Presented research on the experimental psychology and psychopathology of animals at the 14th International Medical Congress in Madrid in 1903 (Nobel Lectures, 1967)

> Defined conditioned reflexes

>> Emphasised the importance of these conditioned reflexes in terms of both physiological and psychological activity

>> Both physical reactions (behaviour) and psychological reactions (thoughts) occur in a reflexive way as a result of conditioning

> Highlighted the importance of the cerebral cortex as the centre of organisation for all organism activity (Babkin, 1949)

Awarded a Nobel Prize for research on digestion in 1904 (Nobel Lectures, 1967) and the Order of the Legion of Honour in 1915

Published *Conditioned Reflexes: An Investigation of the Physiological Activity of the Cerebral Cortex* in 1927 and *Lectures on Conditioned Reflexes: Twenty-Five Years of Objective Study of the Higher Nervous Activity Behavior of Animals* in 1928

> Two books collecting his most famous works to outline his findings relating to conditioned reflexes

> Modern reference to conditioned reflexes regards it as Pavlovian conditioning (in honour of Pavlov) or classical conditioning (because it was the first form of conditioning to be identified)

Death

Died of pneumonia in Leningrad at the age of 86 on 27th February 1936

FOUNDING FATHER OF THE BEHAVIOURAL APPROACH: PAVLOV

Consider the life story of Ivan Pavlov and try to answer the following questions.

1. What was the social and cultural context of the world in which Pavlov developed his theories?
2. How might Pavlov's life experiences have impacted on his perception of human nature?
3. How can this life story contribute to your understanding of the behavioural approach?

Significant learnings

'We must painfully acknowledge that, precisely because of its great intellectual developments, the best of man's domesticated animals – the dog – most often becomes the victim of physiological experiments. Only dire necessity can lead one to experiment on cats – on such impatient, loud, malicious animals. During chronic experiments, when the animal, having recovered from its operation, is under lengthy observation, the dog is irreplaceable; moreover, it is extremely touching. It is almost a participant in the experiments conducted upon it, greatly facilitating the success of the research by its understanding and compliance' (Pavlov, 1893)

'One can truly say that the irresistible progress of natural science since the time of Galileo has made its first halt before the study of the higher parts of the brain, the organ of the most complicated relations of the animal to the external world. And it seems, and not without reason, that now is the really critical moment for natural science; for the brain, in its highest complexity – the human brain – which created and creates natural science, itself becomes the object of this science' (Pavlov, 1928)

Biography of John Broadus Watson

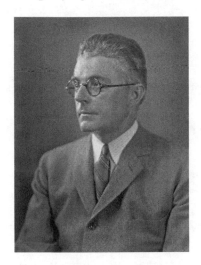

'*Give me a dozen healthy infants, well-formed, and my own specified world to bring them up in and I'll guarantee to take any one at random and train him to become any type of specialist I might select – doctor, lawyer, artist, merchant-chief and, yes, even beggar-man and thief, regardless of his talents, penchants, tendencies, abilities, vocations, and race of his ancestors. I am going beyond my facts and I admit it, but so have the advocates of the contrary and they have been doing it for many thousands of years.*'
—Watson (1930)

Who was John Broadus Watson?

John Broadus Watson established the concept of behaviourism and the Behaviorist Manifesto and this formed the foundation for the behavioural approach

> Pavlov and Skinner also made critical contributions to this approach

>> Pavlov established classical conditioning

>> Skinner established operant conditioning

Early years

Born 9th January 1978 in Greenville, South Carolina

> Father (Pickens Watson) was a farmer and mother (Emma) helped on the farm

Difficult childhood (Buckley, 1989)

> Mother was a strict Baptist who demanded that her children abstain from sinful activities such as drinking

> Father was a heavy drinker with a history of law breaking who had extramarital affairs and eventually left Watson's mother when he was only 13

Education

Absence of a father led him to rebellion against his mother and teachers (Buckley, 1989)

> Occasionally in trouble with the law and had little respect for authority

> Described himself as a poor student with no motivation for academia

> However, his attitude towards education improved significantly when he was accepted to study at Furman University at the age of 16

Graduated with a Master's degree from Furman University in 1899 and earned a doctorate in psychology from the University of Chicago in 1903

Career

Taught at the University of Chicago from 1903 to 1908 and was associate professor at Johns Hopkins University from 1908 to 1920

Delivered a seminal presentation followed by a publication entitled 'Psychology as the behaviorist views it' in 1913

> Regarded as the Behaviorist Manifesto

> Outlined the founding principles of the behavioural approach

> Argued that psychology was the science of human behaviour and thus it should be studied scientifically in laboratory conditions

> 'Psychology as the behaviorist views it is a purely objective experimental branch of natural science. Its theoretical goal is the prediction and control of behavior. Introspection forms no essential part of its methods, nor is the scientific value of its data dependent upon the readiness with which they lend themselves to interpretation in terms of consciousness. The behaviorist, in his efforts to get a unitary scheme of animal response, recognizes no dividing line between man and brute. The behavior of man, with all of its refinement and complexity, forms only a part of the behaviorist's total scheme of investigation' (Watson, 1913)

Published *Behavior: An Introduction to Comparative Psychology* in 1914

> Established himself as the 'founder of behaviourism'

> Proposed that human behaviour could be explained by generalising from animal research into conditioned responses

Elected President of the American Psychological Association in 1915

Published *Psychology from the Standpoint of a Behaviorist* in 1919

Published *Conditioned Emotional Reactions* with Rayner in 1920

> Famous Little Albert study

> Applied the concept of Pavlovian classical conditioning to the development of phobias by conditioning a fear of rats in the child

> Albert was raised in a hospital environment by his mother (wet nurse at the hospital)

> > He was a healthy child with no reported emotional disturbances

> Nine-month-old Albert was tested for natural fear reactions

> > Initial tests revealed no fear of white rats, rabbits, dogs, monkeys, masks, cotton wool, etc.

> > Fear responses (starting, crying, falling over) were recorded for sudden loud noises (striking a steel bar out of sight)

> Eleven-month-old Albert was then exposed to series of pairings between the sudden appearance of a white rat and the loud noise

> > Tests revealed fear responses (withdrawal from the stimuli, whimpering, crying) to the presentation of the white rat alone

> > Further tests found that this conditioned fear had generalised to some extent to visually similar objects (including rabbit, dog, fur coat, white hair) but not dissimilar objects (such as blocks, table, etc.)

> Concluded that human fear can be conditioned

> > Criticised the Freudian perspective of sexual trauma in infancy to argue that adult fear is probably due to conditioning at a young age

> Study was not criticised at the time of publication, but it has been criticised in more recent years and it was used to evidence the need for ethical guidelines (Buckley, 1989)

> > Criticisms focus predominantly on the ethics of inducing fear in a child and the validity of the conclusion that all phobias must have been conditioned at some time

> > Efforts to find the adult Albert concluded that he was likely to have been Douglas Meritte (Beck et al., 2009) – if Douglas was Albert, he passed away in 1925 from hydrocephalus at the age of six and there is no evidence to suggest that he suffered any ill effects from the experiments (although he was never deconditioned, no family stories indicate that he retained a fear of white furry objects)

Forced to resign from Johns Hopkins University in 1920

> Record of indiscretions with women had caused problems through his career

> > He was described as a 'ladies' man' with a history of sexual conquests and voted 'handsomest professor' in 1919 (Benjamin et al., 2007)

Affair with his graduate assistant Rosalie Rayner and subsequent divorce from his wife finally resulted in dismissal from his post (Buckley, 1989)

Although rumours have suggested that his dismissal was related to sexual experiments conducted within the department, this is unlikely to be the case (Benjamin et al., 2007)

Pursued a career in advertising after leaving academia

Unable to find work in academia despite his incredible career to date (Benjamin et al., 2007)

Vice President of J Walter Thompson Agency from 1924 to 1945

Applied behavioural principles to consumerism with impressive results and involved in some of the largest advertising campaigns of his time

Published *Behaviorism* initially in 1925 and revised in 1930

Maintained an interest in psychology despite no longer working in academia

Contained the oft quoted 'Give me a dozen healthy infants . . .' (see start of this biography)

Quote is often misrepresented with the final line omitted – this makes him appear controlling and obsessive

In reality, he recognised that his comments were extreme but made the point that it was no different to the extreme opinion taken by those who argue that we are born into our position in society

He actually recognised and valued the role of both nature and nurture

Retired in 1945

Awarded by the American Psychological Association for his contribution to psychology in 1957

Son collected his award in his place as he did not feel able to attend

Family

Married Mary Ikes in 1904

Mary was one of his students at the University of Chicago

Raised one son and one daughter with Mary

Watson reportedly had several extramarital affairs with students and the marriage ended in divorce in 1920 after Mary discovered his affair with Rosalie Rayner (Benjamin et al., 2007)

Married Rosalie Rayner

Rosalie was his graduate assistant at Johns Hopkins University and their affair caused controversy within the institute (Benjamin et al., 2007)

Raised two sons with Rosalie

Remained married to Rosalie until her premature death in 1935

Experienced difficulties in his later life (Buckley, 1989)

> Watson struggled with his grief following the death of his second wife

> Difficult relationship with his children which worsened after the death of his second wife

> After retirement in 1945, he withdrew from society to live as a recluse on a farm in Connecticut

Death

Died in New York City on 25th September 1958

> Reportedly died of liver cirrhosis

> Burnt all of his unpublished work shortly before his death

>> 'When you're dead, you're all dead' (Watson quoted in Buckley, 1989)

FOUNDING FATHER OF THE BEHAVIOURAL APPROACH: WATSON

Consider the life story of John Watson and try to answer the following questions.

1. What was the social and cultural context of the world in which Watson developed his theories?
2. How might Watson's life experiences have impacted on his perception of human nature?
3. How can this life story contribute to your understanding of the behavioural approach?

Significant learnings

'The Freudians twenty years from now, unless their hypotheses change, when they come to analyze [Little] Albert's fear of a seal skin coat – assuming that he comes to analysis at that age – will probably tease from him the recital of a dream which upon their analysis will show that Albert at three years of age attempted to play with the pubic hair of the mother and was scolded violently for it' (Watson & Rayner, 1920)

Biography of Burrhus Frederic Skinner

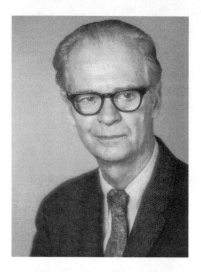

'Society attacks early, when the individual is helpless.'
—Skinner (1948)

Who was B.F. Skinner?

Skinner established the concept of operant conditioning and this formed the foundation for the behavioural approach

> Pavlov and Watson also made critical contributions to this approach
>> Pavlov established classical conditioning
>>
>> Watson introduced the concept of behaviourism

Early years

Born on 20th March 1904 in Pennsylvania, USA

> 'Warm and stable' home environment (Skinner quoted in Vargas, 2005)
>
> Father (William Skinner) was a lawyer and mother (Grace) was a housewife
>
> Eldest of two children
>> Brother Edward died of a cerebral aneurysm at the age of 16

Intellectually advanced from a young age

> Active inventor (Vargas, 2005)
>> Designed a flotation system to identify ripe berries to aid his door-to-door elderberry selling business during his teens

Education

Graduated with a BA in English from Hamilton College in New York in 1926

> Did not enjoy the college lifestyle or the religious persuasion of the school

Dreamed of success as a writer between 1926 and 1928

> Returned home to live with parents while trying to write fiction

Spent a 'dark year' writing short newspaper articles before eventually deciding that his literary skills lacked life experience (Vargas, 2005)

Lived the life of a bohemian by travelling and working in New York City

Studied psychology at Harvard University between 1928 and 1931 (Smith & Morris, 2004)

Returned to school to study psychology after being motivated by books written by Pavlov and Watson

Completed his Master's in 1930 and PhD in 1931

Family

Married Yvonne Blue in 1936

Raised two daughters

Career

Researcher at Harvard University between 1931 and 1936 (Skinner, 1987)

During his PhD and post as a researcher, he worked jointly under the departments of psychology and physiology

Each department assumed that the other was engaged in active supervision, but in reality he was 'doing exactly as I pleased' (Vargas, 2005)

Developed the concept of operant conditioning while a graduate student between 1931 and 1936 (Smith & Morris, 2004)

Designed the operant conditioning chamber 'Skinner Box' for training animals using schedules of reinforcement

Chamber contains a food dispenser, response lever, loudspeaker and lights

Stimulus is presented through the loudspeaker and lights and animal must produce a specific response in order to receive reinforcement through the food dispenser

Alternative versions might include LCD screens to present specific forms of stimuli or electrified floors to deliver punishment

Experimented with rat behaviour using this apparatus to record responses to stimuli

Discovered that behaviour did not appear solely dependent on preceding or co-existing stimulus (classical conditioning), but was also dependent on the consequences of behaviour

Reinforcement and punishment occurring after the behaviour had an impact on the future occurrence of the behaviour

Labelled this new type of conditioning 'operant conditioning'

Lecturer in psychology at the University of Minnesota in Minneapolis between 1936 and 1945 (Smith & Morris, 2004)

Published first book *The Behavior of Organisms* in 1938

>   Outlined the principles of operant conditioning and the impact of reinforcement on behaviour

Created the baby tender or Aircrib for the birth of his second child in 1944 (Skinner, 1987)

>   Baby crib designed to reduce problems associated with a traditional crib
>
>>   Risk of baby trapping legs between bars
>>
>>   Risk of suffocation from blankets
>>
>>   Problems with cradle cap and nappy rashes
>
>   Produced a fully enclosed, temperature-controlled, Plexiglass 'baby box'
>
>>   Highly praised by his daughter Deborah who spent some time in the crib as an infant
>
>   Received a critical reception
>
>>   Critics compared it to the Skinner Box and suggested that he intended to raise a baby in a controlled environment
>>
>>   Unfounded rumours circulated that his daughter was raised entirely inside the box and eventually committed suicide
>>
>>   In reality, the baby tender was a substitute for a cot only – the baby still spent most of life outside the crib
>
>   Despite experimental evidence highlighting the success of the baby tender, it never sold well as it seemed too much like a baby aquarium

Ran Project Pigeon (Project Orcon) for the National Defence Research Committee during World War Two (Skinner, 1960)

>   Project Pigeon was pigeon-guided missiles
>
>   During World War Two, Skinner became aware that the use of bombs was limited by the lack of missile guidance systems
>
>   Received funding to train pigeons to guide bombs to their correct destination
>
>>   Three pigeons in separate boxes in the nose cone of the missile
>>
>>   Each pigeon is presented with an image of what is located in front of the missile and trained to peck the target
>>
>>   Averaged direction of the pecks would guide the movement of the missile
>
>   Highly effective method
>
>>   Pigeons are easily trained and demonstrate consistent responses
>>
>>   Pigeons continue pecking despite surrounding noise and falling sensation
>>
>>   Experimental trials found it to be a reliable technique for missile guidance
>
>   Controversial method was not used by the military
>
>>   Funding was cancelled in 1944

No one was able to take seriously the idea of a bird guiding a missile, and most authorities found it difficult to place trust in such an unusual method (despite the reliable evidence)

Chair of psychology at Indiana University between 1945 and 1948 (Smith & Morris, 2004)

First meeting of the Society of the Experimental Analysis of Behavior was held here in 1946

Tenured professor at Harvard University between 1948 and 1990 (Smith & Morris, 2004)

Highly prolific in teaching, researching and writing

Devised a teaching machine in 1958 (Skinner, 1958)

Experience with his own daughters prompted him to explore applications for operant conditioning in education

Visit to his daughter's maths class made him realise that teaching violated every principle of conditioned learning

'Through no fault of her own, the teacher was violating almost everything we knew about the learning process' (Skinner quoted in Vargas, 2005)

Returned home to begin work on a teaching machine to improve established skills and a programme of instruction to develop new skills

Teaching machine randomly presented questions followed by immediate feedback

Essentially, this machine followed the same principles as the operant conditioning chamber – child was instantly rewarded for desirable behaviour

Programme of instruction presented material broken down into small steps and gradually reduced tutor support over time

Behaviour shaping technique helped the student to learn new skills

Retired in 1974

Death

Diagnosed with leukaemia in 1989

Fought valiantly against the progression of the disease and remained active in his career throughout the last year of his life

Delivered a talk for the American Psychological Association (APA) ten days before his death (Vargas, 2005)

Died on August 18th 1990

Completed his final article (based on the APA talk) on the day he died (Vargas, 2005)

Awarded the Lifetime Achievement Award by the APA in 1990

FOUNDING FATHER OF THE BEHAVIOURAL APPROACH: SKINNER

Consider the life story of B.F. Skinner and try to answer the following questions.

1. What was the social and cultural context of the world in which Skinner developed his theories?
2. How might Skinner's life experiences have impacted on his perception of human nature?
3. How can this life story contribute to your understanding of the behavioural approach?

Significant learnings

'Education is what survives when what has been learned has been forgotten' (Skinner, 1964)

'We shouldn't teach great books; we should teach a love of reading' (Skinner quoted in Evans, 1968)

'The real problem is not whether machines think but whether men do' (Skinner, 1969)

'A failure is not always a mistake, it may simply be the best one can do under the circumstances. The real mistake is to stop trying' (Skinner, 1972)

SUMMARY

Pavlov: established concept of classical conditioning; *early years*, born 1849 in Russia, religious family expected him to join priesthood but he pursued science, educationally advanced from a young age; *education*, doctorate in medicine in 1883 (thesis focused on principles of central nervous system); *family*, married and raised five children; organised and directed the Department of Physiology at the Institute of Experimental Medicine, explored psychic secretion to discover conditioned reflexes in dogs (classical conditioning), won Nobel Prize for research; *death*, died of pneumonia in 1936

Watson: established Behaviorist Manifesto; *early years*, born 1978 in South Carolina, difficult childhood characterised by rebellion after his father left the family; *education*, absence of father led to early rebellion against education, attitude improved after acceptance at university, doctorate in psychology from University of Chicago; *family*, married his student and raised two children, involved in a sex scandal when he divorced his wife following an affair with his graduate assistant Rayner, married Rayner and raised two children, recluse in later life after death of his wife; *career*, associate professor at Johns Hopkins University, presented the Behaviorist Manifest establishing himself as the founder of behaviourism, argued that psychology was the science of human behaviour so it should be studied scientifically in lab conditions, president of the APA, conditioned fear in Little Albert, sex scandal meant he was forced to resign and he could not find a position in academia so worked in advertising, delivered the oft quoted 'Give me a dozen healthy infants . . .', awarded by APA for work in psychology (award collected by son); *death*, died of liver cirrhosis in 1958, burnt his unpublished work before his death

Skinner: established concept of operant conditioning; *early years*, born 1904 in Pennsylvania to a warm and stable family environment, intellectually advanced from young age; *education*, studied English and wanted to be a writer, PhD at Harvard working in psychology and physiology; *career*, discovered behaviour not dependent on co-existing stimuli and introduced concept of reinforcement and punishment to shape behaviour through experimentation with a Skinner Box while a graduate student at Harvard University, designed the baby tender 'Aircrib' after his daughter was born, ran Project Pigeon during WW2, tenured professor at Harvard, devised a teaching machine using operant conditioning principles, retired but continued writing until death; *death*, died due to leukaemia in 1989, lifetime achievement award by APA

BEHAVIOURAL THEORIES OF HUMAN NATURE AND PERSONALITY

LEARNING OUTCOMES

After reading this section, you will be able to:

- describe the stimulus–response model of classical conditioning, including explanations of how pure and second-order conditioning can shape behaviour

- describe the antecedent–behaviour–consequence model of operant conditioning, including explanations of how schedules of positive and negative reinforcement and punishment can shape behaviour

Classical conditioning: stimulus–response model (Figure 4.1)

Stimulus–response

Repeated pairings of an unconditioned and neutral stimulus will result in a conditioned response (Pavlov, 1928)

An unconditioned stimulus produces an automatic reflexive unconditioned response

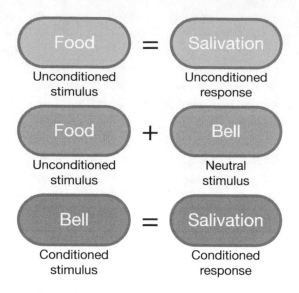

FIGURE 4.1 Classical conditioning in action. Adapted from Pavlov (1928).

For example, food (unconditioned stimulus) will automatically result in salivation (unconditioned response)

A neutral stimulus is repeatedly paired with an unconditioned stimulus to produce a conditioned stimulus

For example, pairing food (unconditioned stimulus) with a bell (neutral stimulus) will teach the individual to associate the two stimuli

A conditioned stimulus will produce the same automatic conditioned response after being paired with the unconditioned stimulus

For example, bell (conditioned stimulus) begins to automatically result in salivation (conditioned response)

S–R model

Stimulus–response

Model suggests that some stimuli are automatically paired with specific responses, and non-automatic responses can be associated with other 'neutral' stimuli through the process of conditioning

Conditioned fear

Fear can be classically conditioned (Watson & Rayner, 1920)

Little Albert was not naturally afraid of rats, but was naturally afraid of sudden loud noises

Little Albert began to demonstrate a fear of rats (cried in response to the sight of a rat) and other similar objects (white fur) after repeated pairings of the rat and a sudden loud bang

Pure and second-order conditioning

All negative human responses can be explained through pure and second-order classical conditioning

> Pure classical conditioning
>
>> Direct pairing between unconditioned and neutral stimulus
>>
>> We have a natural dislike of social disapproval so we will experience an unpleasant emotion (unconditioned response) in response to criticism (unconditioned stimulus)
>>
>> Repeated or a single extreme pairing of criticism (unconditioned stimulus) and an exam (neutral stimulus) will teach a student to associate the two experiences
>>
>> Student will experience an unpleasant emotion (conditioned response) in response to an exam (conditioned stimulus)
>
> Second-order classical conditioning

PAIRING FOR LEARNING . . .

Try to identify the unconditioned stimulus and response and the conditioned stimulus and response in the following examples. Can you predict future behaviour on the basis of this conditioning?

A two-year-old girl is playing with her toys in the garden. Suddenly, her mother notices that the child has found a spider in the grass. She has picked it up and is about to put it into her mouth. Her mother is horrified and screams her name so that she does not eat the wriggling creepy-crawly. The little girl starts at the sound of the scream and drops the spider. She begins to cry so her mother hurries over to comfort her. He mother squashes the 'naughty' spider and cuddles the little girl until she stops crying.

A boy in his mid-teens steals a bottle of bourbon from the kitchen cabinet. He shares the bottle with his friends and, although he does not like the taste, he drinks several glasses. Shortly afterwards, he begins to feel dizzy and he is violently sick. He vomits repeatedly for the next two hours and has a painful headache for the next two days.

A young woman begins working at a local advertising company. Although she tries to talk to the other employees, she feels excluded and she often notices unpleasant comments directed towards her. One of the other women seems to be the ringleader of this nastiness – she constantly undermines her work and occasionally pushes her out of the way when they pass in the corridor. She tries to avoid this horrible woman by hiding in an empty office whenever she smells her strong flowery perfume. Eventually, she leaves the job for work in a different part of town.

Subsequent pairing between conditioned and neutral stimulus

One specific tutor (neutral stimulus) is always present during exams (conditioned stimulus) so the student learns to associate the two stimuli

Student will experience an unpleasant emotion (conditioned response) in response to the tutor (conditioned stimulus)

This could then be generalised to all tutors or all figures of authority

For example, child experiencing a school phobia could be explained in terms of classical conditioning

Operant conditioning: antecedent–behaviour–consequence model (Figure 4.2)

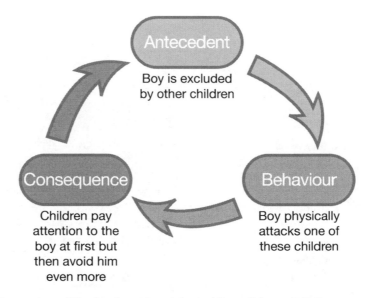

FIGURE 4.2 **Operant conditioning in action. Adapted from Skinner (1938).**

Antecedent–behaviour–consequence

Operant behaviour refers to active behaviours operating on the environment to generate consequences (Skinner, 1938)

All behaviour leads to consequences and these consequences will impact on the likelihood of that behaviour being repeated in the future

A-B-C model

Antecedent–behaviour–consequence

Model suggests that behaviour is prompted by stimuli in the environment (similar to S–R model) and results in specific consequences, then these consequences act as an antecedent for future behaviours

For example, a teenage boy who is excluded by his peers (antecedent) may eventually hit out at one of these other children (behaviour) – this will initially get their attention (rewarding consequence) but will then lead to further exclusion from his peers (consequence forms a new antecedent)

Positive and negative reinforcement and punishment

Hint: think of positive and negative in terms of maths (plus and minus/adding and subtracting) rather than value judgements

All negative human responses can be explained through reinforcement and punishment

Reinforcement

Anything that will strengthen the preceding behaviour

Student is disobedient in class (behaviour) and this results in more attention from the teacher and less ridicule from peers (reinforcement) so he is more likely to be disobedient again in the future

Punishment

Anything that will weaken the preceding behaviour

Student is obedient in class (behaviour) and this results in being ignored by the teacher and mocked by peers (punishment) so he is less likely to be obedient again in the future

For example, child misbehaving in school could be explained in terms of operant conditioning

Reinforcement is anything that will strengthen the preceding behaviour (Skinner, 1938)

Positive reinforcement

Addition of something pleasant results in the behaviour being more likely to be exhibited in the future

For example, giving a child a new toy when he is polite means that he is more likely to be polite again in the future

Negative reinforcement

Removal of something unpleasant results in the behaviour being more likely to be exhibited in the future

For example, reducing the number of sprouts on the plate after the child has been polite means that she is more likely to be polite again in the future

Punishment is anything that will weaken the preceding behaviour (Skinner, 1938)

Positive punishment

Addition of something unpleasant results in the behaviour being less likely to be exhibited in the future

For example, shouting at a child for being rude means that he is less likely to be rude again in the future

Negative punishment

> Removal of something pleasant results in the behaviour being less likely to be exhibited in the future

> For example, taking away a toy after a child has been rude means that she is less likely to rude again in the future

Combination consequences are the most effective

> Punishment is less effective than reinforcement, but a combination of all elements is most effective for behaviour

> For example, children who are disobedient in school may have learnt to exhibit this behaviour because being naughty leads to more attention from the teacher (positive reinforcement) and less ridicule from peers (negative reinforcement) whereas being good leads to bullying from peers (positive punishment) and less attention from the teacher (negative punishment)

Primary and secondary reinforcers and punishers

Reinforcers and punishers have an effect on the recipient

> Effect can be natural or created artificially

Primary reinforcers or punishers

> Naturally result in an automatic response

> For example, food, water, sex, sleep are all natural reinforcers because they aid survival

> Pain, hunger, thirst, tiredness are all natural punishers because they hinder survival

> Secondary reinforcers or punishers

> Need to be paired with a primary reinforcer to create a response

> For example, money is a secondary reinforcer because society has associated money with the ability to gain food, water, sex, etc.

> Poor exam grades are a secondary punisher because society has associated poor academic performance with difficulty gaining a job, thus leading to hunger, thirst, etc.

> Training can utilise secondary reinforcers and punishers to avoid having to constantly provide primary reinforcement or punishment

>> Impractical to provide treats every time a child should be rewarded, so we can use stars on a chart as a secondary reinforcer by first associating with primary reinforcers

> Difficult to distinguish between some primary and secondary reinforcers/punishers

>> Are respect, love and praise primary reinforcers? Or are they secondary reinforcers created as a result of pairing with the ability to gain resources such as food and sex?

Are humiliation, embarrassment and criticism primary reinforcers? Or are they secondary reinforcers created as a result of pairing with the loss of resources such as food and sex?

Answers depend on whether we regard emotional needs as instinctively important for survival

Schedules of reinforcement

Reinforcement (and punishment) can be delivered in two types of schedule

Continuous reinforcement

Partial reinforcement

Continuous reinforcement

Reinforcement is provided every single time the behaviour is exhibited

GETTING WHAT YOU DESERVE . . .

Try to identify the reinforcement and/or punishment in the following examples. Can you predict future behaviour on the basis of this conditioning?

A three-year-old boy throws a tantrum in the supermarket because he wants a chocolate bar. His mother is in a rush because she has to collect her eldest daughter from school and they are already running late. The little boy sits on the floor and refuses to move. He screams until his face turns red and other shoppers begin to stare at him. His mother eventually offers him a chocolate bar and he stops crying in order to eat it. She persuades him to stand up again and they complete the shopping without any further disruptions.

A young woman has a strong fear of travelling in cars. Unfortunately, she is employed in a shop that is a long distance from her home so her husband has to drive her to and from work every day. She spends the journey sitting tensely in the passenger seat with her eyes closed. He is aware of her fear and he tries to comfort her by constantly reassuring her in a gentle voice. Sometimes her fear will become so intense that she will begin to tremble and cry. On those occasions, her husband will pull over the car to hug and soothe her before continuing with the journey.

A father is trying to finish an important report at work, but his wife is sick so he has to take care of their two young daughters. The youngest daughter is drawing pictures in a book without making any noise. He is extremely relieved about this because it means that he can focus on his work. Unfortunately, his eldest daughter is singing noisily and constantly tries to climb on his knee. Eventually, he stops working to give his eldest daughter a lollipop to stop her singing and distract her while he finishes the report.

For example, child is given a sweet every time he scores well on a test in school

Highly effective method for learning behaviours, but can be extremely prone to extinction because the reinforcement has to be maintained constantly

Although effective, it is usually impractical to maintain continuous reinforcement or punishment so schedules will usually revert to partial reinforcement at some point

Partial reinforcement

Reinforcement is provided only at certain times when the behaviour is exhibited

For example, child is sometimes given a sweet when he scores well on a test in school

Highly effective method for maintaining behaviours and extremely resistant to extinction, but can be a slow process for learning behaviours

Four types of partial reinforcement schedule

Fixed ratio schedule: reinforcement is delivered after a set number of responses – for example, child is given a present after passing four tests at school

Variable ratio schedule: reinforcement is delivered after an unpredictable number of responses – for example, child is given a present after passing an unspecified number of tests at school

Fixed interval schedule: reinforcement is delivered after a set period of time has elapsed – for example, child is given a present every Monday provided that they are continuing to pass their tests at school

Variable interval schedule: reinforcement is delivered after an unpredictable period of time has elapsed – for example, child is given a present every so often provided that they are continuing to pass their tests at school

---

SUMMARY

Classical conditioning: stimulus–response model; repeated pairings of an unconditioned and neutral stimulus will result in a conditioned response; conditioned fear, Little Albert; pure and second-order conditioning

Operant conditioning: A-B-C model; active behaviours operating on the environment to generate consequences, positive and negative reinforcement and punishment, primary and secondary reinforcers and punishers, continuous and partial reinforcement (fixed ratio, variable ratio, fixed interval, variable interval)

THERAPEUTIC RELATIONSHIP IN BEHAVIOUR THERAPY

LEARNING OUTCOMES

After reading this section, you will be able to:

* debate the value of focusing on behaviour
* describe and evaluate psychoeducation in the therapeutic process

Behavioural focus

Advantages of behaviourism

No 'mind-reading'

> It is impossible to know the thought processes or emotions experienced by another individual

>> Cognitive therapy claims to know these processes in order to be able to identify distortions or errors in thought and subsequently correct these inaccuracies

>> Psychoanalytic therapy claims to be able to see not just these thought processes, but beyond them into the unconscious processes of which even the client is unaware

>> Person-centred therapy avoids this problem by focusing only on what has already been revealed by the client

> Behaviourism does not require the therapist to guess the inner state of the client – the therapist can simply focus on what the client actually does in relation to problems

Unclear relationship between behaviour, cognition and emotion

> We often assume that we decide to do something (thought), do it (behaviour) and then feel good or bad due to the consequences (emotion)

>> Is this the case?

> Evidence suggests that, at least in some cases, we act first and simply assume that we thought about it in advance

>> Consider an early morning alarm . . .

>> You hit 'snooze' and lie in bed thinking 'I have to get up, I have to get up, I have to get up, I have to get up . . .'

>> You know that you must get out of bed and you keep saying this to yourself and yet you do not move

>> But suddenly you are out of bed and walking to the bathroom!

>> What changed? Could it be that your last thought was slightly more forceful? Or could it be that some behaviours operate entirely independently of thought?

Perhaps we sometimes engage in a behaviour, justify the behaviour to ourselves afterwards, and then on reflection we assume that the thought process came first

This philosophical issue is currently being explored in science

Research evidence has found that neurological activity responsible for the intention to act can precede the conscious decision to act (Libet et al., 1983)

Participants were asked to make a voluntary response while brain activity was compared with the reported decision time

Analysis of the times revealed that the brain activated the intention to move before the participant made a conscious decision to move

These findings have been used to argue against the concept of free will

EDUCATION OR MANIPULATION?

Person-centred therapy would argue that the therapist should not seek to 'educate' the client as this implies that the therapist is an expert and may lead to the client being manipulated into behaving in a certain way. Consider the following cases and reflect on whether behavioural therapy is appropriate for the client. Try to think about the demands and risks of the therapy and those factors that might exclude someone from being able to engage with the treatment. You could also consider which alternative therapies might be more helpful for the client.

Susan has an intense fear of spiders. She is desperate to overcome this fear because she wants to go camping with her new boyfriend. She freezes every time she sees a spider and she had a panic attack last week when she found a spider in her bedroom.

Andrew has recently separated from his wife. He feels incredibly unhappy and frequently begins to cry during the day. He is convinced that he is a failure and he has stopped going to work. His brother is concerned about his wellbeing so he has forced him to see a therapist. Andrew, however, has made it clear that he would prefer to stay in bed – he does not believe that therapy will be helpful for him.

Christopher is a six-year-old boy with autism. He has lived in a residential home throughout his life and he has only limited contact with his birth mother. He does not communicate well with others and he engages in self-harm (banging his head against a wall) if he is introduced to any new people.

Claire is in a relationship with a man who has hit her on three separate occasions. She says that she is in love with him and she does not want to end the relationship. However, her mother is convinced that she needs help so she has persuaded Claire to see a therapist.

Alternative perspective

Cognition and emotion ARE behaviours

> It could be argued that all human actions, including thinking and feeling, are types of behaviour and thus fall under the behaviourist category

> If cognition and emotion are viewed as behaviours, then they can be modified in similar ways to all other behaviours using the core principles of classical and operant conditioning

>> No need to resort to deep analysis or complex interpretations

Therapeutic psychoeducation

Passive and active psychoeducation

Psychoeducation involves the practitioner teaching the client with the aim of improving mental health and wellbeing

Passive psychoeducation

> Therapeutic intervention in which the therapist provides information and educational material (Donker et al., 2009)

> Therapist might give out leaflets or handouts, direct the client towards websites or books, deliver lectures, etc.

> Common form of online therapy

> Evidence suggests that passive psychoeducation alone can have significant benefits on mental health and wellbeing (Donker et al., 2009)

Active psychoeducation

> Therapeutic intervention in which the therapist provides specific advice and guidance in addition to general information and educational material (Donker et al., 2009)

> Therapist might explicitly instruct the client to engage with certain activities or complete certain tasks (sometimes homework) in order to further educate the client on psychological processes

Collaboration between therapist and client

Behaviour therapy is often considered to be a psychoeducational approach (Weishaar, 1993, cited in Mkangi, 2010)

> Therapist adopts a role similar to a teacher and client adopts a role similar to a student

> Therapist collaborates with the client to develop new thinking patterns

Neither an expert nor a novice . . .

> In contrast to the interpretative methods of the psychoanalytic approach and the non-directive methods of the person-centred approach, therapist will not establish him/herself as an expert or a novice with regard to the inner world of the client

Instead, the therapist will educate the client on basic behavioural principles and encourage the client to apply this new knowledge to his or her own life experiences

However, it can be very difficult to avoid being viewed as an expert when educating a client

By definition, teachers are viewed as more expert than students

Client is likely to assume that the therapist is an expert if s/he is using intervention techniques designed to teach the client

One way to avoid being viewed as an expert is to explore some issues in collaboration with the client

For example, therapist could suggest that both parties look for further information as homework between sessions

Education for the future . . .

This educational process will provide the client with the tools needed to address future problems and achieve independence by working towards personal goals without the constant support of a therapist

---

SUMMARY

Focus on behaviour: advantages of behaviourism, no mind-reading, unclear relationships between behaviour and cognition and emotion; arguably, cognition and emotion are behaviours

Therapeutic psychoeducation: passive and active psychoeducation can aid the collaboration between the client (student) and the therapist (neither expert nor novice); educational process provides client with tools to address future problems and achieve independence without the constant support of a therapist

---

THERAPEUTIC TECHNIQUES IN BEHAVIOUR THERAPY

LEARNING OUTCOMES

After reading this section, you will be able to:

- discuss exposure techniques, such as systematic desensitisation and flooding
- discuss contingency management techniques, such as time out and token economy
- describe and evaluate behavioural change programmes, such as personal and social skills programmes and the Nudge programme

Exposure therapy techniques

Reconditioning

Client is exposed to the fear-inducing stimulus in order to extinguish previous unhealthy associations and establish new healthy associations (Abramowitz et al., 2010)

> Unhealthy associations can be extinguished
>
> > Exposure to the associated stimulus without the negative consequences will lead to extinction of the conditioned response
> >
> > Client who has been conditioned to fear dogs because of an early experience associating a dog (neutral stimulus) and a bite (unconditioned stimulus will automatically inspire fear)
> >
> > Client might have this conditioned response of fear of dogs extinguished if he experiences the association between a dog (conditioned stimulus) and no bite (extinction of the association)
>
> Healthy associations can be established
>
> > Exposure to the associated stimulus with positive consequences will lead to establishment of a conditioned response
> >
> > Client who has been conditioned to fear dogs because of an early experience associating a dog (neutral stimulus) and a bite (unconditioned stimulus will automatically inspire fear)
> >
> > Client might have a new conditioned response of calm in the face of dogs if he experiences the association between a dog (conditioned stimulus) and relaxed music (unconditioned stimulus will automatically inspire relaxation)

Reconditioning can address unhealthy maintenance behaviours

> Some clients will adopt safety behaviours to protect themselves from anxiety, fear or other negative emotions
>
> > Avoidance is a common safety behaviour – for example, the client who fears blushing in front of strangers may avoid meeting people by staying at home all of the time
> >
> > Objects and people can be used as safety behaviours – for example, the client who worries about getting lost might refuse to travel unless her husband accompanies her
> >
> > Specific actions or attitudes can also be used as safety behaviours – for example, the client who fears being judged may adopt a brash outward appearance
>
> Safety behaviours are very reassuring in the short term because they offer comfort and reduce the undesirable emotions
>
> However, safety behaviours can work to maintain the problem in the long term
>
> > Individual learns that the problem is reduced only when the safety behaviour is employed

Individual is reinforced for engaging in the behaviour so the safety behaviour is more likely in the future

There is never an opportunity to learn that the safety behaviour is not necessary so the individual never addresses the actual problem

Many forms of 'helping' actually work to establish these counter-productive safety behaviours

For example, the husband who tries to reassure his anxious wife by travelling with her on every trip

Exposure therapy works to expose the client to the fear-inducing stimulus without the presence of safety behaviours so that the client can learn to cope with the problem independently

In some cases, safety behaviours may be permitted at the start of the process and then gradually removed during therapy

Two types of exposure therapy

Systematic desensitisation

Flooding

Systematic desensitisation

Client is systematically exposed to successively more anxiety-inducing stimuli whilst maintaining a stable level of relaxation (Wolpe, 1958)

Three steps to successful systematic desensitisation

Relaxation training

Client is taught a meditative relaxation technique (such as progressive muscle relaxation or internal imagery relaxation) in order to be able to enter a relaxed state on command

Anxiety hierarchy

Client is questioned on the topic of anxiety-inducing stimuli in order to produce a rank order of situations gradually increasing in anxiety severity

Systematic desensitisation proper

Client is placed in a relaxed state then asked to imagine or experience the situation at the lowest rank of their anxiety-inducing scale while remaining relaxed

Once this can be accomplished successfully, client will begin to move up the scale with the aim of maintaining a relaxed state at each stage

Imagined versus in vivo exposure

This technique can use imagined situations or actual stimuli

Both options have costs and benefits

Imagined exposure is safer for the client

In vivo exposure is more realistic

Example of a client with a spider phobia

> Client is taught how to relax using the progressive muscle relaxation technique
>
> Client is asked to rank situations involving spiders according to anxiety – first stage might be seeing a spider at the other side of the room and last stage might be holding a spider in the hand
>
> Client establishes a relaxed state then imagines or experiences a spider at the other side of the room
>
> Client continues until able to maintain this relaxed state in the face of this situation and then moves on to imagine or experience the next stage on the ranked list
>
> Client will eventually get to the final stage and be able to hold a spider while maintaining a relaxed state

Highly successful technique which has been used for a wide range of problems (Spiegler & Guevremont, 2009)

> Phobia, anxiety, anger, asthma, insomnia, nightmares, motion sickness, etc.

Flooding

Client is exposed to the anxiety-inducing stimulus at a maximum level of intensity for a prolonged period of time (Wolpe, 1958)

Client is unable to use avoidance so must face the fear directly

> Clients will often use techniques to avoid their fears so they are never able to learn new associations or extinguish old associations
>
> This technique prevents clients from avoiding the fear or using any anxiety-reducing methods so that they realise that the anxiety-provoking stimulus does not actually lead to any real harm

Client is unable to maintain high levels of anxiety for a prolonged period of time

> Eventually the client will calm down and s/he will then have learnt that the stimulus is not dangerous or threatening

Imagined versus in vivo exposure

> This technique can use imagined situations or actual stimuli
>
> Both options have costs and benefits
>
>> Imagined exposure is safer for the client
>>
>> In vivo exposure is more realistic

Example of a client with agoraphobia

> Client is exposed to the most anxiety-inducing situation in such a way that she cannot escape – perhaps she is deposited in the middle of a crowded supermarket
>
> Client will initially feel intense anxiety, but she is unable to reduce the intensity of the situation or maintain the anxiety for the prolonged period of time
>
> Eventually she will begin to feel calmer and she will learn that she is not in danger in the middle of the supermarket

Highly effective for fear-related disorders (Tryon, 2005), but often requires additional therapeutic support (Spiegler & Guevremont, 2009)

Limited range of disorders can be treated in this way – obviously, the client cannot be exposed to real harm so any excessive fears of genuine danger (such as fears of fire) cannot be treated through flooding

Contingency management techniques

Behaviour shaping

Client is provided with reinforcement and (to a lesser extent) punishment for specific behaviours in order to shape behaviour towards a desirable goal (Skinner, 1938)

Client will sometimes agree to a specific programme of behaviour or set of rules at the start of the treatment and then receive reinforcement or punishment for adhering to this treatment plan

For example, a client suffering substance abuse might devise a plan for reducing substance intake and the therapist will reward positive steps on this plan

Alternatively, clients who engage in inappropriate or self-damaging behaviours might not be specifically involved in devising the programme

For example, a client with severe intellectual disabilities might be encouraged to behave in a socially acceptable way by being rewarded for appropriate behaviour

Two types of contingency management

Time out

Token economy

Time out

Client is punished for failure to adhere to the programme or rules by being isolated from activities or people to some extent for a short time

Often used in cases of overexcitation or aggression in order to give the client time to calm down

Highly effective for children ('naughty step') or those with severe intellectual disabilities, but can also be used in other cases when the client can be taught to give him- or herself a time out to reflect on the situation

Contingent attention

Associated with time out, contingent attention programmes involve the client being reinforced or punished by being granted or denied attention

For example, child who is behaving badly is ignored whereas child who is behaving well is praised

Example of a client with anger management problems

Client is taught to recognise the first signs of anger and then remove himself from the situation before losing his temper

Client is encouraged to engage in a distracting time out followed by a reflective time out before returning to the anger-inducing stimulus

Distracting time out will reduce the anger by refocusing the client on a less provocative stimulus

Reflective time out will allow the client to think about the situation (ideally without returning to the angry state) in order to consider how best to handle the problem

Token economy

Client is reinforced with a token for engaging in a desirable behaviour or for adhering to the treatment programme

Tokens have no intrinsic value, but can be exchanged for reinforcing events at a later time

Material reinforcer, such as a chocolate bar

Service reinforcer, such as breakfast in bed

Privilege reinforcer, such as permission to go out for the evening

Eventually, client will be weaned off the tokens as s/he develops an internal guide for behaviour and can reinforce the self internally rather than relying on external rewards

PHYSICAL PUNISHMENT? NO, PSYCHOLOGICAL TORTURE IS MUCH MORE EFFECTIVE . . .

There is currently a wide debate relating to the effectiveness and morality associated with discipline for children. Consider the opposing arguments for corporal punishment versus psychological punishment and try to answer the following questions based on your knowledge of the area. It is inevitable that your personal opinions will influence your answers – this is absolutely appropriate provided that you remain aware of the difference between an answer based on evidence and an answer based on your own feelings.

1. Which type of discipline is most effective in instantly stopping a child from completing an action that is potentially dangerous (such as putting a hand in a fire)?
2. Which type of discipline is most effective in teaching a child right from wrong (such as not stealing)?
3. Is a smack across the bottom or withholding attention likely to have the greatest long-term effect on a child?
4. How does a parent decide which behaviours should be punished and how does the type of discipline relate to this decision?
5. Which type of discipline is most likely to lead to abuse and what are the potential long-term consequences of such abuse?

Highly effective for those with severe intellectual disabilities and has reported some success for children, but can also be used for other cases such as addiction

Example of a client with an addiction to cocaine

Client is asked to provide regular urine samples to indicate a period of abstinence from cocaine use

Client is rewarded with a voucher for a small dose of methadone

Client is eventually weaned off the methadone by reducing the dosage

Behavioural change programmes

Personal and social skills training

Personal and social skills include a wide range of behaviours

Anger management

Assertiveness

Appreciating the perspective of others

Problem solving

Conflict management

Peer negotiation and resistance skills

Active listening and effective communication

Increased acceptance and tolerance of others

These skills can be taught using psychoeducation, exposure therapy, contingency management, etc.

Highly effective in many applied settings

For example, Project ACHIEVE 'Stop and Think' social skills programme for schools in the US (Knoff, 2004)

Nudge

Behaviour can be positively influenced by gentle nudges (Thaler & Sunstein, 2008)

Nudges can be used at an institutional level by introducing policy changes that nudge people in a positive direction

UK government established the Nudge Unit (Behavioural Insights Team) in 2010

Aim of the unit is to find innovative methods of 'encouraging, enabling, and supporting people to make better choices for themselves' (Behavioural Insights Team, n.d.)

Nudges can be described as small actions to encourage positive behaviour change

For example, the Wales Centre for Behavioural Change has implemented a nudge at the local hospital by painting footprints across the floor to direct people towards the hand-washing stations

Nudges work by establishing a desired behaviour, assessing the current behaviour, seeking to reduce barriers to the behaviour, addressing logical errors and biases against the behaviour, then giving a small prompt to steer the individual towards the better behavioural option

For example, in 2010 the UK government offered subsidies for loft insulation but few people took advantage of the offer – analysis by the Nudge Unit revealed that the main barrier was laziness because people did not want the hassle of clearing the loft, so the Unit suggested that the insulation firm offer to clear the lofts themselves and this action increased uptake by 300% (Bell, 2013)

Nudges are used on a large scale to promote positive public actions

Nudges have been used to encourage the following behaviours

Public have been encouraged to pay their income tax on time by changing the wording on the letters

Drivers have been encouraged to park in their garages to reduce the risk of car theft by placing free skips on the street to allow people to empty their garages of rubbish

Walkers have been encouraged to recycle their rubbish by moving the recycling bin onto the actual footpaths

Patients have been discouraged from missing doctors' appointments by asking them to complete their own appointment cards

Drivers have been encouraged to donate to state parks by introducing an opt-out (rather than an opt-in) donation system

Jobseekers have been encouraged to seek work by establishing a commitment contract in the initial interview at the Jobcentre

Nudges are generally preferable to legislation because they still allow the individual to make a choice rather than enforcing a specific behaviour, thus impinging on individual freedom (Thaler & Sunstein, 2008)

However, if people are unaware that they are being nudged, it is debatable as to whether they really have a free choice

SUMMARY

Exposure therapy: reconditioning, unhealthy associations can be extinguished, new healthy associations can be formed, reconditioning addresses unhelpful maintenance behaviours; systematic desensitisation, relaxation training, anxiety hierarchy, systematic desensitisation proper, imagined versus *in vivo*, highly successful for range of problems (phobia, anxiety, anger, asthma, insomnia, nightmares, motion sickness); flooding, exposure to anxiety-inducing stimuli at maximum intensity for prolonged time, unable to avoid or maintain high anxiety so must eventually face the fear calmly, imagined versus *in vivo*, highly successful for fear-related disorders but additional therapeutic support is needed

Contingency management: behaviour shaping, reinforcement and (to a lesser extent) punishment for specific behaviours to shape behaviour towards a desirable goal; time out, punished for inappropriate behaviour by exclusion from people or activities, contingent attention; token economy, reinforced for appropriate behaviour with a token to be exchanged for treats

Behavioural change programmes: personal and social skills progammes, Project ACHIEVE 'Stop and Think' social skills programme for schools in the US; nudge, behaviour can be positively influenced by gentle nudges, Nudge Unit (Behavioural Insights Team) use nudges on a large scale to promote positive public actions, preferable to legislation because they still allow choice (but is it choice if the individual is being subtly manipulated?)

CASE STUDY DEMONSTRATING BEHAVIOUR THERAPY

LEARNING OUTCOMES

After reading this section, you will be able to:

* appreciate the application of behaviour therapy from the behavioural approach in a therapeutic setting

Recorded session: therapy in action

This chapter is accompanied by a recorded therapy session which is available for viewing.

This session lasts for one therapy hour (50 minutes) and it is presented as the initial session in a new therapeutic relationship. Prior to this session, the client will have completed an initial assessment questionnaire and the therapist will have read this paperwork to ensure familiarity with the case. This completed assessment and a full transcript of the recorded session are available.

No actors are used in this session. The client was one of the authors and the problem presented was genuine. The therapist is an experienced practitioner in the field. The only 'fake' aspect of this recorded session is that the client did not really seek therapy and this is not really the first session of a series of therapeutic contacts.

After the conclusion of the session, the therapist is invited to answer a few key questions about the session. This question and answer session lasts no longer than 10 minutes. The transcript of this session is available.

Presentation of Fay Short: history and symptoms

Fay Short has an acute fear of heights. She has recently experienced high levels of stress at her workplace and some associated physical symptoms (including headaches and backache). However, her primary reason for seeking therapy is a desire to overcome an intense fear of heights. She has previously experienced person-centred therapy for a short space of time over ten years ago, but this was unrelated to her current fears. She would like to overcome these fears during therapy so that they no longer impact on her ability to take part in activities that involve heights.

Therapy session: analysis

The therapy session can be sectioned as follows.

Introduction

Introduction outlining basic contractual details, especially the limits of confidentiality

Focus specifically on the problem presented by the client and an outline of the intended coverage in the session (map of the session)

Invitation to ask questions

Story

Client is invited to explain how the problem began, how the problem has developed over time, and how the problem impacts on current life

Focus on actions carried out during experiences of the problem, including specific behaviours that are maintaining the problem

Goals

Behaviour therapy is explained in terms of how reinforcement and punishment can shape and maintain behaviour

Explained how exposure to problem situations and structured reinforcement of appropriate behaviour can reduce problems

Identified a specific goal for therapy in the near future

Ending

Summary of the session by the therapist

Reflection on how the session was experienced by the client

Explanation of how behavioural problems will be addressed in future sessions, including homework and treatment plan

Invitation to return for future sessions

Key questions to consider in relation to this therapy session

How could the nature of this client be understood from the behavioural perspective?

- What is the current behaviour that is causing a problem for the client?
- Has any previous classical conditioning established the current problem behaviour?
- Has the client experienced a pairing between a neutral experience and an emotive experience leading to the natural invocation of the problem behaviour?
- Are there any stimulus–response associations currently maintaining the problem behaviour?
- Has any previous operant conditioning established the current problem behaviour?
- Has the client experienced reinforcement or punishment to shape the current problem behaviour?
- Are there any consequences currently maintaining the problem behaviour?

What is the nature of the therapeutic relationship in this behaviour therapy session?

- Does the therapist focus on behaviour?
- Does the therapist explore thoughts and feelings and, if so, are these discussed in behavioural terms?
- Does the therapist adopt the role of an expert?
- Does the therapist use passive or active psychoeducational strategies?
- Does the therapist collaborate with the client to solve the current problem?

Which behaviour techniques are demonstrated in this therapy session?

- Does the therapist introduce any exposure techniques, such as systematic desensitisation or flooding?
- How does the therapist encourage reconditioning in the client?
- Does the therapist introduce any contingency management techniques, such as time out, token economy or contingent attention?
- How does the therapist encourage the reinforcement of positive change in the client?
- Does the therapist recommend or advise any specific programme of training to unlearn the old problem behaviours and learn new solution-focused behaviours?

Personal experience of the client

I was very anxious about this session because it was my first experience of behavioural therapy and my first experience of receiving therapy while being filmed. Keith reassured me in the first few minutes and I did manage to forget about the camera after we began talking.

I feel that the rapport with Keith was very positive. I felt comfortable talking to him about my experiences and I felt that he listened to me in an empathic manner. This was rather surprising because I had expected behaviour therapy to be less empathic than my previous experience of person-centred therapy. I did feel that I talked too much, especially at the start of the session. I felt that this did not fit my expectation of a behaviour session – he was less directive than expected and I was somewhat relieved to find that he was not going to demand that my fears were immediately flooded!

This session focused specifically on my behaviour during and after my scary experience in Cambodia. In particular, we explored those behaviours that I use to 'protect' myself and I realised that these behaviours have actually been maintaining my problem. For example, Keith explained that my tendency to avoid heights helps to reduce the discomfort and anxiety in the moment, but will actually teach me to avoid in the future because I am being reinforced for my avoidance. This was a surprise to me because I had never considered my behaviour in this way before – in fact, I always thought that it was very sensible for me to avoid heights given that I am so afraid. Keith also explained that my use of my husband as a support network could also be maintaining my problem – I had never considered that his comfort might be reinforcing my fears, but this made sense when it was explained in the session. On reflection, I feel that I learnt an awful lot about myself during this session.

I was very happy that Keith took the time to explain exactly what I could expect from behavioural therapy. This was very reassuring and his descriptions sounded considerably less scary than I had anticipated. He explained how the behaviours that had been maintaining my fear could be changed to reduce my fears in the future, and this gave me confidence to try out the exercises that he suggested. I left the session feeling reassured and optimistic about working with Keith on my phobia.

—Fay Short

REFERENCES AND BIBLIOGRAPHY

Abramowitz, J.S., Deacon, B.J. & Whiteside, S.P. (2010) *Exposure Therapy for Anxiety: Principles and Practice.* New York: Guilford Press.

Asratyan, E.A. (1953) *I.P. Pavlov: His Life and Work.* Moscow: Foreign Languages Publishing House.

Babkin, B.P. (1949) *Pavlov: A Biography.* Toronto, Canada: University of Chicago Press.

Beck, H.P., Levinson, S. & Irons, G. (2009) Finding Little Albert: a journey to John B. Watson's infant laboratory. *American Psychologist,* 64(7), 605–614.

Behavioural Insights Team (n.d.) Retrieved from http://blogs.cabinetoffice.gov.uk/behavioural-insights-team/

Bell, C. (2013) Inside the Coalition's controversial Nudge Unit. Retrieved from www.telegraph.co.uk/news/politics/9853384/Inside-the-Coalitions-controversial-Nudge-Unit.html

Benjamin, L.T. Jr, Whitaker, J.L., Ramsey, R.M. & Zeve, D.R. (2007) John B. Watson's alleged sex research: an appraisal of the evidence. *American Psychologist,* 62, 131–139.

Buckley, K.W. (1989) *Mechanical Man: John Broadus Watson and the Beginnings of Behaviorism.* New York: Guilford Press.

Buckley, K.W. (1994) Misbehaviorism: the case of John B. Watson's dismissal from Johns Hopkins University. In: Todd, J.T. & Morris, E.K. (eds) *Modern Perspectives on John B. Watson and Classical Behaviorism. Contributions in Psychology,* 24. Westport, CT: Greenwood Publishing Group.

Donker, T., Griffiths, K.M., Cuijpers, P. & Christensen, H. (2009) Psychoeducation for depression, anxiety and psychological distress: a meta-analysis. *BMC Medicine,* 7(1), 79.

Evans, R.I. (1968) *B. F. Skinner: The Man and His Ideas.* New York: Dutton.

Knoff, H.M. (2004) Inside Project ACHIEVE: a comprehensive, research-proven whole school improvement process focused on student academic and behavioral outcomes. In: Robinson, K. (ed.) *Advances in School-Based Mental Health: Best Practices and Program Models.* Kingston, NJ: Civic Research Institute, Inc.

Libet, B., Gleason, C.A., Wright, E.W. & Pearl, D.K. (1983) Time of conscious intention to act in relation to onset of cerebral activity (readiness-potential): the unconscious initiation of a freely voluntary act. Brain, 106(3), 623–642.

Mkangi, A. (2010) Rational emotive behaviour therapy (REBT): A critical review. Journal of Language, Technology and Entrepreneurship in Africa, 2(1), 54–65.

Nobel Lectures (1967) Physiology or Medicine 1901–1921. Amsterdam: Elsevier Publishing Company.

Pavlov, I.P. (1893) Vivisection. Reprinted in Todes, D.P. (2001) Pavlov's Physiology Factory: Experiment, Interpretation, Laboratory Enterprise. Baltimore, MD: Johns Hopkins University Press.

Pavlov, I.P. (1927) Conditioned Reflexes: An Investigation of the Physiological Activity of the Cerebral Cortex (trans. and ed. G.V. Anrep, 2003). Mineola, NY: Dover.

Pavlov, I.P. (1928) Lectures on Conditioned Reflexes: Twenty-Five Years of Objective Study of the Higher Nervous Activity Behavior of Animals. New York: Liverwright Publishing Corporation.

Skinner, B.F. (1938) The Behavior of Organisms. Cambridge, MA: B.F. Skinner Foundation.

Skinner, B.F. (1948) Walden Two. Cambridge, MA: Hackett Publishing Company.

Skinner, B.F. (1958) Teaching machines. Science, 128(3330), 969–977.

Skinner, B.F. (1960) Pigeons in a pelican. American Psychologist, 15(1), 28–37.

Skinner, B.F. (1964) New methods and new aims in teaching. New Scientist, 22(392), 483–484.

Skinner, B.F. (1969) Contingencies of Reinforcement. New York: Appleton-Century-Crofts.

Skinner, B.F. (1972) Beyond Freedom and Dignity. New York: Bantam Books.

Skinner, B.F. (1987) The first baby tender. Reprinted in 2004 in Behaviorology Today, 7, 3–4.

Smith, N.G. & Morris, E.K. (2004) A tribute to B.F. Skinner at 100: his awards and honors. European Journal of Behaviour Analysis, 5(2), 121–128.

Spiegler, M.D. & Guevremont, D.C. (2009) Contemporary Behavior Therapy. Belmont, CA: Wadsworth Publishing Company.

Staats, A.W. (1968) Learning, Language, and Cognition. New York: Holt, Rinehart and Winston.

Staats, A.W. (1996) Behavior and Personality: Psychological Behaviorism, New York: Springer.

Stampfl, T.G. & Levis, D.J. (1973) Implosive Therapy: Theory and Technique. Morristown, NJ: General Learning Press.

Thaler, R. & Sunstein, C.R. (2008) Nudge: Improving Decisions about Health, Wealth, and Happiness. New Haven, CT: Yale University Press.

Thorndike, E.L. (1898) Animal intelligence: an experimental study of the associative processes in animals. Psychological Monographs: General and Applied, 2, 4.

Tryon, W.W. (2005) Possible mechanisms for why desensitization and exposure therapy work. Clinical Psychology Review, 25(1), 67–95.

Vargas, J.S. (2005) A brief biography of B.F. Skinner. Retrieved from http://bfskinner.org/about-b-f-skinner-2/

Watson, J.B. (1913) Psychology as the behaviorist views it. Psychological Review, 20, 158–177.

Watson, J.B. (1914) Behavior: An Introduction to Comparative Psychology. New York: H. Holt.

Watson, J.B. (1919) Psychology from the Standpoint of a Behaviorist. Philadelphia, PA: Lippincott.

Watson, J.B. (1930) Behaviorism. Chicago: University of Chicago Press.

Watson, J.B. & Rayner, R. (1920) Conditioned emotional reactions. Journal of Experimental Psychology, 3(1), 1–14.

Watson, J.B. (1930) Behaviorism. Chicago: University of Chicago Press.

Wolpe, J. (1958) Psychotherapy by Reciprocal Inhibition. Stanford, CA: Stanford University Press.

Chapter 5
Cognitive approach and cognitive therapy

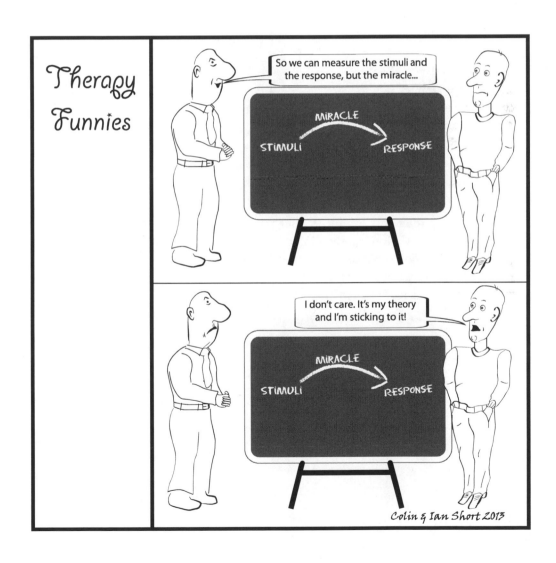

CHAPTER CONTENTS

- Introduction to cognitive approach and cognitive therapy
- Development of the cognitive approach
  - Cognitive revolution
  - Major advances in the cognitive approach
  - Key figures in the cognitive approach
- Personal and professional biographies of Ulric Neisser and Aaron Beck
  - Biography of Ulric Neisser
  - Significant learnings
  - Biography of Aaron Beck
  - Significant learnings
- Cognitive theories of human nature and personality
  - Cognitive schemata
  - Cognitive triad
  - Cognitive distortions
  - Cognition and behaviour
- Therapeutic relationship in cognitive therapy
  - Client–therapist rapport
  - Problems with cognitive therapy
- Therapeutic techniques in cognitive therapy
  - Validity testing cognitions
  - Socratic questioning
- Case study demonstrating cognitive therapy
  - Recorded session: therapy in action
  - Presentation of Fay Short: history and symptoms
  - Therapy session: analysis
  - Personal experience of the client

INTRODUCTION TO COGNITIVE APPROACH AND COGNITIVE THERAPY

This chapter aims to introduce the reader to the cognitive approach to counselling and psychotherapy. Cognitive therapy will be explored as one example of a therapeutic method under the cognitive approach.

LEARNING OUTCOMES

By the end of this chapter, you will be able to:

* describe the development of the cognitive revolution in psychology
* acknowledge the relative impact of Ulric Neisser and Aaron Beck on the development of the cognitive approach
* discuss the core theories of human nature and personality from the cognitive perspective
* discuss the nature of the therapeutic relationship between therapist and client in cognitive therapy
* outline the main therapeutic techniques utilised in cognitive therapy
* appreciate the application of cognitive therapy in a real-world setting

DEVELOPMENT OF THE COGNITIVE APPROACH

LEARNING OUTCOMES

After reading this section, you will be able to:

* list the three main forces in psychology and the subsequent revolution
* discuss the development of the cognitive approach in a historical context
* acknowledge the main contributors to the development of the cognitive approach

Cognitive revolution

Three forces in psychology

> Behavioural theory
>
> Psychodynamic theory
>
> Humanistic theory

And then . . . a cognitive revolution

Revolution began in the 1950s as a response to the three main forces in psychology

> Behaviourist psychology focused too heavily on behaviour, thus failing to appreciate the importance of cognitive mediation
>
> Psychodynamic psychology focused too heavily on unconscious drives, thus failing to account for the possibility of testing cognitions empirically
>
> Humanist psychology relied too heavily on introspection, thus failing to allow for expert guidance and understanding

Revolution was supported by advances in information technology

> Cognitive approach adopted an information-processing approach

> This approach assumed that we could explore the human mind using the analogy of the computer system because humans are essentially active information processors

Cyclical nature of research in psychology

Psychology was initially defined as the study of the human mind

> However, animal research in the early 1900s produced results that could be generalised to human behaviour

> This led to psychology being redefined as the study of human behaviour

Cognitive revolution brought psychology back to the mind

> Psychology began to be defined as the scientific study of mind again

Major advances in the cognitive approach

Initial interest in the cognitive approach

Early psychology explored issues relating to the inner workings of the mind

> Wundt explored immediate experiences of conscious processes (perception and attention)

> Titchener explored the structures of the conscious mind (perception and attention)

> Ebbinghaus explored verbal memory (memory)

> James explored the functions of consciousness (memory)

Early psychological research sought to use scientific methods to study the human mind

> However, it was not always scientific in the way that modern research would regard science

>> Wundt advocated introspection as a method for scientific observation, whereas today we would argue that an objective outsider should complete scientific observations

>> Titchener insisted on rigorous training for all subjects, whereas today we insist on naive participants

> These methods were, however, scientific in the sense that they adopted empirical measures to explore human thought processes

>> Ebbinghaus developed methods to study memory that are still used in memory research today

Focus on the mind was lost when the behavioural approach dominated psychology

> Behaviourism focused exclusively on observable and measurable behaviour

> Concept of the mind was either ignored or regarded as another (less measureable) form of behaviour

Behaviourism dominated psychology during the early 1900s

Work by Thorndike (1898), Pavlov (1928), Watson (1913) and Skinner (1938) emphasised the importance of controlled research measuring observable behaviours

Behaviourism lost favour during the 1950s

Research into the limits of human performance was essential during the Second World War

Understanding how pilots react to large control panels or how snipers attend to potential targets under pressure was a crucial contribution to the war effort

Research focus returned to the investigation of mental processes and these could not be studied effectively within the behavioural paradigm

Computer science provided a new understanding of information processing and proposed the possibility of the human mind as a type of information processor (computer analogy)

Information is encoded

Registering stimuli through your senses (eyes, ears, nose, etc.) and converting this information into a mental representation of reality

For example, hearing sounds emitting from the lips of a person and converting them into meaningful words and sentences

Similar to typing code into a computer

Information is stored

Holding information for a period of time in preparation for when it may need to be retrieved

Similar to storage in the hard drive of a computer

Information is retrieved

Recovering the stored information

Some information may be easy to retrieve

Some information may be difficult to retrieve

Similar to printing or bringing information up on the screen of a computer

'The magical number seven, plus or minus two' published by Miller in 1956

Miller provided empirical evidence for computational processes in the mind

Found that the human short-term memory is limited to seven plus or minus two chunks of information

This means that we can hold between five and nine chunks at any one time inside our heads

For example, you can remember seven digits (1, 4, 2, 6, 3, 9, 4) but the number of digits can be increased substantially if you chunk them (14, 28, 38, 24, 35, 41, 92)

Findings suggest that the human brain processes information and cannot be explained simply through the behaviourist paradigm

'A review of BF Skinner's *Verbal Behavior*' published by Chomsky in 1959

> Chomsky proposed language as an example of human activity that cannot be explained through a stimulus–response paradigm

> > Impossible to condition every word, phrase and expression so language provides evidence for active cognitive processes

> Turning point in the cognition-behaviour debate

A Study of Thinking published by Bruner in 1956

> Bruner proposed a paradigm for studying human thoughts, feelings and behaviours that differed from the accepted behavioural approach

Pinker (2002) identified five major assumptions of the cognitive approach that contributed to the move away from traditional behaviourist, psychodynamic and humanistic approaches

> Mental activity in the mind works through physical activity in the brain through a process of information, computation and feedback

> It is not possible for the mind to be a blank slate because blank slates do not do anything

> Finite combinatorial programs in the mind can generate an infinite range of behaviour

> Although there is some superficial variation in mental processes across cultures, basic mental mechanisms are universal

> The mind is a complex system composed of many interacting parts

Formal establishment of cognitive approach

Cognitive Psychology published by Neisser in 1967

> Neisser argued that perception (in particular, pattern recognition) was input, attention and problem solving were processing, and memory was output

> > 'The term "cognition" refers to all the processes by which the sensory input is transformed, reduced, elaborated, stored recovered, and used' (Neisser, 1967)

> Book had a huge impact on the field

> > Cognitive psychology became a common name and journals, courses and conferences were established in the field

Modern cognitive approach

Cognitive psychology is a thriving research field

> Rapid advancements in computer systems and artificial intelligence continue to influence the development of cognitive theories

Interdisciplinary work is common in modern cognitive psychology

> Cognitive neuropsychology is a common synthesis of research in cognition and research in neuroscience

Key figures in the cognitive approach

Albert Ellis (1913–2007)

Impact on the approach

> Founded rational therapy – original form of cognitive therapy

> Eventually developed rational therapy into rational emotive behaviour therapy (REBT) – earliest form of cognitive-behaviour therapy

> Emphasised the importance of rational thought processes and the dangers of thinking in terms of absolutes

Selected works

> 'Rational psychotherapy and individual psychology' published in 1957

Jerome Bruner (1915–current)

Impact on the approach

> Educational psychologist

> Introduced the concept of scaffolding for supporting the development of learners in education

> Found that poorer children overestimated the physical size of coins (but not similar-sized discs) due to their interpretation of the coins as high value ('New Look' experiments)

> Emphasised the importance of interpretation in reactions to stimuli and noted that this could not be explained with behavioural theories

> Formally established the study of cognitive psychology

Selected works

> 'Value and need as organizing factors in perception' published in 1947

> A Study of Thinking published in 1956

George Miller (1920–2012)

Impact on the approach

> Linguist and computer scientist

> Worked with Chomsky to critique the behavioural approach

> Argued that complex human processes (such as memory) could not be explained by measuring only the behavioural response

> Identified the magical number 7 (human short term memory holds +/- 7 chunks of information)

> Memory research supported the theory of cognitive processes

Selected works

> 'The magical number seven, plus or minus two' published in 1956

Aaron Beck (1921–current)

Impact on the approach

> Applied concepts from cognitive psychology to mental health
>
> Devised the Beck Depression Inventory
>
> Established the cognitive triad and cognitive distortions to explain depression and developed a cognitive approach to treatment

Selected works

> *Cognitive Therapy and the Emotional Disorders* published in 1975
>
> *Depression: Clinical Experimental and Theoretical Aspects* published in 1967

Noam Chomsky (1928–current)

Impact on the approach

> Linguist and political activist
>
> Worked with Miller to critique the behavioural approach
>
> Argued that the concept of learned verbal behaviour (Skinner) was an impossible application of behavioural theory and claimed that behaviourism was both simplistic and superficial as an explanation for human language
>
> Criticisms of the behavioural approach paved the way for the cognitive revolution

Selected works

> 'A review of BF Skinner's *Verbal Behavior*' published in 1959

Ulric Neisser (1928–2012)

Impact on the approach

> Often identified as the founding father of cognitive psychology
>
> Combined work in the fields of perception, attention, problem solving and memory to produce a comprehensive information-processing theory
>
> Highlighted the importance of ecological validity in cognitive research
>
> Challenged behaviourist assumptions

Selected works

> *Cognitive Psychology* published in 1967
>
> *Cognition and Reality* published in 1976
>
> *Memory Observed* published in 1982

Donald Meichenbaum (1940–current)

Impact on the approach

> Focused on changing cognitions by modifying the 'inner dialogue' through psychotherapy

Integrated cognitive and behavioural theories to form cognitive-behaviour modification – original form of cognitive-behaviour therapy (alternative to REBT proposed by Ellis)

Selected works

Cognitive-Behaviour Modification: An Integrative Approach published in 1977

SUMMARY

Cognitive revolution: behavioural, psychodynamic, humanistic; cognitive revolution supported by advances in information technology

Major advances: initial ideas focused on cognition (Wundt, Titchener, Ebbinghaus, James) using semi-scientific methods, then behaviourism dominated the field in the early 1900s, computer science and WW2 reinspired research interest in the mind, Miller and Chomsky and Bruner highlighted problems with radical behaviourism and proposed cognitive alternative in 1950s, Pinker gave five major assumptions leading to the move from behaviour to cognition (mental activity in mind worked through physical activity in brain, mind is not a blank slate because blank slates do not do anything, finite programs create an infinite range of behaviours, superficial variation across cultures but basic mental mechanisms are universal, mind is a complex system composed of many parts); formally established in 1960s with publication of *Cognitive Psychology* by Neisser; modern approach is an interdisciplinary thriving research field

Key figures: Ellis' rational therapy, Bruner's scaffolding for learning, Miller's magical number seven, Beck's cognitive triad, Chomsky's critique of behaviourism, Neisser as the founding father of cognitive psychology, Meichenbaum's cognitive-behaviour modification

PERSONAL AND PROFESSIONAL BIOGRAPHIES OF ULRIC NEISSER AND AARON BECK

LEARNING OUTCOMES

After reading this section, you will be able to:

* outline the personal and professional biography of Ulric Neisser (1928–2012)

* outline the personal and professional biography of Aaron Beck (1921–current)

* appreciate the impact of these key figures on the development of cognitive therapy

Biography of Ulric Neisser

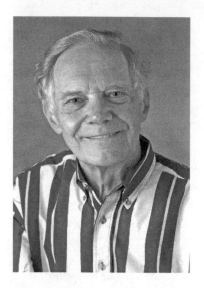

'I was not "the father of cognitive psychology", just the godfather who named it.'
—Neisser (2002)

Who was Ulric Neisser?

Neisser is regarded as the father of the modern cognitive approach

> Challenged the behavioural approach to produce a comprehensive information-processing theory

> Highlighted the importance of ecological validity in cognitive research

Early years

Born on 8th December 1928 in Kiel, Germany

> Father (Hans Neisser) was an economist and mother (Charlotte) was active in the women's movement

Left Germany for the US when he was four years old

> Father came from a distinguished Jewish family and was an anti-Nazi Social Democrat so he moved his family out of Germany for their own safety shortly after Hitler established power

> Father took a position at the University of Pennsylvania

Happy childhood in Swarthmore, Pennsylvania

> Father earned a good salary as an academic

Minor difficulties during his teens due to German heritage

> Academically advanced (good grades, member of the Honor Society), but poor with sports, peers and girls

> Described himself as a 'weird outsider' (Neisser, 2002)

> Determined to be '100% American' to distance himself from the German enemy of the war (Neisser, 2002)

Adopted the name Dick or Dickie because Ulric was too German

Led to his rejection of the cultural and academic values of his German parents

Failed to really appreciate his own heritage – did not even know that his father was Jewish or understand that he could have ended up in a concentration camp if they had remained in Germany (Neisser, 2002)

Expected to pursue a career in science

Parents were highly academic and he felt in competition with his 'all-knowing' father (Neisser, 2002)

Although he performed well academically, he did not really understand scientific theory and had never heard of psychology until he started university (Neisser, 2002)

Education

Studied psychology major at Harvard University from 1946 to 1950

Changed his major to psychology after taking a course covering sensation, perception and learning

Decided to become an experimental psychologist

Sought to 'fight the good fight against behaviourism' (Neisser, 2002)

Also intrigued by parapsychology and the study of extrasensory perception

Established the Harvard Society for Parapsychology (Neisser, 2002)

Although he did not continue research in this area, he did attribute his love of controversial experiments to this early experience

Graduated with a Bachelor's degree *summa cum laude* in 1950

Studied postgraduate psychology at Swarthmore College from 1950 to 1952

Attracted by the recent appointment of Wolfgang Kohler which appealed to his appreciation of Gestalt psychology (perceived to be in opposition to behavioural)

Little contact with Kohler during his degree, but did establish friendship with George Miller and moved away from Gestalt theories

George Miller introduced him to information theory

Graduated with a Master's degree in 1952

Studied postgraduate psychology at MIT from 1952 to 1954

Followed Miller to MIT, but he was not interested in the research

Instructor at Swarthmore from 1953 to 1954

Returned to MIT to complete studies in 1954, but was still unhappy so decided to transfer to nearby Harvard

Studied postgraduate psychology at Harvard from 1954 to 1956

Graduated with a doctorate in psychology in 1956

Family

Married Anna Pierce in 1952

> Raised three sons and one daughter

> > Divorced in 1964

Married Arden Seidler in 1964

> Arden already had three children who lived with the couple (Neisser's four children remained with their mother Anna)

> Raised one son alongside Arden's three children

> Remained married until her death

Career

Research and instructor fellowship at Harvard from 1956 to 1957

> Taught sensation and perception

Associate professor at Brandeis University from 1957 to 1965

Published *Searching for Ten Targets Simultaneously* in 1964

> Explored the fundamentals of human pattern recognition

> Provided evidence for parallel processing by demonstrating parallel visual search

> > Participants could search for ten letters as quickly as one letter

Sabbatical followed by position at the Unit for Experimental Psychiatry from 1965 to 1967

> Sabbatical was taken to complete his seminal book *Cognitive Psychology*

Published *Cognitive Psychology* in 1967

> Combined work in the fields of perception, attention, problem solving and memory to produce a comprehensive information-processing theory

> > Differed from the traditional model of information processing because it argued for parallel rather than linear processing

> Argued that perception (in particular, pattern recognition) was input, attention and problem solving were processing, and memory was output

> > 'The term "cognition" refers to all the processes by which the sensory input is transformed, reduced, elaborated, stored, recovered, and used' (Neisser, 1967)

> Challenged behaviourist assumptions without aggression

> Book had a huge impact on the field

> > Cognitive psychology became a common name and journals, courses and conferences were established in the field

> > Neisser became known as 'the father of cognitive psychology' (Neisser, 2002)

Professor of psychology at Cornell University from 1966 to 1983

> Introduced to Gibson who highlighted the importance of ecological validity and realism in research studies

Published *Cognition and Reality* in 1976

> Started while on sabbatical at the Center for Advanced Study in the Behavioral Sciences in Palo Alto in 1973

> Highlighted the importance of ecological validity in cognitive research

>> Direct opposition to the controlled lab studies of the behavioural approach

> Introduced the concept of the perceptual cycle

>> We hold schemata of information created by input of information which then influence the way that future information is input

>> For example, we hold a schema about how to behave in a restaurant based on our experiences in restaurants – this schema will then influence how we behave when we next visit a restaurant and this experience will reaffirm or conflict with our established schema

Delivered a revolutionary keynote address at the first Practical Aspects of Memory conference in Wales in 1978

> Emphasised the importance of addressing real-world problems using ecologically valid methods

> Argued that psychology typically failed to study anything that is interesting or socially important (Neisser, 2002)

Published *Memory Observed* in 1982

> Emphasised the importance of the ecological study of everyday memory

> Briefly covered the concept of false memories, leading to an invitation to serve on the Board of Scientific Advisors for the False Memory Syndrome Foundation

Chaired professorship at Emory University from 1983 to 1996

Published *Affect and Accuracy in Recall: Studies of 'Flashbulb' Memories* in 1992

> Flashbulb memories are vivid recollections of specific moments in time

>> Almost as though a camera flashbulb has gone off in the head to capture the event on film

>> Usually associated with major events, such as your own wedding or a national disaster

>> For example, most people can vividly recall first hearing the news about the September 11th terrorist attack

> Explored the types of errors common to flashbulb memories

> Reported on a study which compared memories for a major event over time

>> Questioned students immediately after the explosion of the Challenger space shuttle in 1986

>> Questioned students again three years later to find huge discrepancies in memory

>> Students often held inaccurate memories and, in some cases, entirely false memories for the event

For example, one student claimed to recall a girl screaming about the disaster in the corridors at her dorm yet her original report indicated that she discovered the news from friends at lunch

Argued that the past is not stored like a video tape or photograph, but is instead distorted and reshaped based on subsequent experiences

For example, the student mentioned above may have subsequently experienced someone shouting about the Challenger disaster and modified her memory of her first exposure to the news to include this new experience

Chaired an American Psychological Association task force to address the concerns raised in response to the controversial book *The Bell Curve* in 1995

Produced a comprehensive overview of knowledge on IQ testing

Retired from Emory University to work as an emeritus faculty member at Cornell University in 1996

Death

Died on 17th February 2012 at the age of 83 following a long battle with Parkinson's disease

---

FOUNDING FATHER OF THE COGNITIVE APPROACH: NEISSER

Consider the life story of Ulric Neisser and try to answer the following questions.

1. What was the social and cultural context of the world in which Neisser developed his theories?
2. How might Neisser's life experiences have impacted on his perception of human nature?
3. How can this life story contribute to your understanding of the cognitive approach?

Significant learnings

'Most of our oldest memories are the product of repeated rehearsal and reconstruction' (attributed to Neisser, n.d.)

'Cognitive processes surely exist, so it can hardly be unscientific to study them' (Neisser, 1967)

Biography of Aaron Beck

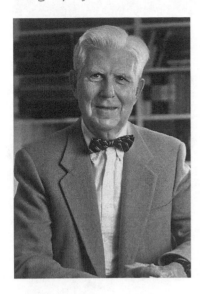

'Don't trust me, test me'
—Beck (cited by Blenkiron, 2005)

Who is Aaron Beck?

Beck founded cognitive therapy in the 1960s

> Cognitive therapy was built on the foundations of cognitive psychology laid down by Ulric Neisser

> Applied cognitive principles to the study of depression to formulate a new theory of depression and a new method of treatment

Early years

Born on 18th July 1921 in Providence, Rhode Island

> Father (Harry Beck) was a printer and mother (Elizabeth Temkin) was a housewife

> Youngest of three children (plus two children who passed away at a young age before his birth)

Depression marred his family

> Parents were Jewish immigrants from Russia

> Mother suffered with depression (Weishaar, 1993)

>> She lost two children prior to his birth and suffered with depressive mood swings

>> Her depression eased following his birth, but still existed to an extent throughout his life

>> Beck believed that he was a replacement for his deceased sister, but still felt proud that he had been able to cure his mother's depression by being born (Weishaar, 1993)

Life-threatening infection following an injury at the age of eight (Weishaar, 1993)

> Missed a great deal of school due to his illness

Experience left him with intense feelings of inferiority and fears of hospitals

Developed the ability to overcome these negative emotions by thinking rationally — first experience of the value of cognitive therapy

Education

Studied English at Brown University from 1938 to 1942 (Weishaar, 1993)

Elected member of the Phi Beta Kappa Society

Associate editor of the Brown Daily Herald

Awarded the Francis Wayland Scholarship, Bennett Essay Award and Gaston Prize for Excellence in Oratory

Graduated *magna cum laude* majoring in English and political science in 1942

Yale Medical School from 1942 to 1946

Initially interested in specialising in psychiatry, but was dissuaded by the irrational nature of theories in psychoanalysis

Graduated with a medical doctorate in 1946

Family

Married Phyllis Whitman in 1950

Met during his internship at Brown University (she was a student at the associated girl's school, the Hillel Foundation)

She matched Aaron Beck in her own career by completing a law degree and serving as a superior court judge in Pennsylvania

Raised two girls and two boys

Alice Beck — followed the career path of her mother and served as court judge

Judith Beck — followed the career path of her father and is now Director of the Beck Institute

Career

Resident in Pathology at Rhode Island Hospital from 1946 to 1948

Resident in Psychiatry at Cushings Veterans Administration Hospital from 1948 to 1949

Fellow in Psychiatry at the Austin Riggs Center from 1950 to 1952

Assistant Chief of Neuropsychology at Valley Forge Hospital in Pennsylvania from 1952 to 1954

Instructor then Associate in the Psychiatry Department of the University of Pennsylvania from 1954 to 1958

Assistant Professor then Associate Professor in the Psychiatry Department of the University of Pennsylvania from 1958 to 1971

Established the Depression Research Clinic focusing on empirical research into the causes and treatment of depression

Designed the Beck Depression Inventory in 1961

> Currently the most widely used assessment scale for the clinical diagnosis of depression
>
> Twenty-one items each presenting four options indicating current and recent emotional and cognitive states – each item is rated and the total score indicates the level of depression
>
> For example:
>
> | | |
> |---|---|
> | 0 | I do not feel sad |
> | 1 | I feel sad much of the time |
> | 2 | I am sad all of the time |
> | 3 | I am so sad or unhappy that I can't stand it |
>
> Diagnosis points vary, but are generally regarded as follows:
>
> 0–10 = Normal
>
> 11–16 = Mild mood disturbance
>
> 17–20 = Borderline clinical depression
>
> 21–30 = Moderate depression
>
> 31–40 = Severe depression
>
> 40+ = Extreme depression

Published *Depression: Clinical Experimental and Theoretical Aspects* in 1967

> Introduced the cognitive triad and cognitive distortions

Professor of Psychiatry at the University of Pennsylvania from 1971

Cognitive revolution during the 1970s led to academic acceptance of cognitive therapy (Weishaar, 1993)

> In psychology, shift from behavioural measures only towards acceptance of internal cognitive processes
>
> In therapy, shift from psychoanalysis towards evidence-based methods
>
> Beck was invited to give lectures in cognitive psychology at many institutions and is regarded as the founding father of cognitive therapy

Published *Cognitive Therapy and the Emotional Disorders* in 1975

> Seminal book formalising the concept of cognitive therapy
>
> Established the theories of automatic negative cognitions and explored their impact on a wide range of mental disorders: depression, eating disorders, drug addiction, anxiety disorders, etc.
>
> Outlined clear methods for treating mental disorders

Founded the Beck Institute for Cognitive Therapy and Research in Philadelphia with his daughter in 1994

> Aim of this institute is to provide training for therapists and treatment of clients using cognitive (today predominantly CBT) methods in order to encourage the growth of this field across the world

Currently retired, but remains Professor Emeritus of Psychiatry at the University of Pennsylvania and President Emeritus of the Beck Institute for Cognitive Therapy and Research

---

FOUNDING FATHER OF THE COGNITIVE APPROACH: BECK

Consider the life story of Aaron Beck and try to answer the following questions.

1. What was the social and cultural context of the world in which Beck developed his theories?
2. How might Beck's life experiences have impacted on his perception of human nature?
3. How can this life story contribute to your understanding of the cognitive approach?

Significant learnings

'Some authors have conceptualized depression as a "depletion syndrome" because of the prominence of fatigability; they postulate that the patient exhausts his available energy during the period prior to the onset of the depression and that the depressed state represents a kind of hibernation, during which the patient gradually builds up a new story of energy' (Beck, 1967)

SUMMARY

Neisser: Father of cognitive psychology; *early years*, born 1928 in Germany but raised in US, happy childhood but some rebellion during teens due to a desire to be 'all-American' rather than German; *education*, expected to pursue a career in science, introduced to psychology at Harvard University and graduated with a doctorate; *family*, married twice and raised five children; *career*, taught at Harvard then Brandeis University, published evidence for parallel processing, published *Cognitive Psychology* which outlined the foundation of the cognitive approach, professor at Cornell University, emphasised the importance of research with ecological validity, highlighted nature of schemata, professor at Emory, explored errors in flashbulb memories and worked to address problems of false memory syndrome, chaired a task force to address controversy about the bell curve and outlined key findings in intelligence, retired but remained emeritus; *death*, died from Parkinson's disease in 2012

Beck: founded cognitive therapy; *early years*, born 1921 in Rhode Island to Jewish Russian immigrants, mother suffered depression (eased somewhat after his birth), sick as a child so missed a lot of school; *education*, graduated *magna cum laude* in English and political science, graduated with an MD from Yale Medical School; *family*, married once and raised four children; *career*, interested in psychiatry but not psychoanalysis, worked in several psychiatry departments before becoming professor at Pennsylvania, devised Beck Depression Inventory, introduced the concepts of the cognitive triad and cognitive distortions, cognitive revolution led to academic acceptance of his theories, outlined cognitive methods from treatment of mental disorders, founded the Beck Institute for Cognitive Therapy and Research with his daughter, currently retired but remains emeritus at Pennsylvania and the institute

COGNITIVE THEORIES OF HUMAN NATURE AND PERSONALITY

LEARNING OUTCOMES

After reading this section, you will be able to:

* discuss cognitive schemata
* describe the cognitive triad
* explain how cognitive distortions can influence thoughts, feelings and behaviours
* explain the link between cognition and behaviour

Cognitive schemata

Cognition

Cognition refers to the mental processes mediating between stimuli (external world) and response (our behaviour)

> Cognition is a higher-level function of the brain

> Cognition is similar to thought

>> Thought is usually a conscious process

>> Cognition is often unconscious and automatic

Cognition involves the following

> Inputting – gaining information from the world

>> Example: noticing that people avoid eating with you and often make an unusual facial expression if they see you eating

> Processing – interpreting this information for meaning

Example: interpreting the facial expression as disgust and realising that people do not like the way that you eat

Responding – behaving in an appropriate manner in response to social cues

Example: closing your mouth when you eat (or never eating in public again)

Cognitive schemata

Cognitive schemata are 'cognitive structures that represent knowledge about a concept or type of stimulus, including its attributes and the relations among those attributes' (Fiske & Taylor, 1991)

Thoughts, attitudes and beliefs about specific stimuli, such as other people, objects, events, situations, etc.

For example, our thoughts, beliefs and attitudes about school teachers

Schemata are created through experience

Our experiences will give us content to build up a schema for future use

For example, our experiences of teachers in school will combine to create a 'teacher schema' outlining our expectations for the teacher role

Four types of schemata

Person schema

Knowledge structures about specific people

Example: my dad is kind and generous, but he is not very good at telling jokes

Role schema

Knowledge about certain roles, including appropriate activities and boundaries for these roles

May be interpreted as stereotypes

Example: police officers can restrain and handcuff you, but they cannot kick or bite you

Event schema or script

Knowledge about events, including appropriate activities and behaviour

Example: you can shout and scream at a football match, but you cannot shout and scream in a lecture (well, not usually . . .)

Self-schema

Knowledge about the self

Example: I work as a lecturer and I love films

Self-schemata are complex because they are often multifaceted

Different theories argue that the self-schema is separated into different parts

Self-concept theory

> Two types of self-schema

>> Existential self – understanding that the self is an entity separate from others

>> Categorical self – understanding the various aspects of the self according to the schemata (knowledge) that we hold about the self

Self-discrepancy theory

> Three types of self-schema

>> Actual self – schema containing knowledge about how we are at the present time

>> Ideal self – schema containing knowledge about how we would like to be

>> Ought self – schema containing knowledge about how we should be

Social theory

> Three types of self-schema

>> Individual self – self as an individual with idiosyncratic traits (personal identity): schemata contain knowledge of things that make you different from every other person in the world

>> Relational self – self as human being who interacts with others: schemata contain knowledge of your personal relationships

>> Collective self – self as a member of the wider world (social identity): schemata contain knowledge of your wider associations

Schemata can operate as heuristics

Heuristics are cognitive short-cuts

> Information in the world is often limited, yet we are expected to make an appropriate response most of the time

>> Heuristics provide us with a simple judgement operation to avoid the complexities of dealing with each instance individually

> Schemata act as heuristics to provide us with a set of cognitions to allow us to quickly interpret a person or situation in order to determine a response

>> For example, our restaurant schema gives us a clear script outlining how to behave in a restaurant – we do not need to treat each restaurant as a novel experience because we can use the schema that has been already created through experience

Heuristics will not always lead to a correct inference, but it is fast and simple method for making an inference that is usually correct

> However, although heuristics can be effective in making accurate inferences in most situations, they are subject to certain errors and biases

Common errors

Overreliance on schemata

> Assumption that every situation will match our schema can lead us to generalise too widely

> Example: assuming that a dress code for one event will be similar in another event – this can lead to social anxiety

Overinfluence of extreme examples

> Schemata based on extreme examples taken from individual cases or small samples can cause us to falsely generalise to the rest of the population

> Example: media coverage of a few airplane accidents can lead us to infer that all airplanes are likely to crash – this could cause us to feel unnecessarily anxious about travelling in a plane

Ease-of-use errors

> Recently digested information is likely to have a strong impact on our schemata, thus influencing our interpretations of future information

> Example: your friend jumps out from behind a door shortly after you have finished watching a scary film so you are more likely to interpret the sudden event as a 'monster' because that thought is at the front of your mind (perhaps even unconsciously) – this could lead to high levels of anxiety

Ignoring base-rate information

> Factual statistical information may be ignored if it is uninteresting or appears irrelevant resulting in inaccurate conclusions

> Example: media images of ordinary people would be less likely to sell products, so the media present the 5% of people who are extraordinarily beautiful and we fail to appreciate the statistic, so conclude that everybody is beautiful – this could lead to low self-esteem by comparison

Schemata are both helpful and dangerous

Schemata are helpful in providing a clear and concise knowledge base for making judgements and decisions

> We can respond quickly and efficiently to similar situations and people

>> For example, my general schema about firemen means that I can react quickly in response to the orders of a fireman even though I have never met him before

> We can generalise to display appropriate behaviour in apparently novel situations

>> For example, my general schema about restaurants means that I will know how to behave in a new venue

> We can guess the internal motivations of people around us based on prior information

>> For example, my schema about my 'funny dad' means that I know why he asked me why the chicken crossed the road

Schemata are also potentially dangerous

We can commit social faux pas by making assumptions

For example, dressing in the wrong way for a nightclub because my schema is based on a different type of venue

We can form stereotypes leading to discrimination

For example, believing that a young black male is going to try to steal my wallet because my schema is based on biased crime dramas

We can make false judgements about ourselves and the world around us

For example, refusing to leave the house because my schema is based on exaggerated media reports

Cognitive triad (Figure 5.1)

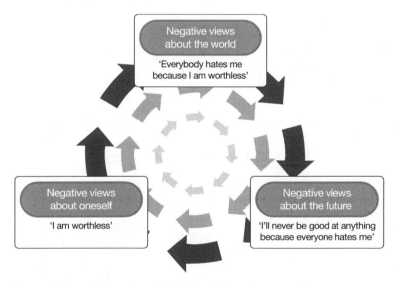

FIGURE 5.1 The cognitive triad. Adapted from Beck (1967).

The cognitive triad explains the nature of depression (Beck, 1967)

Thoughts relate to three domains

Self

World

Future

Depression occurs when these three domains are viewed negatively

The self is worthless

The world is unfair

The future is hopeless

Cognitive distortions

Three levels of cognition (Beck, 1967)

Level 1

Negative automatic thoughts

For example, 'I've got an exam tomorrow and it will be awful'

As the term 'automatic thoughts' suggests, these thoughts happen without any conscious effort

Often when clients are asked what they were thinking that caused them to feel and respond in a certain way to an event, they answer 'I don't know'

However, once they think about the thoughts they had experienced, they can remember them

Automatic thoughts are. . .

Negative, if they result in negative feelings

Closer to the surface than other levels of cognition

Usually specific to an event

Relatively easy to change

Level 2

Dysfunctional assumptions

For example, 'I always do badly at exams'

Dysfunctional assumptions are . . .

More general than automatic thoughts

Feed for automatic thoughts

More difficult to access and change than automatic thoughts

Level 3

Core beliefs

For example: 'I am worthless'

Core beliefs are . . .

Very general and affect the individual at identity level

Very difficult to access and change

Faulty negative automatic thoughts (Beck, 1975)

Distortions lead to faulty thinking

Negative cognitive triad is usually due to cognitive distortions

Many different types of cognitive distortion

Dichotomous thinking

Arbitrary inferences

      Selective abstraction

      Overgeneralisation

      Magnification

      Minimisation

      Personalisation

      Labelling and mislabelling

Dichotomous thinking

    Viewing the self, others and the world in extreme categories

    All-or-nothing thinking

      Focusing on absolute terms, such as 'always', 'every', 'never', 'must', etc.

For example, assuming that you always fail exams and never succeed in your studies and everyone else is always getting better grades than you

Arbitrary inferences

    Drawing conclusions on the basis of limited evidence

    Mind reading and fortune telling

      Assuming that others think badly of you and predicting that things will turn out badly in the future

For example, assuming that your lecturer thinks that you are stupid because you asked a question or predicting that you will get terrible questions in your final exam

Selective abstraction

    Focusing on one specific detail to the exclusion of all other information

    Mental filter

      Paying attention to one negative aspect of a situation and ignoring all of the possible positive aspects of the same situation

For example, ignoring all of the positive comments on your marked assignment and focusing only on the one critical comment

Overgeneralisation

    Generalising from a single stimulus to all stimuli

    Sweeping generalised conclusions

      Concluding that things will always be this way or that things will never change or that these things will always happen or . . .

For example, faulty thought that you will fail all of the exams on your degree because you failed one midterm

Magnification

    Magnifying negative components

    Making a mountain out of a molehill

      Overestimating or exaggerating problems and difficulties

For example, overestimating how much work is required for your next assignment so that it seems like an impossible task

Minimisation

Minimising positive components

Playing down the positive

Underestimating or ignoring positives and benefits

For example, underestimating the value of the high grades obtained in your previous assignments

FIND THE DISTORTION

Identify which cognitive distortions are being demonstrated in each of the following examples.

Simon has recently separated from his girlfriend. He feels very angry – he describes his ex-girlfriend as a 'witch' and claims 'women are only after your money'. He insists that his relationships have always ended badly and says that he will never find a woman to be able to settle down.

Julie has not been out of her house for seven months. She believes that she is ugly and thinks that people will judge her. Before she withdrew into her home, she went to the local shop and felt that the person behind the counter was staring at her. She claims that this person was probably thinking that she looked deformed – she felt nauseous so had to leave the shop immediately. She wants to be able to go out again, but she does not feel that she will ever be able to face strangers without feeling dizzy and nauseous.

Karen was planning a trip to the seaside with her niece at the weekend. Unfortunately, it is raining heavily when she wakes up on Saturday morning. She is disappointed that she will not be able go on the trip and she feels as though she has let her niece down. She states that it is all her fault that they cannot go and explains that nothing ever seems to go right for her.

John has just returned from an annual review at work. Although his boss had stressed that his sales figures had been excellent and that his customer service was exemplary, John is particularly concerned because she also mentioned that there is room for improvement in his written reports. John feels that he is not capable of doing his work any more and thinks that he should begin to look for another post before he is dismissed.

Paul has been invited to a party on Saturday night. Although he would like to go out, he has decided not to attend the party because he thinks that it will be boring. He is certain that people will ignore him and he will feel uncomfortable. He decides to stay home instead, but then feels lonely and unhappy all evening.

Personalisation

Assuming personal attributions for negative events

It's all my fault . . .

Holding the self personally responsible for uncontrollable events

For example, blaming yourself for being stupid when you fail an exam (ignoring the fact that you were sick on the day)

It's all their fault . . .

Holding others personally responsible for uncontrollable events

For example, blaming your tutor for lecturing badly when you fail an exam (ignoring the fact that you did not revise)

Labelling and mislabelling

Assigning absolute and unchangeable labels

Hard to climb out of a box

Giving the self or others or situations labels which suggest that they will always exist in that particular way

For example, labelling yourself as 'stupid' so that you no longer even try to learn or labelling an assignment as 'impossible' so that you do not even attempt to complete it

Cognition and behaviour

Are thoughts, feelings and actions inevitably linked?

If we assume that cognition leads to behaviour . . .

We can predict emotions and behaviour based on cognition

We can change emotions and behaviour by changing cognition

However, this assumption is challenged in two ways

Cognition can follow (rather than precede) behaviour in some circumstances

Cognition can be entirely disassociated from behaviour in some circumstances

Cognition can follow (rather than precede) behaviour

Research evidence has found that neurological activity responsible for the intention to act (behaviour) can precede the conscious decision to act (cognition) (Libet et al., 1983)

Participants were asked to make a voluntary response while brain activity was compared with the reported decision time

Analysis of the times revealed that the brain activated the intention to move before the participant made a conscious decision to move

These findings have been used to argue against the concept of free will

Cognition can be disassociated from behaviour

There appears to be a big difference between what people think and how people behave

Early sociology study of establishments found that many places in the US claimed that they did not serve Chinese customers, but actually did when visited by the researcher accompanied by three friends from China (LaPiere, 1934)

Little link between attitudes about alcohol and alcohol consumption (Gregson & Stacey, 1981)

Only 9% of variability in behaviour can be explained by attitudes (Wicker, 1969)

Cognitive dissonance

Cognitive dissonance is a clear example of the divide between thoughts and behaviour

Although people may not always think and do the same thing, people do like to feel that their behaviours are consistent with their attitudes

Discrepancy between thoughts and behaviour can result in cognitive dissonance

Festinger (1957) claimed that cognitive dissonance is an unpleasant state of psychological tension generated by two or more inconsistent cognitions

Two or more bits of information do not fit together so the individual feels uncomfortable

People seek harmony in their attitudes and behaviours so they will often try to reduce cognitive dissonance by changing either the thought or the behaviour

Change behaviour to fit with thoughts

Change thought to fit with behaviour

Greater cognitive dissonance will result in greater attempts to change either behaviour or thought

For example, Simon does not like his job (thought) yet he continues to go to his work place every day (behaviour) – these two experiences are in conflict (cognitive dissonance) so he will change one cognition by either quitting his job (changing behaviour) or deciding that he actually likes his job (changing thought)

Susan is aware that smoking damages your health (thought) yet she continues to smoke (behaviour) – these two experiences are in conflict (cognitive dissonance) so she will either quit smoking (changing behaviour) or begin to argue that smoking is not really too damaging (changing thought)

Link between cognition, emotion and behaviour

Absence of a direct link between cognition and behaviour leads to questions about the appropriateness of seeking to change cognition in order to change negative emotions and behaviours

Often clients may recognise their own faulty automatic thoughts and acknowledge the alternative logical thoughts, but this awareness does not lead to an improvement in emotion and behaviour

For example, an individual might be aware that he is exaggerating when he says that he cannot cope with the loss of his job, but this awareness may not reduce the depression associated with this loss

---

SUMMARY

Schemata: cognition is the mental process mediating between stimuli (external world) and response (our behaviour); schemata are thoughts, beliefs and attitudes relating to specific stimuli, based on experience, four types (person, role, event/script, self); heuristics are cognitive short-cuts, can help process information efficiently but can be dangerous due to errors; common schema errors include overreliance on schemata, extreme examples, ease-of-use errors, ignoring base-rate information

Negative cognitive triad: self is worthless, world is unfair, future is hopeless

Cognitive distortions: three levels of cognition (negative automatic thoughts, dysfunctional assumptions, core beliefs); automatic faulty thoughts are caused by cognitive distortions; distortions include dichotomous thinking, arbitrary inferences, selective abstraction, overgeneralisation, magnification, minimisation, personalisation, labelling and mislabelling

Cognition and behaviour: if cognition leads to behaviour then we can predict and change behaviour by focusing on cognition, but evidence suggests that this link is not direct; cognition can follow (rather than precede) behaviour; cognition can be dissociated from behaviour, cognitive dissonance; absence of link between cognition and behaviour raises questions about trying to change cognitions; sometimes individual is aware that cognition is faulty but still cannot change behaviour

---

THERAPEUTIC RELATIONSHIP IN COGNITIVE THERAPY

LEARNING OUTCOMES

After reading this section, you will be able to:

- describe and evaluate client–therapist rapport in the therapeutic process
- debate the potential problems associated with cognitive therapy

Client–therapist rapport

Rapport is necessary but not sufficient

Rapport is necessary

> Core conditions of humanistic approach are important for establishing a positive working relationship

> Positive relationship is vital if the client is going to collaborate with the therapist to work towards therapeutic change

> Core conditions provide a firm foundation for cognitive therapies

>> Empathy, unconditional positive regard and congruence are crucial to the success of therapy

>> Young and Beck (1980) note that an effective cognitive therapist should communicate genuineness, sincerity and openness alongside warmth and concern – they also advise using and encouraging humour to establish positive rapport

Rapport is not sufficient

> Simply providing warmth, congruency, empathy and unconditional positive regard is not sufficient for effective change

> Cognitive techniques are essential for making lasting changes

Rapport is a desirable therapist strategy for developing a collaborative therapeutic relationship (Young & Beck, 1980)

> Rapport is described as a 'harmonious accord between people' (Young & Beck, 1980)

> In terms of cognitive therapy, rapport refers to the teamwork of the therapist and client working together in comfort and security

> Rapport requires the therapist to go beyond simply showing warmth and empathy – the therapist must also be flexible enough to adapt the therapy to suit the needs of each individual (Young & Beck, 1980)

Collaborative empiricism is crucial

Some clients may have the impression that the therapist can offer a 'fix' for their problems

> In reality, however, the process of cognitive therapy is exploratory with the aim of setting goals and moving towards those goals in collaboration

Effective therapy depends on the client and therapist collaborating to identify and correct faulty cognitive processes

> 'Collaborative empiricism means that the patient and the therapist become co-investigators both in ascertaining the goals for treatment and investigating the patient's thoughts. Methods of guided discovery are used to help patients to test their own thinking through personal observations and experiments rather than via cajoling or persuasion' (Beck & Dozois, 2011)

Two benefits of collaborative empiricism in the therapeutic relationship (Hutton & Morrison, 2012)

> Clients are more engaged when treated as an equal partner by therapists

> Clients who are involved in the decision-making processes during therapy will learn how to make better decisions in the future outside therapy

COLLABORATIVE EMPIRICISM OR MANIPULATION?

Imagine that you are a therapist working with a client who makes the following statement.

> *'I'm just feeling really confused about everything at the moment. I mean, I love my wife but we argue about starting a family all of the time. We only just got married but it feels like I never want to be around her. I find myself trying to get out of the house whenever I can. Me and John go to the game or the pub or just chill out on the sofa at his place. I can just be myself with him. I can talk to him and he really seems to get me. I don't know. I don't think that I am ever going to be happy.'*

Consider the questions that you might now ask in order to work with your client to identify faulty thinking (cognitive distortions), set goals and establish an action plan.

Imagine that you suspect that your client is attracted to his friend but refusing to accept his own feelings. What questions could you ask to test the theory that he might be gay?

Imagine that you suspect that your client loves his wife but is afraid about starting a family. What questions could you ask to test the theory that he might have a fear of commitment?

Consider the manipulative potential in the questions that you have devised. Your work with this client has the potential to steer him in specific directions and this is a huge risk for any type of therapy, but particularly those that seek to alter cognitive processes. It is essential that all therapists are aware of this risk so that they can structure their practice towards collaborative empiricism rather than manipulation.

Problems with cognitive therapy

Who decides which cognitions should be tested?

Many people hold cognitions which are arguably irrational and/or illogical without experiencing psychological problems

For example, many religious people hold beliefs that could be interpreted as irrational (indeed, Ellis concluded that religion was irrational)

It would not be appropriate for the therapist to decide that these cognitions must be tested and corrected if found to be illogical

Many people also hold cognitions that are undeniably irrational and/or illogical without experiencing psychological problems

For example, many people who play the lottery hold the belief that they will win one day but the statistical evidence suggests that this is illogical

It would not be appropriate for the therapist to decide that all cognitions must be tested and corrected if found to be illogical

Much cognition is based on subjective, rather than objective, factors

For example, cognitions about whether a person is attractive or unattractive are based on subjective opinions rather than unbiased logic

It would be very difficult for the therapist to address the logic of subjective opinion – instead, the therapist should focus on exploring counter-opinions

Therapists must ensure that they only address cognitions if these cognitions are causing problems for the client

What happens when a cognition contributing to the negative emotion is found to be logical?

Some cognition may be found to be accurate, but may still contribute to the problem

For example, cognitions relating to the loss of a loved one may be absolutely correct ('he is never coming back, I will always miss him, etc.') and these cognitions may be contributing to the depression of the client

Therapist may need to accept that these cognitions are logical, but explore any underlying implicit cognitions that lack logic

Therapist could instead address the implicit cognition 'I cannot cope with this' by focusing on how the client has managed to cope with this situation (or similar situations) up until this point

Is it ethical for a therapist to try to change minds?

Padesky (1993) acknowledges that changing beliefs can be therapeutic, but argues that the use of cognitive therapy for this sole purpose might undermine the empirical basis of the approach

Therapists who decide that a thought is illogical and guide the client towards changing their thoughts in that direction are arguably manipulating the mind of the individual in their own preferred direction

For example, the therapist who believes that abortion is morally wrong could guide the client towards an unwanted birth by questioning the logic of 'I will not be able to cope with a child right now'

Evidence for false memory insertion has often been associated with psychodynamic therapy, but there is a case to suggest that the process of changing cognitions could lead to similar problems

> For example, the therapist who repeatedly questions the logic of the client who runs away from home could force the client to assume a defensive position by justifying the actions with a belief about abuse

Alongside individual ethical concerns, there are social concerns related to the potential for cognitive manipulation on a wider scale

> Cognitive therapy (and CBT) are strongly promoted as the primary solution to many psychological problems

>> National Institute for Health and Clinical Excellence stated that computerised CBT should be offered to patients meeting the criteria for mild depression and individual CBT with antidepressant medication should be offered to patients meeting the criteria for moderate or severe depression (NICE, 2004, amended 2007)

>> UK government has highlighted CBT as the treatment of choice for those diagnosed with depression or anxiety and Health Secretary Alan Johnson promised a budget of £170 million in 2007 for the expansion of mental health therapies with the specific proviso that only evidence-based treatments such as CBT would be funded (Vaughan, 2007)

>> Given the widespread popularity of this therapeutic method, many (vulnerable) individuals are exposed to these cognitive techniques

Cognitive therapy has the potential to encourage individuals to think in ways that are more beneficial to society

>> Positivity, happiness and wellbeing have all been promoted as major targets for the government and cognitive therapy could be used as a method of encouraging these emotional states

>> Arguably, this could be interpreted as a means to control a dissatisfied general public in the face of increasing global and national difficulties

---

SUMMARY

Client–therapist rapport: core conditions are critical, rapport is a desirable strategy for developing a collaborative therapeutic relationship, but cognitive techniques are also essential because relationship rapport alone is necessary but not sufficient; collaborative empiricism is crucial to correct faulty cognitive processes experienced by the client

Problems with cognitive therapy: who decides which cognitions to test? What happens when problem cognitions are logical? Is it ethical to change minds?

THERAPEUTIC TECHNIQUES IN COGNITIVE THERAPY

LEARNING OUTCOMES

After reading this section, you will be able to:

*   discuss methods used to validity test cognitions
*   discuss the use of Socratic questioning in guided discovery

Validity testing cognitions

Cognitive validity refers to the accuracy of the thought

Some people hold cognitions that are demonstrably inaccurate

> For example, a clinically underweight woman who believes that she is overweight holds an inaccurate cognition

> In these cases, the validity of the cognition can be tested directly

Some people hold cognitions that are subjective and inconclusive

> For example, a woman of average appearance who believes that she is ugly

> In these cases, the validity of the cognition may not be tested directly, but weight can be added to the opposing argument

In therapy, the client is encouraged to test cognitions for validity to identify distortions (Beck, 1975)

Identifying distortions for validity testing

Distortions are not problematic *per se* but can cause problems in some cases

> For example, an individual who believes that he has heard the voice of God offer words of comfort during difficult times might be classed as someone who is harbouring an irrational or illogical cognition; however, this belief is psychologically healthy because it does not lead to problems

> In contrast, an individual who believes that he has heard the voice of God order him to kill someone might also be classed as someone who is harbouring an irrational or illogical cognition and this belief is likely to be dangerous and lead to problems

Cognitive therapy is used only for those cognitions that may be causing some problems

> For example, a client suffering depression who holds the cognition that everybody hates him might benefit from testing this cognition for validity with the aim of reducing depressive symptoms

Defending the thought

Cognitions can be tested for validity by asking the client to defend the thought

> Client must provide evidence to support their belief in that cognition
>
> > For example, a client suffering depression who holds the cognition that everybody hates him might be asked to show evidence that everyone hates him
>
> The therapist will constantly question client to reveal the distortions and faulty logic until eventually the client must accept that the cognition is invalid
>
> > For example, a client suffering depression who holds the cognition that he is useless and everybody hates him might be asked 'what about your mum/ girlfriend?', etc.
>
> Invalid cognitions can be discarded and new valid cognitions can take their place

TESTING COGNITIONS

Consider the following examples of potentially faulty cognitions and try to devise methods for testing these ideas against reality. It is important to consider the potential outcomes of these tests and how the client could be assisted in understanding these outcomes.

I need to drink to get through my day. I have a really stressful job and a couple of glasses of wine in the evening help me to wind down. Nothing else really does the trick. If I don't drink, I am going to be even more stressed and I won't be able to cope.

I can't go out because everyone will stare at me. And they will think that I look stupid and ugly. They will know that I am a freak and they will laugh at me. It is safer for me to stay at home.

I don't give presentations. I am just too nervous. If I try to talk in front of people, I will start to panic. I will go bright red and then my voice will go squeaky. I will start to feel hot and dizzy and I might pass out. That would be horribly embarrassing.

If I go up something high, I will start to panic and then I will definitely fall. My legs are not strong enough to support me and they will start to shake. I will not be able to stay safe and I could end up dying.

People think that I am stupid. I don't want to go to school because the teachers think that I'm thick. They talk down to me and treat me like an idiot. There's no point anyway because I'm not going to pass any of my exams.

I am rubbish at everything. I always mess it up. The world would be a better place if I was not here at all.

Experimentation

Cognitions can be tested for validity by asking the client to conduct an experiment

> For example, a depressed client might be encouraged to test his belief that he always fails at everything in order to replace this faulty and irrational cognition with a more logical and rational cognition

>> Client who has recently lost his job might suffer depression because he believes that he is a failure

>> Therapist might encourage the client to test this belief that he is a failure by exploring past experiences and trying new experiences

>> He might be asked to consider previous tasks and list times when he has succeeded in order to determine whether he really does always fail at everything

>> He might be asked to try a new skill (such as cooking a particular meal) to determine whether he really does fail at everything

Socratic questioning

Socrates the teacher

Socrates was an educator in ancient Greece

> Socrates taught Plato and Aristotle

>> Plato wrote much of his work because Socrates rarely committed his methods and theories to paper

Socrates appreciated the value of making the pupil find his or her own answers

> Socratic questions are designed to encourage the learner to discover the answers by engaging in deeper thought about the issue in question

> Socratic questions will help to establish critical thinking skills

Types of Socratic question

Six types of Socratic question

> Questions aiming to clarify thinking

>> Ask the speaker to explain in more detail

>> For example, can you rephrase that?

> Questions aiming to probe assumptions

>> Ask the speaker to question his or her own assumptions

>> For example, how could you verify or disprove that?

> Questions aiming to establish evidence

>> Ask the speaker to provide real evidence or rationale

>> For example, can you give me an example of this?

Questions aiming to explore alternative perspectives

> Ask the speaker to consider the argument from the viewpoint of another person

> For example, what is the counter-argument for this?

Questions aiming to investigate possible implications

> Ask the speaker to consider the possible outcomes

> For example, what are the possible consequences of that?

Questions aiming to question the question

> Ask the speaker to consider why that question was asked in the first place

> For example, why was that question important?

SOCRATIC DINNER PARTY

Imagine that you are hosting a dinner party. Choose six guests from history, literature, film, etc. and list their names in the table below. Now try to think of some questions that you would like to pose to each of your guests. How could you use the Socratic method to explore these areas of interest?

Guest	Questions

Consider how your questions could guide the speaker towards disclosure. Is there a risk to this level of guidance?

Guided discovery in therapy

Socratic questioning can be used to guide discovery during the therapeutic process

Effective guided discovery uses Socratic questions that the client has the knowledge to answer, draws the attention of the client to relevant information that exists outside current focus, and shifts the client from the concrete to the abstract so that the new conclusions can be used to re-evaluate previously held cognitions (Padesky, 1993)

Padesky (1993) identifies the following 'good' Socratic questions for therapy

Have you ever been in similar circumstances before?

What did you do?

How did that turn out?

What would you do now that you didn't know then?

What would you advise a friend to do?

Padesky (1993) highlights the importance of Socratic questions in guided discovery

Four stages to the guided discovery process

1. Gaining information
2. Listening
3. Summarising
4. Synthesising

This cycle can be repeated throughout a session in order to guide the client towards discovering more about his own cognitions

Client: My kids hate me. I am just rubbish at everything.

Therapist: You sound really angry about that. Have you managed to do anything at all this week? (Gaining information to validity test the cognition)

Client: Not really. I was at work all week so I couldn't get to do anything with them at all.

Therapist: So did you go to work every day this week? (Listening has led the therapist to pick up on the fact that the client has been to work all week)

Client: Yeah. I had to finish a project for a customer so I was in every day until late. It meant that I couldn't get home before eight all week.

Therapist: So you successfully went to work every day and managed to complete a project for a customer? (Summarising to draw attention to the main points of the revelation)

Client: Yeah.

Therapist: I am just feeling a little confused about how this all fits together. You mentioned earlier that you are rubbish at everything but how does this fit with your success in getting this project done? (Analytical questions to encourage the client to apply the new information to the original cognition)

Client: Okay, I guess it doesn't. I am not rubbish at everything. I am just finding it hard to balance work and home.

The overgeneralisation distortion has now been identified and corrected to allow the client to now focus on the real problem

SUMMARY

Validity testing cognitions: cognitive validity is the accuracy of thoughts, some thoughts are demonstrably inaccurate, some thoughts are subjective; therapy identifies distortions for validity testing (only those causing problems); validity testing is done by working to logically defend the thought (indefensible thoughts must be faulty) or experimentation (experiments to test the thought)

Socratic questioning: questions aiming to clarify thinking, probe assumptions, establish evidence, explore alternative perspectives, investigate possible implications, and question the question; guided discovery to lead the client to their own answers; Socratic questions used to aid guided discovery by gaining information, listening, summarising and synthesising

CASE STUDY DEMONSTRATING COGNITIVE THERAPY

LEARNING OUTCOMES

After reading this section, you will be able to:

- appreciate the application of cognitive therapy from the cognitive approach in a therapeutic setting

Recorded session: therapy in action

This chapter is accompanied by a recorded therapy session which is available for viewing.

This session lasts for one therapeutic hour (50 minutes) and it is presented as the initial session in a new therapeutic relationship. Prior to this session, the client will have completed an initial assessment questionnaire and the therapist will have read this paperwork to ensure familiarity with the case. This completed assessment and a full transcript of the recorded session are available.

No actors are used in this session. The client was one of the authors and the problem presented was genuine. The therapist is an experienced practitioner in the field. The only 'fake' aspect of this recorded session is that the client did not really seek therapy and this is not really the first session of a series of therapeutic contacts.

After the conclusion of the session, the therapist is invited to answer a few key questions about the session. This question and answer session lasts no longer than 10 minutes. The transcript of this session is available.

Presentation of Fay Short: history and symptoms

Fay Short has an acute fear of heights. She has recently experienced high levels of stress at her workplace and some associated physical symptoms (including headaches and backache). However, her primary reason for seeking therapy is a desire to overcome an intense fear of heights. She has previously experienced person-centred therapy for a short space of time over ten years ago, but this was unrelated to her current fears. She would like to overcome these fears during therapy so that they no longer impact on her ability to take part in activities that involve heights.

Therapy session: analysis

The therapy session can be sectioned as follows.

Introduction

> Introduction outlining basic contractual details, especially the limits of confidentiality
>
> Focus specifically on the problem presented by the client and an outline of the intended coverage in the session (map of the session)
>
> Invitation to ask questions

Story

> Client is invited to explain how the problem began, how the problem has developed over time, and how the problem impacts on current life
>
> Focus on thoughts experienced during experiences of the problem, including rating the strength of the cognition

Goals

> Cognitive therapy is explained in terms of how thoughts can influence our feelings and behaviours
>
> Explain how thoughts can be tested for validity to reduce problem cognitions
>
> Identify a specific goal for therapy in the near future

Ending

> Outline the expected duration and content of future sessions (map of the sessions)
>
> Explain that homework will be set each session, such as experiments to test validity of thought processes and diaries to record thoughts
>
> Set readings as an initial homework
>
> Reflection on how the session was experienced by the client
>
> Invitation to return for future sessions

Key questions to consider in relation to this therapy session

How could the nature of this client be understood from the cognitive perspective?

* What does the client appear to think about herself?
* What does the client appear to think about the world?
* What does the client appear to think about the future?
* Does the client hold a positive or negative view of herself, the world and the future?
* Does the client hold thoughts based on available evidence?
* Is there any indication of any cognitive distortions?
* How do the thoughts held by the client impact on her feelings and behaviours?

What is the nature of the therapeutic relationship in this cognitive therapy session?

* Is the therapist honest and open?
* Does the therapist have a good rapport with the client?
* Does the therapist challenge any cognition held by the client?
* Are there any positive or negative effects of challenges to the cognition held by the client?
* Does the therapist suggest any experiments to test cognitions?

Which cognitive techniques are demonstrated in this therapy session?

* Which Socratic questions does the therapist use?
* How does the client respond to Socratic questions?
* How does the therapist encourage the client to identify cognitive distortions?
* How does the therapist encourage the client to defend the cognitive distortions?
* Does the therapist test any cognition for validity and what is the outcome of this test?

Personal experience of the client

I felt a little bit anxious about this session because it was my first experience of cognitive therapy as a client (and I was a little worried about being filmed disclosing potentially personal information!). However, my fears began to reduce as soon as I started talking to Keith. We established a good rapport and I felt comfortable sharing my experiences with him. He seemed to be genuinely interested in my story, and this was contrary to my expectations (I had previously experienced person-centred therapy and thought that cognitive therapy might be less relationship focused and more business-like).

I shared my story with Keith at the start of the session and I quickly forgot about the camera. I found his questions both engaging and frustrating at times – I often wanted to talk about how something 'felt' but he kept drawing me back to my thought processes. Although this was initially rather challenging, I did begin to see the value of this focus as he started to explain the way that my thoughts can impact on my feelings. His explanations in the later part of the session were particularly helpful and I think that I gained a good understanding of how my thoughts are helping to maintain my problem.

During this session, I realised several things for the first time. In particular, I realised that one of my primary concerns about heights relates directly to my own self-confidence. I have a firm belief about myself – I will look stupid if I panic – and this thought leads me to evaluate myself in a negative way. This means that I feel a strong need to constantly maintain control over myself and the wider world, and I recognised that this is both irrational and impossible. This increased understanding of my own fears has helped me to understand my anxiety a little better, and I now realise that it is only by facing this fear that I might be able to 'prove' to myself that it is not always 'stupid' to lose control. Alongside my low self-confidence and need for control, I also realised that I hold a more legitimate fear of falling. This seemed very sensible to me at the start of the session (and I guess that I believed that this was why my phobia was justified). However, during the session, it became clear to me that my fear is far more exaggerated than is reasonable in the circumstances.

At the end of the session, I had a clear understanding about cognitive therapy and a road plan for the future sessions. I was confident about my ability to tackle my concerns and I actually felt quite eager to get started on some of the readings suggested in the session.

—Fay Short

REFERENCES AND BIBLIOGRAPHY

Anderson, J.R. (2009) *Cognitive Psychology and Its Implications*. New York: W.H. Freeman.

Beck, A.T. (1967) *Depression: Clinical, Experimental, and Theoretical Aspects*. Philadelphia, PA: University of Pennsylvania Press.

Beck, A.T. (1975) *Cognitive Therapy and the Emotional Disorders*. Oxford: International Universities Press.

Beck, A.T. & Dozois, D.J. (2011) Cognitive therapy: current status and future directions. *Annual Review of Medicine*, 62, 397–409.

Blenkiron, P. (2005) Stories and analogies in cognitive-behaviour therapy: a clinical review. *Behavioural and Cognitive Psychotherapy*, 33(1), 45–59.

Bruner, J.S. (1956) *A Study of Thinking*. New York: Wiley.

Bruner, J.S. & Goodman, C.C. (1947) Value and need as organizing factors in perception. *Journal of Abnormal and Social Psychology*, 42(1), 33.

Chomsky, N. (1959) A review of B.F. Skinner's *Verbal Behavior*. *Readings in the Philosophy of Psychology*, 1, 48–63.

Ellis, A. (1957) Rational psychotherapy and individual psychology. *Journal of Individual Psychology*, 13(1), 38–44.

Festinger, L. (1957) *A Theory of Cognitive Dissonance*. Stanford, CT: Stanford University Press.

Fiske, S.T. & Taylor, S.E. (1991) *Social Cognition*. New York: McGraw-Hill.

Gregson, R.A. & Stacey, B.G. (1981) Attitudes and self-reported alcohol consumption in New Zealand. *New Zealand Psychologist*, 10, 15–23.

Hutton, P. & Morrison, A.P. (2012) Collaborative empiricism in cognitive therapy for psychosis: a practice guide. Cognitive and behavioral practice. Retrieved from http://dx.doi.org/10.1016/j.cbpra.2012.08.003

LaPiere, R.T. (1934) Attitudes vs actions. *Social Forces*, 13, 230–237.

Libet, B., Gleason, C.A., Wright, E.W. & Pearl, D.K. (1983) Time of conscious intention to act in relation to onset of cerebral activity (readiness-potential): the unconscious initiation of a freely voluntary act. *Brain*, 106(3), 623–642.

Meichenbaum, D. (1977) *Cognitive-Behavior Modification: An Integrative Approach*. New York: Springer.

Miller, G.A. (1956) The magical number seven, plus or minus two: some limits on our capacity for processing information. *Psychological Review*, 63(2), 81.

National Institute for Health and Clinical Excellence (NICE) (2004, amended 2007) Clinical Guidelines for Depression in Adults. Retrieved from http://guidance.nice.org.uk/CG90

Neisser, U. (1967) *Cognitive Psychology*. New York: Appleton-Century-Crofts.

Neisser, U. (1976) *Cognition and Reality: Principles and Implications of Cognitive Psychology*. San Francisco, CA: W.H. Freeman.

Neisser, U. (ed) (1982) *Memory Observed: Remembering in Natural Contexts*. New York: W.H. Freeman.

Neisser, U. (2002) Ulric Neisser: an autobiography. Reprinted in Lindzey, G. & Runyan, W.M. (eds) (2007) *A History of Psychology in Autobiography*, 9. Washington, DC: American Psychological Association.

Neisser, U., Novick, R. & Lazar, R. (1963) Searching for ten targets simultaneously. *Perceptual Motor Skills*, 17, 955–961.

Padesky, C.A. (1993) Socratic Questioning: Changing Minds or Guiding Discovery? Invited keynote address at the 1993 European Congress of Behaviour and Cognitive Therapies, London.

Pavlov, I.P. (1928) *Lectures on Conditioned Reflexes: Twenty-Five Years of Objective Study of the Higher Nervous Activity Behavior of Animals*. New York: Liverwright Publishing Corporation.

Pinker, S. (2002) *The Blank Slate: The Modern Denial of Human Nature*. London: Penguin Books.

Skinner, B.F. (1938) *The Behavior of Organisms*. Cambridge, MA: B.F. Skinner Foundation.

Thorndike, E.L. (1898) Animal intelligence: an experimental study of the associative processes in animals. *Psychological Monographs: General and Applied*, 2, 4.

Vaughan, J. (2007) Mental health therapies: £170 million expansion. Retrieved from www.cnwl.nhs.uk

Watson, J. (1913) Psychology as the behaviorist views it. *Psychological Review*, 20, 158–177.

Weishaar, M.E. (1993) *Aaron T. Beck*. London: Sage Publications.

Wicker, A.W. (1969) Attitudes vs actions: the relationship of verbal and overt behavioural responses to attitude objects. *Journal of Social Issues*, 25, 41–78.

Winograd, E. & Neisser, U. (1992) *Affect and Accuracy in Recall: Studies of 'Flashbulb' Memories*. New York: Cambridge University Press.

Young, J. & Beck, A.T. (1980) Cognitive therapy scale: rating manual. Unpublished manuscript retrieved from http://81.31.167.73/consultant/sharif/Instruments/Clinical%20Form/CBT%20Rating%20Scale%20Manual.pdf

Chapter 6
Integrative and eclectic therapies

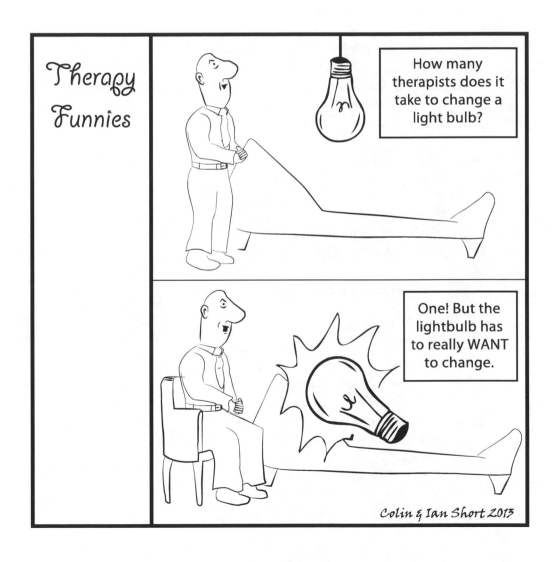

CHAPTER CONTENTS

- Application of cognitive therapy and behaviour therapy techniques
- Structure of therapeutic sessions
- Empirical evidence for CBT
- Computerised CBT
- Third Wave cognitive-behaviour therapies
- Case study demonstrating cognitive-behaviour therapy
- Multimodal therapy
  - Multimodal therapy: eclectic
  - Development of multimodal therapy
  - Basis of psychological problems
  - Assessment process
  - BASIC ID
  - Profiling
  - Tracking and bridging
  - Case study demonstrating multimodal therapy
- Neurolinguistic programming
  - Neurolinguistic programming: eclectic
  - Development of neurolinguistic programming
  - Representation systems
  - Meta model
  - Anchoring and swishing
  - Controversies in NLP
  - Case study demonstrating neurolinguistic programming

INTRODUCTION TO INTEGRATIVE AND ECLECTIC THERAPIES

This chapter aims to introduce the reader to several integrative and eclectic therapies currently practised across the world. The terms 'integrative' and 'eclectic' are used here to describe any therapy that combines two or more approaches in order to produce a novel therapeutic method (please refer to Chapter 1 for more information on integration and eclecticism).

LEARNING OUTCOMES

By the end of this chapter, you will be able to:

- describe and evaluate a range of different counselling and psychotherapy methods and techniques
- explain the origin of each therapy and indicate how they relate to the core approaches in psychology

GESTALT THERAPY

LEARNING OUTCOMES

After reading this section, you will be able to:

* explain that Gestalt therapy is an integrative therapy combining psycho-dynamic and humanistic approaches

* discuss the history of Gestalt therapy with a brief biography of Friedreich 'Fritz' Perls

* explain the importance of holism and completion

* discuss phenomenological, field and existential perspectives

* explain how we have awareness of ourselves and the environment

* discuss the disturbances of the contact boundary

* explain the paradoxical theory of change

* discuss the dialogical relationship between therapist and client

* explain how language can be grounded in the here and now

* describe and evaluate experiential learning used in therapy

* appreciate the application of Gestalt therapy in a therapeutic setting (case study)

Integration of humanistic and psychodynamic approaches

Gestalt therapy is founded in the humanistic approach, but the founder arrived at the therapy through the psychodynamic approach

Integration of person-centred and psychoanalysis therapies

Often described as an existential-humanistic approach

Awareness, choice and responsibility are the underlying aims

While Gestalt therapy is not goal directed in the same way as some other approaches (for example, cognitive-behaviour or solution-focused therapy), it does have some general aims

Fritz Perls focused on raising awareness

Awareness of self, others and the environment

Awareness of self will lead to natural change

Awareness in the here and now of experiencing will ultimately lead to greater choice

Awareness of the present will also allow for previous unfinished business to emerge, and this can be brought into the present and worked with through experiments and exercises in the therapeutic exchange

Laura Perls focused on contact and support

Modern Gestalt therapists focus on the development of the relationship, as this is the vehicle through which change is achieved

> Fritz did Gestalt therapy a disservice in his years of 'hot seat' confrontation

>> The infamous session documented with Gloria is interesting, but not representative of modern Gestalt therapy

Modern Gestalt therapy encourages clients to take responsibility for what they think, what they feel and how they behave

> Client encouraged to be mature enough in relationships to be responsible for themselves and not to take on responsibility for others (thoughts, feelings and behaviours)

> Client encouraged to be able to ask for what s/he wants and to be able to help others

Development of Gestalt therapy

History of Gestalt therapy

Established in the 1940s by Friedreich and Laura Perls

> 'Gestalt' is from the German for shape/pattern/configuration

> Gestalt therapy originated from the psychodynamic approach (Perls was trained in psychoanalysis and the first book introducing Gestalt was described as a revision of Freud's theory)

>> Use of dream analysis and focus on the disturbances of the contact boundary draws from the psychodynamic approach

> However, Gestalt is essentially an existential humanistic approach

>> Focus on the subjective experience of the individual in the here and now with recognition of the client draws from the humanistic approach

> 'Gestalt therapy is an existential-phenomenological approach and as such is experiential and experimental' (Perls, 1992)

>> Focus on the process (what is happening here and now in the therapeutic situation)

>> Focus on awareness of self, others and what lies between

First book to introduce Gestalt therapy was written by Perls in 1942 as *Ego, Hunger, and Aggression: A Revision of Freud's Theory and Method* – subtitle was changed in 1966 to *The Beginning of Gestalt Therapy*

The term 'Gestalt therapy' was coined by Perls, Hefferline and Goodman (1951) in their book *Gestalt Therapy: Excitement and Growth in the Human Personality*

New York Institute for Gestalt Therapy was established for workshops and seminars in the home of Fritz and Laura Perls in New York in 1951

> Workshops and seminars were then established throughout the country and the APA convention held a special intensive Gestalt workshop in 1954

Laura was an often-overlooked major influence in the development of Gestalt therapy

While Fritz was the charismatic showman, Laura was the organiser and supporter

'Without the constant support from his friends, and from me, without the constant encouragement and collaboration, Fritz would never have written a line, or founded anything' (Perls, 1990)

Brief biography of Friedreich 'Fritz' Perls (1893–1970)

'I do my thing and you do your thing; I am not in this world to live up to your expectations; and you are not in this world to live up to mine; you are you, and I am I, and if by chance we find each other, it's beautiful; if not, it can't be helped'
—Perls (1969, Gestalt Prayer)

Who was Friedreich 'Fritz' Perls?

Perls founded Gestalt therapy with his wife in the 1940s

Emphasised the importance of the 'here and now' within the therapeutic relationship

New type of existential humanism

Early years

Born on 8th July 1893 in Berlin, Germany

Raised in a 'disturbed' family surrounded by fighting

He claims that his mother beat him with carpet-beating rods, but she failed to break his spirit (instead, he broke the rods)

Education

Expected to study law (following in footsteps of uncle) but actually studied medicine before and after serving time in the army in WW1

Qualified with an MD and worked with injured soldiers

Career

Trained in psychoanalysis in Vienna, and undertook analysis with William Reich

Reich went on to develop Reich body analysis

Focused on psychoanalysis and established a psychoanalytic training institute in South Africa after Hitler came to power

Travelled for some time as a psychiatrist but eventually settled in the US to write up his theories of therapy

Published *Gestalt Therapy* in 1951

Co-founded the New York Institute for Gestalt Therapy with Laura Perls in 1952

Moved from New York to Big Sur, California, and was involved at the Esalen Institute

Incorporated many Zen concepts into the therapy after staying at a monastery in Japan

Established a Gestalt community in Canada

In San Francisco in the 1960s, he became famous for his work and demonstrated his confrontational style in workshops

> People were either very impressed or saw him as manipulative and meeting his own needs

> He certainly seemed to enjoy the limelight!

Family

> Married Laura Perls in 1930

> > Raised two children

> As well as being his wife, Laura Perls also worked alongside her husband to develop and promote Gestalt therapy (Leibig, 1990)

> > Laura Perls was born on 15th August 1905 in Pforzhein, Germany

> > She became interested in psychology, aged 16, after reading about dream work in literature by Freud

> > She earned a doctorate in Gestalt psychology at Frankfurt University, then studied existential philosophy as a student of Buber and worked alongside Kurt Lewin

> > She was a member of the Berlin group of Gestalt psychologists

> > She was instrumental in keeping the New York Institute for Gestalt Therapy going while Fritz travelled the world demonstrating and promoting Gestalt

> > After the death of Fritz, she continued making contributions and promoting Gestalt therapy until her own death in 1990 at the age of 85, close to her birthplace in Germany

> 'I [Laura] was a Gestalt psychologist before I got into psychoanalysis. Fritz was an analyst before he got into Gestalt psychology. Sometimes it set us an insoluble conflict' (Perls, cited by Leibig, 1990)

Death

> Died of heart failure on 14th March 1970 in Chicago, USA

Significant learnings

> 'Lose your mind and come to your senses' (Perls, 1970)

> 'Our dependency makes slaves out of us, especially if this dependency is a dependency of our self-esteem. If you need encouragement, praise, pats on the back from everybody, then you make everybody your judge' (attributed to Perls, n.d.)

> 'The only difference between the wise man and the fool is that the wise man knows he is playing' (attributed to Perls, n.d.)

> 'I am not in this world to live up to other people's expectations, nor do I feel that the world must live up to mine' (attributed to Perls, n.d.)

Holism and completion

'Gestalt' is a German word that has no direct equivalent in English. The closest words in English are *form, configuration* or *pattern*

Gestalt has a *wholeness*, a completion, about it

In order to understand something or someone, all aspects of the experience need to be taken into account and seen from the individual's perspective

Humans do not see things in isolation, but in context, and they have a predisposition to form patterns

We seek to complete 'Gestalts' and organise their experiences into meaningful 'wholes'

Anything not completed becomes 'unfinished business'

For example, we see a series of dots and we fill in the gaps to perceive it as a square

```
*    *    *    *

*                   *

*                   *

*    *    *    *
```

Or we see two familiar people shopping together, but we have never seen them spending time together before, so we fill in the gaps to make sense of the situation ('you'll never guess who I saw with . . .')

Figure and ground (Figure 6.1)

Rubin's vase (Rubin, 1915) is a well-known example of figure and ground

Depending on whether you see black or white as the 'figure', you will either see a vase or the profiles of two people

Figure comes to the forefront while the ground remains as the backdrop

Theory of figure and ground demonstrates how our attention works

This highlights how some things become important (figure) until they are completed when they can fade back into unimportance (ground)

For example, we see two familiar people shopping together, but we have never seen them spending time together before, so we fill in the gaps to make sense of the situation ('you'll never guess who I saw with . . .')

Seeing these two people together becomes the figure and everything else becomes the ground

Before seeing the two people, we might have been aware of being hungry (a previous 'figure')

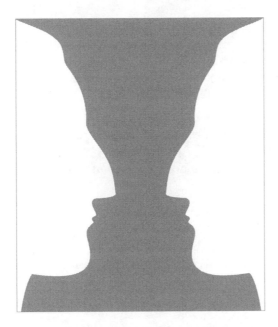

FIGURE 6.1 Figure and ground vase. Adapted from Rubin (1915).

But we are then distracted by them and forget about being hungry for a while

After we fill in the gaps (e.g. they must be in a relationship), we can go back to being aware of being hungry

Putting hunger on hold was temporary because, since we did not eat, it was an incomplete Gestalt (unfinished business)

Perspectives

Phenomenological perspective

Fritz and Laura Perls were greatly influenced by the works of phenomenological philosophers like Husserl, Heidegger and Sartre

Phenomenology looks at subjective experience from the first-person view (Woldt & Toman, 2005)

Each individual experiences the world through his or her senses

Experience is subject and creates individual realities

The best way to understand a client is to help explore his or her view of the world and to raise awareness in the present

The phenomenological perspective underpins humanistic therapy as it relies on understanding the client's world (empathy) rather than interpreting that world

This attitude towards the therapeutic encounter requires the therapist to be aware of her beliefs, attitudes, assumptions, etc. and to *bracket* off these personal experiences

Therapist must put personal experiences to one side to be available to meet the clients in their world, and to share the meanings they make of their moment-by-moment experience in the therapeutic encounter

The client is active in creating meaning, and the client and therapist together are active in co-creating the meaning of the 'what' and the 'how' of the relationship

Field theory perspective

Field theory is a concept developed by Lewin in the 1940s (Lewin, 1943)

Field theory explores interactions between an individual and the environment (total field)

The field is 'dynamic' in the sense that each part depends upon all other parts (Woldt & Toman, 2005)

This theory underpins the principle of holism – the therapist should view the client not as separate parts or separate from the environment

The client is the sum total of thoughts, feeling, behaviours, physical sensations, past and current experiences, social and cultural influences

We are not separate from our environment; we are part of it and influence it as it influences us

In Gestalt therapy, the immediate field is the therapeutic relationship in the moment-by-moment experience

Existential perspective

Existentialism states that the starting point of philosophical thinking must be the experiences of the individual (Woldt & Toman, 2005)

Existential choice lies at the heart of what it means to be human

We choose what we think, what we feel and how we behave

Therefore we have choice, maybe not for our situation but in how we respond to that situation

Individuals have to deal with four major themes or ultimate concerns in life (Yalom, 1980)

Isolation

Social beings have the need for interaction

Interactions give a sense of belonging

This interaction is important for self-esteem

Meaningless

The big 'meaning of life' question

We strive to make sense of, and give meaning to, our lives

Having a meaning provides the motivation to live fully

Mortality

We need to come to terms with the inevitability of death

Some people turn to religion with the belief of an afterlife

Family and friends may surround us, but we die alone

Freedom

We give up some freedom in order to have relationships, thus we avoid isolation

But we still have freedom to choose the way we respond to situations (how we think, feel and behave)

Individuals have to act and take responsibility for their actions

Existential therapy places the subjective experience of the client central to the therapeutic process

Awareness of self and environment

Zones of awareness

There are three zones of awareness (Perls, 1969)

The division of awareness into three zones is useful in helping the client focus on all aspects of self and identify the location of the focus of attention at any one time

However, Gestalt therapy is holistic, thus it is noted that these zones are interconnected

Inner zone

This is our inner world

It includes bodily sensations, tension, relaxation, emotions, etc.

It may not be within the awareness of the individual

In therapy . . .

This information is not available to the therapist

But the therapist may help a client focus on this awareness by directing her to focus on what she can become aware of

For example, the therapist might say 'spend a minute becoming aware of what is going on for you inside – notice how you are sitting – notice where you have any points of tension – focus on your breathing – pay attention to your emotional state . . .'

Middle zone

This is our thinking zone

It includes our images, fantasies and reactions

It makes sense of our experiences, giving meaning and understanding

In therapy . . .

Therapist may help a client focus on this awareness by asking for specific client thoughts

For example, the therapist might say 'what are you thinking now?', 'what do you think of being asked to focus on what is happening inside?', 'notice any images you have, etc . . .'

Outer zone

This is about our contact with, or withdrawal from, the outside world

This is where an individual meets the environment

We need to be aware of what is going on in the world and how we relate to the world

In therapy . . .

Therapist may help a client focus on this awareness by directing focus towards the environment

For example, the therapist might say, 'be aware of what you can see around you – notice what sounds you can hear – how are you present in this relationship?'

Freedom of movement

In order to experience all aspects of life fully, we need to be able to move freely between these different zones

For example, we might be aware of how something in the environment (negative behaviour of a loved one) is affecting us internally (tightening in the stomach) and then make a decision (I need to challenge that behaviour)

However, it is possible to be predominantly focused in one area and this can lead to problems

For example, a teenager may be incapable of making decisions without knowing what other people would say about him or a woman may be obsessed with body image

Gestalt cycle

Also known as the cycle of awareness or cycle of experience

Gestalt cycle has seven stages (Clarkson, 1989) (Figure 6.2)

1. Sensation

Something emerges from the background and draws our attention

We sense and feel things

2. Awareness

These feelings and sensations come into awareness

Our awareness is raised

We become interested and notice the sensation

This then becomes a new figure

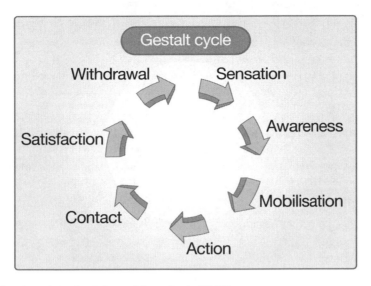

FIGURE 6.2 The Gestalt cycle. Adapted from Perls (1969).

3. Mobilisation

  We prepare ourselves to take action in order to satisfy the need

  Decisions are made and action is planned

4. Action

  We engage in activity in order to satisfy the need

  Action occurs at the boundary between self and the environment

  It precedes full contact

5. Contact

  We become fully involved in the action

  We are fully engaged with others or the environment

  At some point we become aware of a sense of completion

6. Satisfaction

  We become more aware that the need for action has been satisfied. We can identify and enjoy the sense of satisfaction and completion

  There is acceptance and integration and we are ready to withdraw

7. Withdrawal

  We finish with the action and feel satisfied

  We lose interest and let go of that particular figure

  There is a move back to equilibrium

  The next figure can now emerge for the cycle to begin again . . .

Cycles of Gestalt can be small or large and can run over a short term or long term

> For example, as you sit reading, you may become aware of a sensation in your body, maybe your back is stiff from sitting reading too long – you decide it is time for a break, maybe time to get up and walk around, stretch a little – you get up, engage in the activity of moving and after a few minutes feel ready to sit down again and resume reading – this is a complete simple Gestalt

> For example, a couple have been married for 22 years but the woman has slowly become aware of a growing dissatisfaction with the relationship. Having tried to ignore it, she now pays attention to the feeling, thinks and plans to do something about it – she may choose to leave the relationship, take action and fully engage in that process. This is a major life-changing event but is ultimately a good move for her and, after a time, she sees herself as a single woman again

If we move through all seven stages, we will complete the Gestalt and be available for the next figure to emerge

> This process of completion, or the desire to complete, is a key principle of Gestalt therapy, known as 'organismic self-regulation' (Yontef, 1993)

> However, at any stage, the cycle could become blocked by one of the boundary disturbances

>> If this happens, then the Gestalt is not completed and becomes unfinished business, retaining a hold over the individual

EXPERIENCING THE GESTALT CYCLE – PART 1

Stop reading for a minute and pay attention to what emerges from the temporary equilibrium.

Work through an example of a complete Gestalt – go through the seven stages and back to equilibrium, then try to describe your experiences below.

Sensation	
Awareness	
Mobilisation	
Action	
Contact	
Satisfaction	
Withdrawal	

Contact boundary

Distinction between self and environment

'A person exists by differentiating self from other and by connecting self and other'
—Yontef (1993)

Boundary between the self and the rest of the world allows us to . . .

Establish a healthy sense of independence by acknowledging the boundary limits

Make contact with the rest of the world by consciously reaching across the boundary

Firm yet permeable contact boundary

Boundary must be firm enough to allow autonomy of thoughts, feelings and behaviours

Boundary must be permeable enough to allow exchanges to occur between self and others

Disturbances of the contact boundary

Boundary can become too firm (impermeable) or too permeable (infirm)

An impermeable boundary may lead to isolation

Isolation involves a loss of contact between the individual and the rest of the world

For example, the woman who insists that she does not need anyone in her life might be experiencing isolation

An infirm boundary may lead to being unclear about the sense of self in relation to other

Blurred sense of self involves a tendency to blindly accept the opinions, beliefs and values of others

For example, the man who believes that he is stupid because his high school teacher once accused him of stupidity might have a blurred sense of self

Seven patterns of boundary disturbance (Polster & Polster, 1988)

Retroflection

Introjection

Projection

Confluence

Deflection

Desensitisation

Egotism

Conceptually similar to the ego defence mechanisms described in psychoanalysis

Retroflection involves resisting the impulse to take action in the environment

Behaviour is internalised so that the individual behaves towards the self in the way that s/he would like to behave towards another OR in the way that s/he would like others to behave towards them

For example, self-harming in response to anger towards your boss

Introjection involves the internalisation of the environment without critical evaluation

Thoughts, attitudes and opinions of others are accepted and internalised without consideration of whether they are accurate and these introjected values are then imposed on the self

For example, student who believes that he is stupid because his high school history teacher once told him that he was stupid

Projection involves the attribution of unacceptable aspects of the self to the environment

Elements of the self which do not fit with the acceptable self-image are disowned and attributed to other people

For example, man who insists that everyone else is 'gay' because he is refusing to accept his own sexuality

Confluence involves a loss of the distinction between the individual and the rest of the world

Individual feels obligated or constrained to certain elements of the environment

For example, the woman who lives only for her children might be experiencing confluence

Deflection involves a failure to recognise or acknowledge aspects of the environment

Avoiding contact with or awareness of someone or some situation

For example, woman who wants to avoid confronting a colleague so instead does not look at her, talks about her rather than to her, remains vague when asked about the problem, and changes the subject when the disagreement is raised

Desensitisation involves a failure to attend to feelings and sensations

Feelings and sensations are neglected

This might be a bad thing; for example, we may ignore a chest pain because we are fearful of what it might mean

This might also be a positive thing; for example, when running a marathon we might become desensitised to the tiredness in our legs or a blister on our foot

Egotism involves dissociation with the environment to become a neutral observer

Egotism 'is characterised by the individual stepping outside of himself and becoming a spectator or a commentator on himself and his relationship with the environment' (Clarkson, 1989)

We are not truly in the experience if we are observing it from the outside

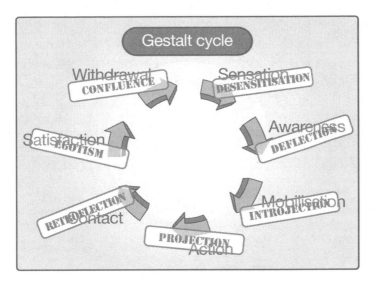

FIGURE 6.3 Boundary disturbances in the stages of the Gestalt cycle. Adapted from Perls (1969).

For example, people on holiday who only experience things through a video camera – they are so busy recording the holiday that they miss out on the first-hand experience of it

Disturbances at the contact boundary will interrupt a Gestalt from completing the Gestalt cycle

Seven boundary disturbances correspond to the seven stages of the Gestalt cycle (Figure 6.3)

Sensation may be interrupted by desensitisation

Awareness may be interrupted by deflection

Mobilisation may be interrupted by introjection

Action may be interrupted by projection

Contact may be interrupted by retroflection

Satisfaction may be interrupted by egotism

Withdrawal may be interrupted by confluence

Any incomplete Gestalts represent unfinished business

Many small Gestalts will be attended to in the short term

For example, we can delay going to the toilet when we are stuck in traffic by distracting ourselves for a short time, but the sensation will come back stronger to remind us that we need to take action

Other Gestalts are more complex

For example, we can delay the experience of bereavement by staying busy with funeral arrangements and this complex Gestalt takes a lot of energy to suppress while it remains incomplete

EXPERIENCING THE GESTALT CYCLE – PART 2

Think back to the previous activity – you stopped reading for a minute and paid attention to what emerges from the temporary equilibrium by working through an example of a complete Gestalt.

Consider the seven boundary disturbances – how could these have blocked your completion of this Gestalt?

How would it feel to be blocked in the completion of this Gestalt and how could you overcome the disturbances to ensure successful completion?

Go back through the seven stages with consideration of possible blocks at each stage, then write your experiences below.

Sensation blocked by desensitisation	
Awareness blocked by deflection	
Mobilisation blocked by introjection	
Action blocked by projection	
Contact blocked by retroflection	
Satisfaction blocked by egotism	
Withdrawal blocked by confluence	

Paradoxical theory of change

'Change occurs when someone becomes what he is, not when he tries to become what he is not'

—Beisser (1970)

This concept is about having respect for the self in the here and now

> Acceptance of the self as it is right now, without any demand for change

> Rather than trying to change to meet some preconceived idea of self, we need to become more aware and more accepting of ourselves in the present

> Once we do this, we will have already have made a significant change and other changes will follow naturally

Change is not possible unless the individual is truly aware of the self as it currently exists

> Awareness and acceptance of who you are now open the possibility of future change

We cannot change through coercion or pressure from others

> Acceptance of the individual as we exist at that moment is essential in order for us to change

> Consider attempting to move a stubborn donkey – the more you pull on his reins, the more he will insist on staying still

>> However, if you stop pulling and accept that he will stay as he chooses, then he will probably choose to move because he now has the freedom in which to make that choice

In therapy, the therapist must promote acceptance by focusing on the here and now

> The therapist should demonstrate respect for who the client is at this moment in time, yet recognise his or her potential for growth and change

> The therapist should provide a safe and non-judgemental environment focusing on how the client is at the present time in order to encourage the client to accept the self and open the possibility for future change

Topdog/underdog

Perls used the Gestalt terms 'topdog/underdog' to refer to intrapersonal conflicts similar to the Freudian concept of superego and ego

> Clients come into therapy because they want to make changes in their lives, to overcome or manage problems, or to live life more fully

Gestalt therapists resist taking on the role of the instigator of the change process, as this sets them up as expert when they want to develop a relationship of equals

> It would create a topdog/underdog relationship between therapist and client

> 'The Gestalt therapist believes that the topdog/underdog dichotomy already exists within the patient, with one part trying to change the other, and that the therapist

must avoid becoming locked into one of these roles. He tries to avoid this trap by encouraging the patient to accept both of them. One at a time, as his own' (Beisser, 1970)

Relationship between topdog and underdog shows the nature of internal conflict

The topdog is authoritarian, making demands ('You should/shouldn't' and 'you must/mustn't')

The internal response from the underdog is defensive, sometimes apologetic but always manipulative

The underdog has effective strategies for getting what it wants

The battle between topdog and underdog is ongoing

'The person is fragmented into controller and controlled. This inner conflict, the struggle between the topdog and the underdog, is never complete, because topdog as well as underdog fight for their lives' (Perls, 1969)

Dialogical relationship

Change process in Gestalt occurs through the relationship between client and therapist

Quality of the relationship is determined by the quality of the ongoing contact

Gestalt dialogue embodies authenticity and responsibility (Yontef, 1993)

Gestalt therapist does not manipulate the client towards a goal, but instead engages the client in dialogue

Directing a client towards a goal leads to a lack of responsibility, failure to accept ownership and dependency on others

Dialogue requires the therapist to show his or her true self and be honest (congruent) in the exchange

'Gestalt therapist says what s/he means and encourages the patient to do the same' (Yontef, 1993)

Four characteristics of dialogue (Yontef, 1993)

Inclusion

Inclusion is similar to the Rogerian concept of empathy

It is being aware of the experience of the client from their phenomenological viewpoint

It is without judgement, and so offers unconditional positive regard

This creates a safe place for the client to fully experience his or her own world

Presence

Presence in Gestalt is about the therapist being active in the process

The therapist will use appropriate self-disclosure statements to share thoughts, feelings and experiences, thus modelling to the client how to get in touch with immediate phenomenological experiencing and helping the client to become more aware of self in the process

'In Gestalt therapy the therapist does not use presence to manipulate the patient to conform to pre-established goals, but rather encourages patients to regulate themselves autonomously' (Yontef, 1993)

Commitment to dialogue

Commitment to dialogue is about the contact between therapist and client

The dialogical relationship is central to the Gestalt therapeutic process, and again the therapist can model to the client how to 'do' the relationship

The therapist is committed to the process and to being an equal in that process – not intending to control or manipulate the client

Dialogue is lived

Put simply, the relationship between therapist and client is active and lived out in the here and now

There is immediacy about the ongoing relationship – it is done, not talked about

Along with verbal communication, non-verbal communication is also part of this lived dialogue

Immediate dialogue between client and therapist

'Gestalt therapy emphasizes that whatever exists is here and now and that experience is more reliable than interpretation. The patient is taught the difference between *talking about* what occurred five minutes ago (or last night or 20 years ago) and *experiencing* what is now' (Yontef, 1993)

The client may be talking about past events, but s/he should discuss them in terms of how s/he feels about them in that moment

The therapist does not assume the role of the expert to interpret the expressions of the client, but merely encourages the client to enhance self-awareness by remaining in the present and accepting responsibility for the self

Immediate dialogue within the client

The client may benefit from engaging in dialogue within the self

Two parts of the self may be split and the client can use various techniques to encourage a dialogue between these two halves

For example, the empty chair technique

Language in the here and now

Gestalt therapy aims to ground the client in the here and now

Language can often be used to distance the individual from the fullness of experience

Instead of owning the experience in the here and now, the individual can use language to make the experience seem distant or as though it is happening to someone else

For example, if the client talks of experiencing a feeling in the past, the therapist will invite her to bring it into the present ('Can you feel that anger here and now?') as it is only in the present that the feeling can be processed

Owning the expression

The client may suggest his or her own feelings, thoughts and behaviours, but use language to avoid ownership of these feelings, thoughts and behaviours

For example, in response to the question 'how did you feel when he shouted at you?', the client may say 'well, one often feels a little annoyed when someone is mean' or 'well, you tend to feel annoyed when someone is mean'

The therapist can draw attention to this use of language to encourage the client to change it to 'I' and own the expression

For example, the therapist might say 'who feels annoyed?' and encourage the client to say aloud 'I feel annoyed'

Accepting responsibility for the statement

The client may deny responsibility for an expression by asking the therapist to confirm that the expression is true

For example, the client might say 'but I shouldn't feel jealous, should I?'

The therapist can draw attention to the use of this language to encourage the client to change questions to statements in order to accept that s/he is responsible for the content of that statement

For example, the therapist might respond with 'turn that question into a statement' and the client would say 'I should not feel jealous' – now that they have accepted that statement as their own, they can consider whether they really believe it rather than relying on confirmation from someone else

Avoiding limiters (should and shouldn't/must and mustn't)

We all have our own internal rules and limitations, often introjected by parents and significant others in our childhood

For example, a client might say

> You should work hard
>
> You shouldn't get angry
>
> I must try harder
>
> I mustn't get upset

The therapist can challenge the client to see how this language affects him/her in the present

For example, the therapist might ask in response

> In what ways does saying 'should' affect you?
>
> What would happen if you did? (get angry or upset)
>
> How does using the word 'must' limit you in the present?
>
> Can you change 'you' to 'I'?

Establishing control over actions

The client may insist that external forces are responsible for his or her own behaviour by using words to imply that things are beyond their control

> For example, the client who feels angry that her husband never washes the dishes might say 'I end up washing them because I can't just leave them in the sink'

The therapist can draw attention to the use of this language to encourage the client to change 'can't' to 'won't' in order to accept that she is in control of her own actions

> For example, the therapist might question why the dishes 'can't' be left in the sink and encourage the client to rephrase the expression to 'I won't just leave them in the sink'

INCREASING AWARENESS OF LANGUAGE

Try to record yourself engaged in a natural conversation. This can be a bit tricky as you tend to behave differently when being recorded so it is often a good idea to leave the device recording for a long period of time and then focus on the middle section only.

Listen to the recording and note the number of times that you use language outside the here and now – are there any examples of you avoiding ownership by using second or third person, denying responsibility by asking questions, establishing limitations by asserting shoulds and musts, and claiming that external forces control actions by implying a lack of control?

Experiential learning in therapy

Staying in the moment

In Gestalt therapy, clients are encouraged to stay in the moment and not to escape into the past or the future

> For example, the client may be experiencing uncomfortable thoughts or feelings – rather than avoiding these uncomfortable sensations (maybe by changing the subject), the therapist would encourage the client to stay with the thought or feeling so as to fully experience it

>> Encouraging the client to be in the here and now eliminates anxiety. Perls (1969) argues that 'anxiety is the gap between the *now* and the *then*. If you are in the now you can't be anxious, because the excitement flows immediately into on-going spontaneous activity. If you are in the now, you are creative, you are inventive'

Clients can be encouraged to stay in the here and now by bringing the external issues into the real moment of the therapy

This is experiential learning

Client learns through real experiences in the moment

This can be done through experiments, exercises and dream work

Experiments

Experiments emerge from the dialogue between client and therapist

Therapist might notice something and invite the client to try an experiment on the basis of this observation

For example, the therapist might notice that the client is tense and invite him to try breathing deeply before repeating his previous statement in order to experiment with how that feels

Below is an example of an experiment

Dialogue begins after the therapist notices that the client has folded together his hands and is currently trying to pull them apart

Therapist: What are you doing with your hands?

Client: Well, my fingers are interlocked and I'm trying to pull them apart.

Therapist: Are they both equal or is one hand controlling the other?

Client: Well now you mention it, it feels like the right hand is in control.

Therapist: What would the left hand want to say to the right hand about this?

Exercises

While a Gestalt therapist may be creative and design experiments for the client in the here and now of the therapeutic relationship, there are also well-established techniques that are frequently used

These techniques are known as 'exercises' and trainee therapists are taught how to use these exercises in work with clients

Exercises are ready-made techniques preplanned to encourage therapeutic progress

The therapist can use these techniques with a client if it is deemed appropriate in that moment

Common exercises include internal dialogue exercises, reversal exercises, exaggeration exercises and repetition exercises

Internal dialogue exercises (empty chair)

Instead of running an internal dialogue, the client is encouraged to externalise the dialogue by using an empty chair to house the other person

This technique can be used to allow the client to converse between the different parts of the self, practise talking to someone who is not present, or explore the world from the viewpoint of another person

For example, a client who suddenly lost her mother might be encouraged to imagine that her mother is in the other chair and be given an opportunity to say all of the things she wanted to say to her (and perhaps answer for her mother too)

Reversal exercises

Clients are encouraged to try being the polar opposite of what they feel that they actually are

This technique can be used to encourage the client to accept different parts of the self by letting them try out these unfamiliar roles in a safe environment

For example, a client who insists on always being cheerful might pretend to be sad for a while to experience how it feels

The client may also be asked to try reversing roles

This technique can be used to encourage the client to view the world from different perspectives

For example, the therapist might ask 'if I had your problem, what would you be saying to me?' and the therapist and client could then role play this reversal of roles

Exaggeration exercises

The client is encouraged to exaggerate certain movements, postures or expressions

This technique can intensify the feelings associated with the behaviours and help the client to experience them fully in the moment

For example, a client who is experiencing repressed anger and revealing it subtly by gently clenching her fist might be encouraged to clench her fist even harder in order to accept the feelings

Repetition exercises

The client is encouraged to repeat certain words or phrases

The effect of repetition is similar to exaggeration – this technique can intensify the feelings associated with the behaviours and help the client to experience them fully in the moment

For example, a client might say 'he makes me really angry' and the therapist may then invite the client to repeat the statement over and over, or louder, until the client experiences the feeling in the here and now, can express it and feel some relief and release from it

Below is an example of a combination of exercises

Dialogue begins after the client states that she is angry with her father

Therapist: You say you are angry with him. What do you really want to say to him?

Client: What I *really* want say to him?

Therapist: Why not? It's safe to try it out here.

Client: Well, I think I'd want to say 'Screw you'.

Therapist: Go on then, say it. Imagine that he is sitting over here in this chair. Say whatever you need to say to him.

Client: (*quietly*) Screw you.

Therapist: Louder.

Client: (*louder*) Screw you.

Therapist: Again.

Client: Screw you. Screw you. (*shouting*) Screw you, you bastard.

Dream work

Perls was trained in psychoanalysis so he was influenced by dream work as a way of accessing the unconscious

> In psychoanalysis, dreams are analysed and interpreted

> In Gestalt, dreams are explored, brought into the here and now, and the client is encouraged to give them meaning

>> Through this meaning different aspects of the dream, which are believed to be different aspects of self, may be integrated

Dreams are the royal road to integration

> For example, a client recalls a dream in which he is going to give a talk to a local charity group but cannot get to the venue because of road works – unsure of which way to go, he asks a policeman for directions but, rather than being helpful, the policeman is critical of him not knowing the way, and not being prepared enough by setting off too late. As the dream continues other obstacles prevent the client from making progress

>> *Stage* 1: therapist would first let the client recall the dream as above

>> *Stage* 2: therapist would ask the client to relive the dream as if it were happening now, so the client may start: 'I am going to give a talk for a local group. I am driving along but now see that the road ahead is closed and that there is a diversion. I am aware of feeling anxious that I might be late . . .'

>> *Stage* 3: the therapist may set up dialogues between different characters or different parts of the dream – she could ask the client to expand upon the dialogue with the policeman or ask him to speak as if he were the road works (what would the road works be saying to you? what would you say back to the road works?)

>> *Stage* 4: as the exercise progressed, the client would be encouraged to come to some understanding of the dream from his own (not the therapist's) point of view

> It is important to note that all parts of the dream are parts of the dreamer, so the client is himself and also the policeman, the road works, the diversion, the

other obstacles, etc. Understanding this will give the client the opportunity to become aware of, and to integrate, these different aspects of the self

Below is an example of dream work with a client

Dialogue begins after the client mentions being affected by a dream ('it hasn't left me')

Therapist: Okay, tell me about what happened in your dream.

Client: Well, the dream starts off with me walking along a track, through some pine trees. It was a bright day and I could hear the wind in the trees. Around a bend I came across two oak trees, one fallen across the track. I scrambled over the tree, it was a little difficult but I managed and carried on, but then wondered why they were there, two oaks in a pine forest.

Therapist: Have you any thoughts on what it might mean?

Client: Well, I guess there are some obvious things, the tree blocking the path might mean the things I have to deal with in my job . . . or in my life.

Therapist: Tell me the dream again, this time as if you were reliving it in the present tense.

Client: Okay. I'm walking down a forest track, pine trees on either side. It's a nice day and I can hear the wind in the tree tops, although it is still here on the track. I'm going round a corner and I see a big tree across the path. It is one of two oaks, the other standing next to it. They look out of place in the middle of all the pine trees and I am sad that it's fallen because the other is one left on her own.

Therapist: Talk now as if you were the tree still standing. What would she say?

Client: She would say something like 'I am big and strong. I give shade on sunny days and shelter from the rain. Animals live in me.'

Therapist: And what would she say to you?

Client: She would say 'and you can rest here too'.

Therapist: And you would reply?

Client: 'I can't, I can't stop. I don't have time.'

Therapist: Say that again.

Client: I can't stop. I don't have time. I never have time (*she becomes quiet and reflective*). I never have time (*she begins to cry*).

There is no assumption that doing dream work will lead to any new insights, but this example confirmed for the client the more obvious messages (overcoming obstacles, always busy) and the less obvious (feeling sad about never having time)

Revisiting the dream, the client identified the oak still standing as her mother – her mother lived alone and, remembering the dialogue, the client decided to spend more time with her

FINDING THE MEANING IN DREAMS

As I was starting to write this section on Gestalt therapy, I had a dream that I had entered a marathon. I was not prepared for the start of the race and it began before I arrived. I needed to change, find a safe place for my valuables, and find the starting point. I became increasingly anxious because the race was well under way, and I knew I needed to phone someone to tell them that I had not yet started and that they should not expect me at the finish at the agreed time. I rarely remember my dreams but this was very vivid. The meaning was not lost on me. I spared my co-author the phone call, got my writing shoes on, and started running . . .

Think of a recent dream – try to relive the dream by thinking through all of the different parts and characters. Move around the dream taking on the role of significant parts and setting up dialogues. Stop when you are happy that you have made some sense of the meaning.

Case study demonstrating Gestalt therapy

Susan, 42, came into therapy through the occupational health department of a local company in which she is the marketing manager. She had been advised to visit the therapist due to her difficulties managing her workload and her recent absences due to depression. Her managerial role is 'pressured' and she feels trapped in her day-to-day life. The therapy was limited to six sessions.

In the following exchanges, therapist denotes therapist, client denotes Susan. Confidentiality statement and the contract have been discussed. The session is joined just after the therapist has invited the client to begin talking. However, she seems reluctant to speak and sits staring at her folded hands.

> Therapist: If you do not feel comfortable talking about what brings you here, perhaps you can tell me what you are feeling right now?
>
> Client: I just feel anxious (*client has folded her hands together and begins trying to pull them apart*).
>
> Therapist: What are you doing with your hands?
>
> Client: Well, my fingers are interlocked and I'm trying to pull them apart.
>
> Therapist: Are they both equal or is one hand controlling the other?
>
> Client: Well, now you mention it, it feels like the right hand is in control.
>
> Therapist: What would the left hand want to say to the right hand about this?
>
> Client: I'm not sure. Maybe it would say 'leave me alone'. Just leave me alone.
>
> Therapist: So say it now. Be your left hand and say what you want to say to your right hand.

Client: Leave me alone. Just stop everything and leave me. I need some peace. I need to rest (*client is quiet for a few moments*). It makes me think about a dream that I had. It wasn't really a scary dream, but it hasn't left me since I woke up.

Therapist: Would you be happy to explore this dream a little? We could talk about your dream as though it is happening right now and you could think about what it all means to you.

Client: Yes. I think that I could do that.

Therapist: Okay, tell me about what happened in your dream.

Client: Well the dream starts off with me walking along a track, through some pine trees. It was a bright day and I could hear the wind in the trees. Around a bend I came across two oak trees, one fallen across the track. I scrambled over the tree, it was a little difficult but I managed and carried on, but then wondered why they were there, two oaks in a pine forest. Further on I suddenly felt lost, I could still hear the wind but when I looked up the trees are not blowing. I realised that the sound was not the wind, it was the sea . . . and then I was on a long beach. I could see some people in the distance so I ran, but the beach was so long that it seemed to take hours. When I got to the people I saw that they were statues, standing separately, facing the sea. A bit like those statues by that what's his name . . . you know, he did the Angel of the North. Anyway, the tide was coming in so I walked back up the beach and found a cafe but it wasn't a cafe, it was like an abattoir or maybe a place where they package up meat. It was full of carcasses. I'm a vegetarian. I was just about to leave when an old man came out of a room and said that he knew me. I knew that he didn't, that he was lying, and I got scared and ran away. He was chasing me, and I was running through deep wet sand. I saw a lighthouse in the distance and knew if I could get to it I would be safe. That's it. I woke up. It was so vivid, I don't usually remember my dreams.

Therapist: Have you any thoughts on what it might mean?

Client: Well, I guess there are some obvious things, the tree blocking the path might mean the things I have to deal with in my job . . . or in my life. Having to run for so long, I always feel like I'm running just to keep up at work. But I don't know what the statues or the lighthouse mean, or who the old man was.

Therapist: Tell me the dream again, this time as if you were reliving it in the present tense.

Client: Okay. I'm walking down a forest track, pine trees on either side. It's a nice day and I can hear the wind in the tree tops, although it is still here on the track. I'm going round a corner and I see a big tree across the path. It is one of two oaks, the other standing next to it. They look out of place in the middle of all the pine trees and I am sad that it's fallen because the other is one left on her own.

(*At this point the therapist has choices — he could set up a dialogue between the client and the fallen tree, but as the client has already attached a possible meaning to this, and has indicated an emotional response to the tree still standing, he chooses to explore this.*)

Therapist: Talk now as if you were the tree still standing. What would she (*picking up on the client's use of 'her'*) say?

Client: She would say something like 'I am big and strong. I give shade on sunny days and shelter from the rain. Animals live in me.'

Therapist: And what would she say to you?

Client: She would say 'and you can rest here too'.

Therapist: And you would reply?

Client: 'I can't, I can't stop. I don't have time.'

Therapist: Say that again.

Client: I can't stop. I don't have time. I never have time (*she becomes quiet and reflective*). I never have time (*she begins to cry*).

(*The dream work stops but the client is keen to continue later in the session after exploring issues around the pressures of her job — the dialogue picks up at the point of arriving at the statues.*)

Therapist: Now have a dialogue with one of the statues. What does the statue want to say?

Client: I am always here, always looking to the horizon. I feel nothing but am slowly being eroded by the wind and the sea. I'm rusting with salt water.

Therapist: And what does that mean to you?

Client: I think it's the part of me that is growing old. I've always been me, but I'm aware that some days I feel old, tired. I see younger people coming into the same types of job as mine, and I remember being their age, keen, full of life. I'm scared of rusting, eroding away.

Therapist: And the horizon?

Client: Ah yes, that fits. Always looking for the perfect life, just beyond my sight and out of reach.

Therapist: And the lighthouse?

Client: As I get closer I see it is no longer used, no light. It was once a beacon of safety, now it has outlived its usefulness. And as I say that I'm thinking of the fallen oak, and from nowhere I'm thinking of my dad. He died six years ago. I haven't thought about him for ages, but I know that the lighthouse and the oak are him (*she sobs*). He was wonderful, I still miss him.

Therapist: And the lighthouse would say to you?

Client: (quietly) It's okay. I'm still here in your dreams. I can still light your path, even if others can't see it.

Therapist: And you would say?

Client: I love you dad (*client begins to cry and she is unable to continue for a while*). But also I am just so angry with him.

Therapist: Are you feeling angry right now?

Client: Yes. He let me down. He left me on my own and I had to deal with everything without him.

Therapist: You say you are angry with him. What do you really want to say to him?

Client: What I *really* want say to him? It is hard to say. You shouldn't think that way about your father. Especially when he is gone.

Therapist: Who shouldn't think that way?

Client: I guess . . . I mean, I shouldn't.

Therapist: Can you say that?

Client: I shouldn't think bad things about my father (*she pauses*). But why shouldn't I? If that's how I feel. And that *is* how I feel.

Therapist: If you don't want to say it, then that's okay. But it's safe to try it out here if you want to explore how it feels to say it.

Client: Well, I think I'd want to say 'Screw you'.

Therapist: Go on then, say it. Imagine that he is sitting over here in this chair. Say whatever you need to say to him.

Client: (*quietly*) Screw you.

Therapist: Louder.

Client: (*louder*) Screw you.

Therapist: Again.

Client: Screw you. Screw you (*shouting*). Screw you, you bastard. You left me all alone with her.

The therapist noticed that Susan had referred to her mother for the first time here. Further exploration revealed that Susan had suffered verbal abuse at the hands of her mother throughout her childhood – she would frequently criticise her and this led to her feeling worthless. The therapist tried to keep this discussion in the room (rather than focusing on events in the past) by asking how the she felt today about her mother. Eventually, Susan was able to work through her issues towards her mother by writing her a letter.

ANALYSING THE CASE STUDY

Try answering the following questions using information about Gestalt therapy.

- What type of boundary disturbance might Susan be experiencing?
- Where is Susan being blocked in her cycle of awareness?
- Which parts of Susan are topdog and which parts of Susan are underdog?
- How does the therapist keep the discussion in the here and now?
- How is Susan encouraged to own the expression and assume responsibility for her thoughts?
- What experiments does the therapist use?
- What exercises does the therapist use?
- How is Susan helped through dream work?

SUMMARY

Humanistic and psychodynamic: Gestalt is founded in the humanistic approach but the founder arrived from the psychodynamic approach

Development: established in the 1940s by Perls (Fritz and Laura), first book to introduce Gestalt therapy by Perls in 1942, term 'Gestalt therapy' was coined in 1951, New York Institute for Gestalt Therapy was established for workshops and seminars in the home of Perls in New York in 1951

Holism and completion: see patterns as wholes, seek to complete things to avoid unfinished business; figure and ground highlight how we attend to things (figure) until they are completed then they fade from attention (ground)

Perspectives: phenomenological, field theory, existential

Awareness: zones of awareness (inner, middle, outer), freedom of movement between zones; Gestalt cycle (sensation, awareness, mobilisation, action, contact, satisfaction, withdrawal)

Contact boundary: distinction between self and environment, boundary should be firm yet permeable; disturbances lead to isolation or confluence, seven patterns of disturbance (retroflection, introjection, projection, confluence, deflection, desensitisation, egotism); disturbances correspond to Gestalt cycle

Paradoxical theory of change: must accept self in here and now for change to be possible; topdog/underdog

Dialogical relationship: authentic and responsible; inclusion, presence, commitment to dialogue, dialogue is lived; immediate dialogue within client and between client and therapist

Language in the here and now: owning the expression, change 'it' or 'you' to 'I'; accepting responsibility for statements, change questions to statements; avoiding limiters, change shoulds and musts to wants; establishing control over actions, change 'can't' to 'won't'

Experiential learning: staying in the moment; experiments, born of dialogue; exercises, ready-made preplanned techniques, internal dialogue empty chair exercise, reversal exercise, exaggeration exercise, repetition exercise; dream work, exploring meanings to allow integration of different parts of self, royal road to integration

TRANSACTIONAL ANALYSIS

LEARNING OUTCOMES

After reading this section, you will be able to:

* explain that transactional analysis is an integrative therapy combining psychodynamic and humanistic approaches

* describe the history of transactional analysis with a brief biography of Eric Berne

* discuss the Parent, Adult and Child of the ego-state model

* discuss the roles of positive strokes and negative strokes in reciprocal, crossed and covert transactions

* discuss the payoffs in the games people play

* describe therapeutic methods for creating the antithesis of games

* discuss the life positions and life scripts, highlighting the significance of early childhood messages

* map the process of therapy through the five key stages

* appreciate the application of transactional analysis in a therapeutic setting (case study)

Transactional analysis: humanistic and psychodynamic approaches

Transactional analysis (TA) is grounded in the humanistic and psychodynamic approaches

Integration of person-centred and psychoanalysis therapies

'Transactional analysis is a theory of personality and a systematic psychotherapy for personal growth and personal change' (International Transactional Analysis Association, 2013)

On the difference between TA and other theories, Berne said (with a smile)

'I think most other therapies . . . talk about thinking and feeling. Our question to the patient is not what do you think or how do you feel, but what are you going to do about it? . . . There's a story, that I think is a little unfair, but anyway it sort of illustrates what I mean, where a patient came in one day and said to the psychiatrist "by the way, I killed my wife last night and hid her body in the closet". And some people might say "ah ha, now we've got something to work with, what's your interest in closets?" Whereas we might say "why are you killing your wife?"' (Berne, 1966)

TA has applications in a number of areas

Theory is wide ranging

Theory of personality

Theory of communications

Theory of human development

TA has the main aim of autonomy (Berne, 1961)

This means behaving, thinking and feeling in response to the reality of the here and now rather than responding to script beliefs

In order to move towards autonomy we need to consider three connected areas: awareness, spontaneity and intimacy

Awareness

In order to behave, think and feel in response to the here and now, we need to be able to live in the present

We often spend time remembering the past and anticipating the future, not fully engaged in the present

We bring the past into the present though transactions, games and replaying familiar patterns

We are playing to gain strokes – these reinforce our life position and our early childhood script decisions and, when we have these scripts, we are not fully engaged in the present

Spontaneity

Being spontaneous involves exercising choice in the present

It may feel risky because we are not playing out familiar games

Once we become aware of the present, we need to respond to it with awareness and through choice

Intimacy

Intimacy involves being real in relationships

Being open and honest and not hiding behind the mask that we often present to the outside world

Speaking our real thoughts and showing our true feelings exposes us to others and makes us vulnerable, so we rarely do it

However, when we do show our true selves, we experience a richer, more meaningful relationship

For example, when we fall in love

This also happens in the intimacy of the therapeutic relationship

Autonomy is a desirable aim but the journey towards it is challenging

It challenges us to become aware of the way our childhood decisions influence us in the present

It challenges us to break free from these old ways of behaving, thinking and feeling and to respond more appropriately to the here and now

It challenges us to take risks, to make ourselves vulnerable in order to achieve more meaningful, intimate relationships with self and others

Development of transactional analysis

History of transactional analysis

Introduced by Berne as an 'extra-Freudian' method of treating disturbance

Often regarded as a logical step forward from psychoanalytic therapy, but the therapy arguably draws more on the humanistic approach

Focus on interactions between people rather than unconscious drives

International Transactional Analysis Association established in 1964

Approach began to be popular amongst practitioners, but still regarded as an offshoot by many researchers and purists

Controversial due to non-technical terminology

Extremely popular with the general public

Games People Play (Berne, 1964) has sold more than five million copies

Often regarded as pseudoscience by critics

Fails to present evidence for ego-states or games

Brief biography of Eric Berne (1910–1970)

'Awareness requires living in the here and now, and not in the elsewhere, the past or the future'

—Berne (1964)

Who was Eric Berne?

Berne founded TA in the 1960s

Emphasised the importance of interactions between individuals and the games that people play within these interactions

Early years

Born on May 10th 1910 and raised in Canada as Eric Bernstein

Father died in 1921 and mother raised her two children alone

Education

Qualified with an MD from McGill University in 1935

Career

Studied psychoanalysis during his residency in psychiatry at Yale

Initially worked at the San Francisco Psychoanalytic Institute under Erik Erikson, but began to diverge from traditional psychoanalysis

Served in the Army Medical Corps during World War II, gaining the rank of major – discharged in 1945

Focused specifically on the nature of intuition and social interactions

Developed the term transactional analysis as a label for his style of therapy in the 1950s

Published *Transactional Analysis in Psychotherapy* in 1961

Published bestseller *Games People Play* in 1964

Founded the International Transactional Analysis Association in 1964

Published *What Do You Say After You Say Hello?* in 1972

Family

Married three times and raised four children

Death

Died on July 15th 1970 following a heart attack

Significant learnings

'The moment a little boy is concerned with which is a jay and which is a sparrow, he can no longer see the birds or hear them sing' (Berne, 1964)

'Each person designs his own life, freedom gives him the power to carry out his own designs, and power gives the freedom to interfere with the designs of others' (Berne, 1972)

Ego-state model of personality

Human personality is composed of three ego-states (Figure 6.4)

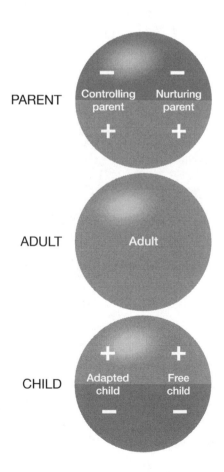

Structural model states that we are always in one of three ego-states at any point in time (Berne, 1964)

Parent

Child

Adult

Functional model states that we are always in one type of that ego-state (i.e. *how* we are in that ego state)

Nurturing Parent

Controlling Parent

Free Child

Adapted Child

Adult

Parent

Known as the exteropsyche state

FIGURE 6.4 **The three ego-states. Adapted from Berne (1964).**

Perceiving reality from the perspective of a parent and responding to others in a parental manner

Influenced by the perceived actions of the real parents

Parent state can be caring and supportive (Nurturing Parent)

> For example, I may adopt the Parent state by encouraging people to wrap up warm and worrying that they may catch a cold

Parent state can be critical and demanding (Controlling Parent)

> For example, I may adopt the Parent state by criticising the way people dress and trying to make them wear something else

Child

Known as the archaeopsyche state

Perceiving reality from the perspective of a child and responding to others in a child-like manner

Influenced by own behaviours as a child

Child state can be spontaneous and fun loving (Free Child)

> For example, I may adopt the Child state by spontaneously singing loudly in my car while waiting at traffic lights

Child state can adapt to rules or the demands of others (Adapted Child)

> For example, I may adopt the Child state by asking permission from my friend before buying a new pair of shoes

Adult

Known as the neopsyche state

Perceiving reality from an objective viewpoint and responding to others in a logical manner unfettered by emotion

Influenced by logic, reason and a scientific understanding of the world

Adult state is usually located in the here and now and involves an appreciation of current feelings and logical interpretations of thoughts and beliefs

> For example, I may adopt an Adult state when I recognise my desire to go to a party the night before a major exam but make a decision to revise at home instead because I know that the grades on the test will be important to me in the future

Adult ego-state is the rational, logical state and does not divide into different types of Adult

Ego-states do not determine actual roles

Ego-states are labels for the way that we behave, think and feel

> Always indicated by a capital letter: Parent, Child, Adult (P, A, C)

> Ego-state model is also known as the PAC model

Our roles indicate our actual relationships with others

> I might be a parent to someone or a child to someone

Ego-states can conflict with our actual roles

> For example, in the television sitcom *Absolutely Fabulous*, Saffy adopts a Parent state towards her actual parent Eddy and Eddy adopts a Child state towards her actual child Saffy

Ego-states are not intrinsically good or bad

Nurturing Parent may appear positive (supportive and caring), but this could become negative if the support was given to the extent that it encourages dependency

Controlling Parent may appear negative (critical and demanding), but this could become positive when we need someone to take charge of a situation

Functional ego-states can be beneficial

> Parent state allows us to care for others

> Child state allows us to relax and have fun

> Adult state allows us to deal with problems logically

Dysfunctional ego-states can be damaging

> Parent state can be controlling and overcritical of the self

> Child state can be demanding and risk-taking

> Adult state can make us overanalyse everything and not let us have any fun

---

GUESS THE EGO-STATE

Look at the scenarios below to identify the ego-states of the protagonists.

- Woman suffering with alcoholism who cannot resist spending all of her money on vodka as soon as she gets paid each week.
- Man scolding an employee in a condescending tone for arriving at work five minutes late.
- Teenager who refuses to go to a party the night before an exam because he wants to get good grades.
- Boy who helps his father into bed when he returns home drunk after a night on the town.
- Girl who looks up through her eyelashes and talks in a baby voice to persuade her boyfriend to buy her a new pair of shoes.
- Elderly person who carefully writes down her expenditure each week to ensure that it is covered by her pension.

We should move freely between different ego-states

Ego-states are not personality types used to categorise individuals

> Instead, they are designed to inform about specific interactions in that moment so our ego-states should change from moment to moment

It is possible for us to move between ego-states internally and externally

> For example, you are being playful by teasing your partner (Child) but you suddenly become concerned when she seems upset (Parent)

> It is cold and dark in the middle of winter and the alarm clock goes off – you lie in bed running an internal dialogue: 'just five more minutes (Child), but I really should get up now (Parent), but it's cold and I'm tired (Child), I've really got to go to work (Parent), okay if I don't get up now I'll be late (Adult)'

Exclusions occur when we exclude one or two ego-states from our interactions

It would be healthy to be able to move freely between ego-states and for us to have access to all ego-states as appropriate

However, we may have a tendency to use one or two particular ego-states most of the time

> For example, a reckless individual may frequently use the Child

We may also have a tendency to use one particular ego-state when we are with certain people or in certain situations

> For example, a normally mature woman might go into the Child whenever she is in the presence of her father

> For example, a confident adult might go into the Child when confronted by a police officer

If a person is mostly in Parent and Adult, with very little Child

> S/he will lack spontaneity and will find it difficult to have fun

> S/he will be serious and logical, and be very aware of the rules

If a person is mostly in Child and Parent, with very little Adult

> S/he will not be able to check reality and balance judgements

> S/he is likely to have wider mood and behaviour swings

If a person is mostly in Adult and Child, with little Parent

> S/he will not have a good awareness of the rules

> S/he may act on impulse but will be able to rationally assess the outcomes

> S/he may make the rules up as s/he goes along

ARE YOU EXCLUDING STATES?

Think about your interaction with someone that you know and try to answer the following questions.

- Do you rely on one or two ego-states a lot of the time?
- Do you use one ego-state when you are with this certain person?
- Do you use one ego-state when you are in a certain situation?
- Do you notice a particular ego-state in that person?
- How does your ego-state impact on your relationships with this other person?
- How does the ego-state of the other person impact on the relationship with you?
- What would happen if you changed your ego-state when relating to this other person?

Contaminations occur when we think that we are in one ego-state but are actually in another

We want to be rational and sensible so we assume that our responses are Adult

However, we frequently respond in Parent or Child but justify our actions/thoughts/feelings by believing that we are Adult

If a person thinks s/he is in Adult but is really in Parent

S/he is bringing beliefs that were introjected from parents in childhood into the present and thinks they are true

For example, the belief that all Scotsmen are mean, all blondes are dumb, love will only hurt you, you cannot trust anyone, etc.

If a person thinks s/he is in Adult but is really in Child

S/he is bringing beliefs that were formed in childhood into the present and thinks they are true

For example, the belief that I am no good at maths, I will never get on in life, I must keep trying, they are all laughing at me, etc.

Therapy enhances understanding and control of our own ego-states

When we analyse our own ego-state in therapy, we can begin to understand some of our unhealthy behaviours, thoughts and feelings

For example, a client who has a tendency to revert to Child state when dealing with an authority figure might benefit from recognising this in order to strengthen his or her own Adult state

Using the ego-state model to understand different aspects of a person's personality is known as 'structural analysis'

Therapy also gives us choices about moving into and between ego-states, rather than going into them automatically

It would be healthy to be able to move freely between ego-states and for us to have access to all ego-states as appropriate

Transactions and strokes

Transactions refer to the interactions between people

Transactions involve the communication between two or more people

People communicate in one of the ego-states

Transactions are based on whether the state addressed is the state that eventually responds

Three types of transactions

Complementary (or reciprocal)

Crossed

Covert (or ulterior)

Complementary transactions

Each individual is addressing the ego-state of the other individual

Child to Child: Let's skip this lecture and have lunch instead

Child to Child: Okay, shall we get a burger?

Does NOT mean that the states have to match – simply means that the other person is in the state that you are addressing

Parent to Child: You have to get this work done at once

Child to Parent: But I want to go out tonight

Complementary transactions are often simple transactions

Adult to Adult: Hi, how are you?

Adult to Adult: Fine thanks, and you?

First person invited the second person to respond from Adult and the second did respond from Adult so the transaction is complementary

Ego-state addressed is the one that responded

Communication feels comfortable and may continue

Crossed transactions

Each individual is addressing a different ego-state to the one held by the other individual

Child to Parent: Shall I buy some new shoes?

Adult to Adult: It is your money so you can make your own decision

Crossed transactions can have a negative impact on relationships

> Child to Child: Let's skip this lecture and have lunch instead

> Parent to Child: You're always doing that, do you want to fail?

> Student invited her friend into Child, but the response was from Parent so the transaction is crossed

> Communication is not comfortable, unless one person changes ego-states to get the communication back to complementary

> For example, since the friend responded in Parent and invited the student into Child, the conversation could only become complementary again if the student replies from Child ('Aw but I don't want to go')

When we have a communication that does not feel good, it is likely that there has been a crossed transaction

Covert transactions

Each individual has a different implicit ego-state and explicit ego-state

> Explicit Adult to Adult: We will need to stay late at the office tonight to finish this work

> Explicit Adult to Adult: That is a very sensible idea

> Implicit Child to Child: Let's stay behind and have sex

> Implicit Child to Child: That sounds like fun

Covert transactions occur when the message is on the explicit (or social) level but the real meaning is on an implicit (or psychological) level

> Mother comes home from work to find a mess, points to a pair of shoes in the middle of the room and says 'What are these here?'

> The answer, of course, is 'a pair of shoes' but the real meaning of the communication is 'pick these up and put them away'

> It is likely that the person who receives the question ('what are these?') will respond by tidying the shoes away

> Behavioural response holds the key to the real meaning of the transaction

Covert communications are the basis for the playing of games

GUESS THE TRANSACTION

Look at the transactions below to identify which ego-states are being used and whether the transaction is complementary, crossed or covert (if covert, try to identify the underlying meaning).

Manager: You're late.
Worker: Sorry, it won't happen again.

Person 1: It's awful – the mess the bankers have got us into and they are getting bonuses!
Person 2: Yes, they should be ashamed of themselves.

Husband: I've had a heck of a day.
Wife: Huh, you should see what I had to put up with.

Wife: The bin's full.
Husband: Is it really?

Car salesman: This one is probably too sporty for you.
Customer: I'll take it!

Husband: Wrap up warm when you go out.
Wife: Aw but I wanted to wear my short skirt.

Wife: The weather is getting colder so we need to fix the boiler this weekend.
Husband: Aw but I wanted to go to the football match.

Strokes refer to the attention gained from other people

Every individual craves recognition, acknowledgement and attention

Often we do not even care what type of attention we receive

Strokes can be verbal or non-verbal

Verbal strokes

Other people give us attention by involving us in their conversation or referring to us when they speak

Non-verbal strokes

Other people give us attention by doing things for us or to us

Strokes can be conditional or unconditional

Conditional strokes

Other people give us attention only if we behave in a certain way

Unconditional strokes

Other people give us attention irrespective of how we behave

Strokes can be positive or negative

Positive strokes

Other people give us praise, compliments, kindness, love, etc. and we experience a positive feeling as a result

Negative strokes

Other people give us criticism, punishment, cruelty, etc. and we experience a negative feeling as a result

We would always prefer to receive positive strokes, but we will settle for negative strokes if there are no other strokes available

> For example, a child wants praise from his mother (positive stroke) but he learns that he is ignored when he is well behaved (no strokes) and receives attention in the form of punishment when he is badly behaved (negative strokes) – since some attention is better than no attention, he is constantly badly behaved

GUESS THE STROKE

Look at the scenarios below to identify whether the stroke is verbal/non-verbal, conditional/unconditional or positive/negative.

- Husband flashes his wife a withering look when she changes the channels on the television.
- Girlfriend receives a bunch of flowers through the mail with a card reading 'just because'.
- Mother spanks her child for misbehaving.
- Friend calls to say 'you are such a kind person' after receiving help moving to a new house.
- Boyfriend leans over to kiss his girlfriend when she brings him a cup of tea.
- Teacher says 'well done on this essay' to a student.

Therapy enhances our understanding of our own transactions and the strokes that we give and receive as a result of these transactions

> When we analyse our own transactions in therapy, we can begin to understand some of the unhealthy patterns of relating

>> For example, a couple frequently engaged in crossed transactions might benefit from trying to create complementary transactions instead

> When we analyse the strokes in our lives, we can begin to understand that some of our unhealthy tendencies are ineffective methods of gaining strokes and we can see how we impact on others by providing strokes

>> For example, client who has a tendency to give negative strokes and withhold positive strokes might benefit from realising how this impacts on her children

Games people play

Games involve a series of transactions leading to a predictable payoff

Games are sets of social behaviours that we habitually play when interacting with others without being consciously aware of our patterns

'A game is an ongoing series of complementary ulterior transactions progressing to a well-defined, predictable outcome. Descriptively, it is a recurring set of transactions . . . with a concealed motivation . . . or gimmick' (Berne, 1964)

Payoffs are the reason why we play games (Berne, 1964)

> We are each seeking a payoff
>
> > Gaining attention
> >
> > Gaining stimulation
> >
> > Gaining confirmation that we are correct
> >
> > Avoidance of anxiety
> >
> > Avoidance of guilt
> >
> > Avoidance of responsibility
>
> Payoffs give us temporary satisfaction . . . but we ultimately feel dissatisfied and frustrated by the game

While games are being played, they are a source of strokes (Berne, 1964)

> Payoff will give us a familiar, but negative, feeling
>
> These 'racket feelings' originate in childhood and we set up a series of transactions (games) outside of awareness in order to experience the feelings
>
> Racket feelings are familiar, predictable and safe . . . but ultimately negative

Different types of games (Berne, 1964)

Why don't you/yeah but

> First player presents a problem and second player offers possible solutions to the problem, but the first player rejects every solution
>
> > *Student*: I'm worried that I'll fail the test.
> >
> > *Lecturer*: Why don't you draw up a revision plan?
> >
> > *Student*: Sounds good, but I never know when I'll be free
> >
> > *Lecturer*: Well, why don't you try to revise for an hour a night?
> >
> > *Student*: Yeah but I'm always tired after college and work.
> >
> > *Lecturer*: Why don't you revise at the weekend then?
> >
> > *Student*: Yeah but I have to work Saturdays and visit my mum on Sunday . . .
>
> Payoff during the game for each player is the feeling that they are working towards a solution to the problem

If it weren't for you

> Each player refuses to accept responsibility for their actions or the results of their actions
>
> > *Wife*: If it weren't for you, I could have a career by now
> >
> > *Husband*: Well, if it weren't for you, I would have gone to university

Payoff during the game for each player is the feeling that their current problems are not their own fault

Now I've got you, you son of a bitch

First player sets up a trap for second player to allow the release of repressed anger

Mother: Where's your uniform?

Son: Upstairs in my room.

Mother: You said you were going to bring it down for the wash!

Son: I forgot.

Mother: You always forget. What about me? Running around after you, do you think I don't have a life too?

Payoff during the game for the first player is the release of emotions

Kick me

First player positions him/herself to receive negative strokes, often due to limited experience with positive strokes in the past

Daughter wears old clothes to go out

Mother: Why don't you make an effort, all your friends do?

Payoff for the first player is the receipt of negative attention

Why does this always happen to me?

First player positions him/herself to suffer multiple misfortunes

Employee takes on more work even though he is already under pressure to meet deadlines

He doesn't complete the task and gets disciplined

Payoff for the first player is inverse pride in the form of knowing that his/her misfortunes are worse than the misfortunes of other people

Karpman (1968) identified three positions in games (Figure 6.5)

Persecutor, Victim, Rescuer form a 'drama triangle'

Each player in a game will start in one position

Just before the end of the game there will be a switch in positions

Each player will end up with a negative feeling

Consider the 'Why don't you/yeah but' game

Player offering possible solutions to the problem is the Rescuer and the player seeking help is the Victim

Student: I'm worried that I'll fail the test.

Lecturer: Why don't you draw up a revision plan?

Student: Sounds good, but I never know when I'll be free

Lecturer: Well, why don't you try to revise for an hour a night?

Student: Yeah but I'm always tired after college and work.

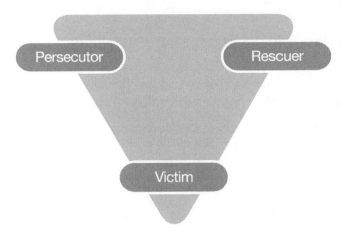

FIGURE 6.5 **The drama triangle. Adapted from Karpman (1968).**

Lecturer: Why don't you revise at the weekend then?

Student: Yeah but I have to work Saturdays and visit my mum on Sunday . . .

Student is the Victim and lecturer is the Rescuer

Both are getting some payoff from the game

Then the switch happens and the first player turns into the Victim and the second player turns into the Persecutor

Lecturer: Well, I don't know what else to suggest.

Student: So you can't help me at all then.

Lecturer is now the Victim and student is the Persecutor

Both feel dissatisfied with the outcome – familiar feelings may be helplessness (student) and uselessness (lecturer)

Antithesis of games

First rule of games

Once you know that you are playing a game, end the game

Refuse to take the opposing role in the game

For example, client adopts the Child ego-state by explaining how much she hates being married and you adopt the Parent ego-state by trying to give advice about improving her relationship – you realise that you are playing the 'why don't you/yeah but' game so you stop the game

How do you stop the game?

Move to the second rule . . .

Second rule of games

Break the game by depriving the actors of the payoff

> Work out which game is being played, determine the payoffs for the actors (sympathy, vindication, etc.) and stop the payoffs

> For example, client adopts the Parent ego-state by explaining that she has to do all of the work at home – you realise that she is playing the 'Kick me' game so you break the game by refusing to offer sympathetic responses

Break the game by responding from a different ego-state

> Work out which ego-state is expected from the other player and adopt a different ego-state in response

> For example, client adopts the Child ego-state by claiming that life is not fair and seems to want you to comfort him from the Parent ego-state – you realise that he is playing the 'Why does this always happen to me?' game so you break the game by adopting the Child ego-state instead

Life positions and scripts

Life positions are the basic views that we take about others and ourselves

Games reinforce our life position

> One reason why we play games is to reinforce our position in life

Life positions are developed in childhood

> We establish our views about others and ourselves based on early experiences

There are four life positions (Harris, 1967)

> I'm OK, you're OK

> I'm OK, you're not OK

> I'm not OK, you're OK

> I'm not OK, you're not OK

I'm OK, you're OK

> A person in this position is confident, optimistic and engages well with life and others

> This is the healthiest position from which to view self and others

> No obvious games or racket feelings

> This is the position that the therapist would assume in the therapy

I'm OK, you're not OK

> A person in this position sees the self as superior to others

> Critical of others (familiar ego-state Controlling Parent)

> Often gets angry (racket feeling) with others

> Starts all games as the Persecutor

I'm not OK, you're OK

> A person in this position sees the self as inferior to others

> Likely to appease and adapt (familiar ego-state Adapted Child)

> Often strives to get away from others and feels depressed or afraid (racket feeling)

> Starts all games as the Rescuer or Victim

I'm not OK, you're not OK

> A person in this position sees the self and others as worthless and everything in the world as hopeless

> Likely to avoid activities or maybe sabotage activities

> Often feels pessimistic and hopeless (racket feeling)

> Starts all games as the Victim

Life positions are important because they determine the racket feelings that we are likely to have, games we play, ego-states that we feel comfortable in, likely transactions that we have, and kind of strokes that we give and receive

> All of these elements serve to consolidate our life script

Life scripts are the story of our lives (Steiner, 1966, 1974)

Life scripts refer to writing a life story with a beginning, middle and end

Much of the theory relating to transactions and strokes fits with a humanistic approach, but life scripts have a foundation in psychodynamic theory since they highlight the significance of childhood events, messages and decisions

Life scripts are created in childhood (Berne, 1964)

> The basis of this script is written in infancy

>> Even before we can talk, we receive preverbal messages from our parents and significant others; for example, we will receive non-verbal strokes by being held close or neglected and we recognise facial expressions

>> When we have only a little language, we receive verbal messages that may reinforce these preverbal messages; for example, we will receive verbal strokes in the form of 'good girl' or 'well done'

> More detail is added as we grow in childhood

> Changes and additions will be made in adolescence

> Scripts developed in childhood impact on adulthood

>> We are not aware of the influence that this script has on our lives

Early messages can be very powerful and hard to identify in adult life (Steiner, 1966, 1974)

> Negative messages are known as injunctions

>> Injunctions will begin 'Don't . . .'

> Positive messages are known as permissions

>> Permissions will begin 'You must/should/can . . .'

Injunctions

Goulding and Goulding (1979) identified 12 injunctions that they saw repeatedly in their work

Don't exist

Don't be you

Don't be a child

Don't grow up

Don't make it

Don't do

Don't be important

Don't belong

Don't be close

Don't be well

Don't think

Don't feel

Injunctions often come from the Child ego-state of the real parents

Like all other people, your real parents will always be in the Child, Parent or Adult ego-state

In the Child state, your parents can give you injunctions

Injunctions start as preverbal messages and are likely to be delivered outside of awareness of the parent(s)

For example, one or both parents may neglect the baby, sending the message 'don't exist' (an infant will not have the ability to make rational decisions the way an adult can, so these decisions are likely to be more 'extreme')

Preverbal messages may then be reinforced by verbal messages later in infancy For example, the parent tells a child 'you were a surprise' or 'you weren't planned' or 'you were a mistake' or 'you were not wanted'

Injunctions influence our life script

We internalise (introject) these messages and they become part of our own Child ego-state

Permissions

There are two types of permissions: rules and attributes

Rules and commands

For example, 'do what you're told', 'you should try harder', 'big boys don't cry', 'do your best'

Attributes

For example, directly to the child 'you're a good girl', 'you're not as clever as your sister'

For example, indirectly to the child 'he's the naughty one', 'she's so good at looking after me', 'she's the quiet one'

Permissions often come from the Parent ego-state of the real parents

Like all other people, your real parents will always be in the Child, Parent or Adult ego-state

In the Parent state, your parents can give you permissions

Permissions start as preverbal messages and are likely to be delivered outside of awareness of the parent(s)

For example, one or both parents may cuddle the baby whenever he is quiet, sending the message 'be quiet' (an infant will not have the ability to make rational decisions the way an adult can, so these decisions are likely to be more 'extreme')

Preverbal messages may then be reinforced by verbal messages later in infancy

For example, the parent tells a child 'be a quiet boy'

Permissions influence our life script

We internalise (introject) these messages and they become part of our own Parent ego-state

Programs

Alongside injunctions and permissions, we also receive information from our parents about how to do things

This information provides us with programs for how to interact with the world

For example, how to read, tie shoe laces, use a knife and fork, etc.

Programs come from the Adult ego-state of our real parents and they are then introjected into our own Adult ego-state

In early childhood we receive thousands of verbal and non-verbal messages from parents and significant others

Injunctions: restrictions and controls sent from the Child state of others and integrated into your own Child state

Permissions: verbal rules, commands and attributes sent from the Parent state of others and integrated into your own Parent state

Programs: useful 'how to . . .' messages sent from the Adult state of others and integrated into your own Adult state

These messages form the basis of the decisions that we make about self and others (life positions) and underpin the life script that we write for ourselves

Scripts developed in childhood impact on adulthood

This life script is played out through our lives

We are not aware of the influence that this script has on our lives

Therapy would help a client become aware of things that are currently outside of awareness through script analysis

We are not always playing out our script – there are times when we are thinking, feeling and behaving appropriately in the here and now

Two factors that make it more likely that a person will enter a script (Stewart & Joines, 1997)

If the here-and-now situation feels stressful to the individual

If there is a similarity between a stressful event in childhood and the events experienced in the here-and-now situation

While the 'what' (the content) of the script is different for each individual, 'how' we live out the script (the process) falls into six main patterns (Berne, 1972; Kahler, 1978)

Always
Never
Until
After
Almost
Open ended

Always

A person with an Always script is likely to play out familiar patterns of behaviours (e.g. relationships) always with the same results ('why does this always happen to me?')

Alternatively s/he may always be doing the same thing (same job, same relationship)

S/he may have received strong consistent permissions in childhood to keep going, try hard to do well, make things work

In therapy, s/he could be challenged to consider how things could be different but, of course, she may also Always be doing therapy

Never

A person with a Never script never gets what s/he wants

S/he makes plans but never carries them out

S/he starts things but never finishes them

S/he may have received the injunctions 'Don't make it' and 'don't (do anything)' in childhood

In therapy, s/he should focus on a specific goal and be stroked for any success

Until

A person with an Until script will put things off

S/he will not enjoy herself until she has finished all her work

S/he will do the things she wants to do when the kids have left home

S/he may have received consistent permissions such as 'be perfect' and 'work hard' (do your homework, then you can play out) in childhood

In therapy she may be reluctant to commit to the process as she might not be a perfect client – she should be encouraged to work in the here and now, not to focus on the future

After

A person with an After script will not enjoy today for fear of tomorrow

His/her fun tonight will be spoiled by the thought that s/he will regret it in the morning

S/he may have good health but worry that s/he will become ill

S/he is likely to start a sentence with a positive then add a 'but' and a negative statement

S/he may have received strong injunctions such as 'Don't have fun' in childhood

In therapy, she should be encouraged to stop sentences (and thoughts) before the 'but' or change the sentence around so it ends with the positive element – therapy sessions should always end on a positive note

Almost

Kahler (1978) built on Berne's theory and divided the Almost script process into Almost Type 1 and Almost Type 2

A person with an Almost Type 1 script will get close to achieving their aim but will not quite do it

S/he will almost make it this time or almost finish this time

S/he will try really hard and will engage in activities to a point

S/he may have received 'try hard' but 'you'll never make it' messages in childhood

A person with an Almost Type 2 script does achieve their aim but does not take time to enjoy the achievement, as s/he has already got a new goal to focus on

S/he may well be very successful, getting promotion after promotion, but is rarely satisfied

In therapy, Type 1 should set small goals and achieve them whereas Type 2 should be encouraged to take time to experience the sense of achievement

Open ended

A person with an Open ended script will experience a lack of direction at a certain point in life

S/he might achieve something in the short term but then have a sense of 'what next?' before something else comes along

Bigger life events (e.g. children leaving home or retirement) may bring a bigger sense of 'what now?' and can result in anxiety or depression

In therapy, s/he would be encouraged to reframe this as a gift – s/he is free to write her own answer to 'what now?' free from the patterns present in the other script processes – s/he should work on small goals linked to larger long-term goals

Therapeutic process

Client–therapist relationship

Psychoeducational approach in which therapist and client take joint responsibility for the work

Therapist takes the life position 'I'm OK, You're OK'

> Provides the support needed for the client to move towards greater autonomy in their life

> Teaches the client about relevant theory

>> For example, the ego-state model, transactions, strokes and games

Clients will become more aware of their processes through this educational process

> With this awareness, they will be encouraged to explore being more spontaneous in relationships both inside and outside the therapy room

> Clients will experience intimacy in the therapeutic relationship

Lister-Ford (2002) identifies five stages in the process of therapy

> Stage 1

>> Client recounts his/her history

>> Therapist listens, reflects, questions to gather relevant information

>> Therapist teaches the relevant parts of theory when appropriate

>> Together they develop a safe, mutual therapeutic relationship

> Stage 2

>> Client becomes more aware of issues and the personal role in maintaining patterns and problems

>> Client notices the feelings that emerge during the process

>> Client begins to take more responsibility in the process

> Stage 3

>> Client begins to work through issues as feelings become stronger

>> Client begins to re-evaluate life

>> Challenging time in the process

> Stage 4

>> Client makes choices about how s/he wants to live with increased awareness

>> Client begins to challenge old script behaviours, thoughts and feelings

>> Client replaces old scripts with ones more appropriate to the here and now

> Stage 5

>> Therapy comes to an end

>> Client has more autonomy over her life

>> Therapist and client review the process and prepare for moving on

Active approach in which the therapist makes an initial assessment of the client's problem and contracts with the client to set effective goals

> Treatment planning has three parts

> > Diagnosis

> > > Assessing the problem and planning interventions

> > Contract

> > > Agreeing the therapeutic goals with the client

> > Treatment direction

> > > What techniques to use, for both short-term and long-term goals

> Planning is ongoing and flexible throughout the process as new information emerges and as the client makes changes

Pragmatic in the interventions

Change in any part of the client's way of being changes the client

> Interventions can be made at any point where they will benefit the client

> For example, if a client has problems in communicating with figures in authority, she may be taught the ego-state model and how transactions work

> > This might bring about significant change for her and she might be happy with this change

> > The therapist will see the value in exploring her way of relating at deeper levels, to analyse script, parental messages, games, etc.

> > The short-term goal of improving relationships may be achieved

> > The long-term goal of becoming free from script is still in place

> > Further short-term interventions will be implemented to help the client become more aware and to spend more time making decisions from the Adult ego-state

> > Eventually the client may be able to remove old scripts and live in the here and now

Case study demonstrating transactional analysis

Roy, 33, came into therapy through the occupational health department of a local county council where he worked in health and safety. It was five months after the break-up of his third marriage. He was 'dissatisfied with life', wondering why 'it always happens to me'. In the aftermath of the ending of the relationship, he had begun to drink heavily again, and was now in danger of losing his job. The therapy was limited to six sessions, with the facility to extend, by agreement, in exceptional cases.

In the following exchanges, therapist denotes therapist, client denotes Roy. Confidentiality statement and the business contract have been discussed. The session is joined as Roy begins his story.

Client: I don't know where to start really. I think I'm here because my boss said that I needed help. I've missed a few days work recently and been late a few times, and she smelled drink on my breath and then made me go to occupational health, and here I am.

Therapist: Sounds like you don't really want to be here.

Client: (*hesitant, voice child-like, body language closed*) I don't really, talking about feelings to a stranger and all that . . . but if she's making me come I might as well give it a go.

Therapist: It's your choice. I don't want to work with someone who feels forced to come. You might find it useful to 'give it a go'. How about we decide at the end of the session?

Client: Okay (*pauses, then begins to talk, almost apologetically . . .*). About six months ago my wife said she was leaving. Right out of the blue. I didn't see it coming, I thought we were doing okay. It's like . . . (*pause*) . . . it's just happened again.

Therapist: So it took you by surprise, but it's happened before.

Client: Yeah, twice. There goes my third marriage down the drain. Why does it always happen to me? I fall in love and then they leave me. I just never learn. I shouldn't trust them. All women are selfish bastards; they don't care about me, only about themselves. I should've listened to my dad. He hated them. 'Never trust a woman with your money or your life' he used to say. Anyway, after she left I just sat there, feeling sorry for myself I suppose. I managed to keep it together but felt crap, all sad and angry at the same time, so I phoned a few mates and we went for a drink. That was just over five months ago, and I've been drinking ever since.

Therapist: And the drinking, has that happened before as well?

Client: Yes, after both my other marriages. Only I don't want it to go the same way. First time, after my first marriage, I lost my job and then my house. I drank really heavily for nearly a year. Second time was shorter but worse. I got into trouble and was sent down. I'm not a violent man, but . . .

The therapist noted the way that Roy was describing his situation. His story was one of being badly treated by cruel and heartless women. The patterns emerging in the story suggested something else was going on in Roy's relationships. Later in the session, it emerged that Roy had actually begun to drink heavily during, not after, the marriages, and that when drinking, Roy would be verbally abusive to his partners. 'But I never hit them' he said. When asked about his childhood, he said his mother was a timid woman who often told Roy 'If it wasn't for you I'd have gone a long time ago.' He said he felt loved but not wanted by his mum. When asked to say more, he became quiet, reflective, almost tearful, and changed the subject. He spoke of being a frightened child. He remembers waiting for his dad to come home and would know his mood by the way he closed the front door. His father could be kind and loving, but could also be verbally abusive to Roy's mother and to Roy. Thursday nights were the worst. Roy's father was paid, in cash, on Thursdays and would come home drunk after the pubs closed. Most Thursdays Roy would lie in bed and listen to his father shouting, and then hitting his mother. 'But he never hit me', he said.

In subsequent sessions more of Roy's story emerged. The therapist encouraged Roy to take responsibility for his work in the sessions, and helped him identify patterns of behaviour, the roles he took in those patterns, the familiar feelings he experienced, the messages he received in childhood that influenced his thoughts, feeling and behaviours, and how all these linked to his script.

After the initial reluctance to engage, Roy found therapy useful, and was keen to gain insights. Translating this new awareness into behavioural change was harder, but Roy was well motivated to change.

Roy had the initial six sessions and then a further four, the maximum allowed under the employer scheme. At the end of the therapy, Roy felt that he had the knowledge and understanding he needed to make immediate changes (short-term management of problems), but knew that there was much to be done in order to free himself from his early childhood influences and decisions (longer term work to be free from script).

ANALYSING THE CASE STUDY

Try answering the following questions using information about transactional analysis.

- What ego-state was Roy in the early exchanges?
- What did the therapist do about this?
- What game is being played out in Roy's relationships?
- What position does he play and what position does he end up in?
- What position have his partners played and what position did they move to?
- What key script messages did he receive that may influence his relationships with women?
- What script process does Roy have?
- What do you think Roy's life position is?

SUMMARY

Humanistic and psychodynamic: main aim is autonomy (awareness, spontaneity and intimacy)

Development: introduced by Berne as an 'extra-Freudian' method of treating disturbance, International Transactional Analysis Association established in 1964, controversial due to non-technical terminology

Ego-state model of personality: Parent (critical and nurturing) perceives reality from the perspective of a parent and responds to others in a parental manner; Child (free and adapted) perceives reality from the perspective of a child and responds to others in a child-like manner; Adult perceives reality from an objective viewpoint and respond to others in a logical manner unfettered by emotion; ego-states are not actual roles and are not good or bad; should have free movement between states; exclusions occur when we lack one or two states; contaminations occur when we are in a different state to the one we think that we are in; therapy enhances understanding and control of states

Transactions and strokes: transactions (complementary, crossed, covert) result in positive or negative strokes (verbal/non-verbal, conditional/unconditional)

Games: series of transactions leading to a predictable payoff; Why don't you/yeah but; If it weren't for you; Now I've got you, you son of a bitch; Kick me; Why does this always happen to me?; drama triangle, persecutor, victim, rescuer

Antithesis of games: first rule is stop the game; second rule is break the game by depriving player of payoffs and responding from a different ego-state

Life positions and scripts: positions include I'm OK, you're OK; I'm OK, you're not OK; I'm not OK, you're OK; I'm not OK, you're not OK; life scripts contain injunctions, permissions and programs; scripts are written in childhood, based on verbal and non-verbal messages received from parents and significant others; six patterns of playing out scripts (always, never, until, after, almost and open ended)

Therapeutic process: joint relationship responsibility, psychoeducational; five-stage process to increased awareness; treatment plan includes diagnosis, contract, treatment direction; pragmatic in interventions

RATIONAL EMOTIVE BEHAVIOUR THERAPY

LEARNING OUTCOMES

After reading this section, you will be able to:

- explain that rational emotive behaviour therapy is an integrative therapy combining the cognitive and behavioural approaches

- discuss the history of rational emotive behaviour therapy with a brief biography of Albert Ellis

- outline the ABCDE model

- discuss the dangers of musturbation: 'neurosis-inciting musts' of irrational beliefs

- describe and evaluate techniques for disputing irrational beliefs

- describe and evaluate techniques for cognitive restructuring

- describe and evaluate techniques for shame-attacking exercises

- appreciate the application of rational emotive behaviour therapy in a therapeutic setting (case study)

Rational emotive behaviour therapy (REBT): cognitive and behavioural approaches

Rational emotive behaviour therapy is grounded in the cognitive and behavioural approaches

> Integration of cognitive and behavioural therapies
>> Cognitive therapy and behavioural therapy are rarely practised independently any more
>> Instead, they are often integrated to produce a new form of therapy
>> Rational emotive behaviour therapy is one of these integrations

Development of rational emotive behaviour therapy

History of rational emotive behaviour therapy

Rational emotive behaviour therapy was founded in the 1950s

> Therapy initially introduced as rational therapy (RT)
> Rational therapy (RT) changed to rational emotive therapy (RET) in 1961
>> Irrational and rational thoughts were linked to emotion
> Rational emotive therapy (RET) changed to rational emotive behaviour therapy (REBT) in 1993
>> Irrational and rational thoughts and emotions were linked to behaviour
>> Earliest form of cognitive-behaviour therapy

History of REBT is the history of Albert Ellis

Brief biography of Albert Ellis (1913–2007)

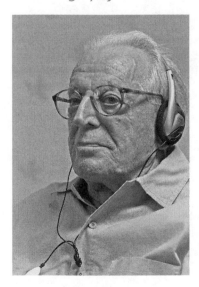

'You largely constructed your depression. It wasn't given to you. Therefore, you can deconstruct it.'
—Attributed to Ellis (n.d.)

Who was Albert Ellis?

Ellis founded rational emotive behaviour therapy in the 1950s

Introduced concept of emotion and cognition alongside behaviour therapy

First type of cognitive-behaviour therapy

Introduced the concept of irrational thoughts (decade before Beck) and explored their impact on a wide range of mental disorders – depression, sexual disorders, procrastination, anxiety, etc.

Established the non-profit Albert Ellis Institute in 1964

Author of over 600 papers and 50 books on REBT

REBT therapy was the earliest form of cognitive-behaviour therapy (CBT) – often described as the grandfather of CBT

Early years

Born on 17th September 1913

Born in Pittsburgh and raised in New York City

Physically and emotionally distant family life

Father was a businessman – often absent from home on business

Mother was a housewife – emotionally absent from her children

Mother often failed in her duties as a mother and Ellis was usually left to care for his siblings

Ellis described his mother as a self-absorbed woman who frequently verbalised strong opinions on most things but failed to support her views with evidence (Ellis et al., 2005)

Ellis was the eldest of three children

Ellis recalls purchasing an alarm clock with his own money so that he could rise early enough to get his brother and sister ready for school (Ellis et al., 2005)

Parents divorced by the time Ellis was 12 years old

Ellis coped with the family tensions by immersing himself in books and became a studious teenage boy

Numerous childhood health problems

Eight hospitalisations (kidney disease, tonsillitis, streptococcus) between the ages of five and eight

Little support from his family during illness – few visits or efforts to console him (Ellis et al., 2005)

Instilled a strong sense of independence in the growing child

Experienced extreme fears of rejection in teenage years

Responded to his shyness and inability to talk to women by desensitising himself to rejection from the opposite sex

'I made verbal overtures to 100 different women sitting on park benches in the Bronx Botanical Gardens, got rejected for dating by all of them (one woman kissed me in the park, and made a date for later that evening, but never showed up!)' (Ellis, 1996)

Education

Graduated with a Bachelor of Arts degree in business from City University of New York in 1934

Initially intended to set up in accounting, make enough money to retire at 30, and then work on becoming a great American novelist

Unfortunately, the Great Depression resulted in poor business ventures and he had little success in fictional writing (Albert Ellis Institute, 2012)

Discovered a talent for non-fiction writing and focused on producing a treatise on sexual liberation – as many friends considered him an expert on sexual matters, he also began informal therapy at this time (Ellis et al., 2005)

Master's degree in clinical psychology from Teachers College, Columbia University in 1943

Doctorate in clinical psychology at Columbia University in 1947

Worked as a psychologist offering sex and family therapy in his own part-time private practice – psychology was unlicensed at that time in the US (Ellis et al., 2005)

Published several articles while working on his PhD

One article was a critique of paper-based personality tests (Ellis, 1946)

Trained as a psychoanalyst under Richard Hulbeck at the Karen Horney Institute

Extremely unusual for a non-MD to be accepted as a trainee

Although initially impressed with the effectiveness of psychoanalysis, he became quickly disillusioned with the lack of scientific support and empirical evidence for the methods (Albert Ellis Institute, 2012)

Career

Lecturer at New York University and Rutgers University in the late 1940s

Senior clinical psychologist at Northern New Jersey Mental Hygiene Clinic in the late 1940s

Chief psychologist of the State of New Jersey in 1950

Still maintained a private part-time practice in New York

Expanded his part-time practice to full time in 1952

His reputation as a sexologist helped increase the client base of his growing practice, and he was even involved as an expert witness in some legal cases (for example, cases against publishers of obscene materials) (Ellis et al., 2005)

However, his reputation as an advocate of sexual liberation also hindered his ability to find a post as a lecturer in several major universities, including his own graduate school (Ellis et al., 2005)

Introduced rational therapy in 1955

Abandoned psychoanalysis and focused on changing behaviour by confronting irrational thoughts and changing them to rational thoughts

First paper presented to the APA convention in Chicago in 1956

Published a seminal paper introducing the approach, 'Rational psychotherapy and individual psychology', in 1957

Established the Institute for Rational Living in 1959 (Ellis et al., 2005)

Non-profit organisation aiming to educate the public

Changed rational therapy to rational emotive therapy in 1961

Irrational and rational thoughts were linked to emotion

Published *Reason and Emotion in Psychotherapy* to integrate emotion into rational therapy in 1962

Purchased a mansion on 65th Street in Manhattan to house the Albert Ellis Institute in 1964

Lived in the top floor of this building and continued working with patients

Dedicated most of the profits from his work back to the institute, allegedly taking only $12,000 a year salary alongside the promise of lifetime accommodation and medical care (REBT Network, 2006)

Changed rational emotive therapy to rational emotive behaviour therapy in 1993

Irrational and rational thoughts and emotions were linked to behaviour

Earliest form of cognitive-behaviour therapy

Published 'Changing rational emotive therapy (RET) to rational emotive behavior therapy (REBT)' to explain the change to include behavioural elements in 1995

Later life was marred with conflict and controversy (REBT Network, 2006)

Unfortunately, following a serious illness, the board of trustees refused to continue paying for medical expenses in 2004 – he was able to continue living and working at home only by using his own savings to continue to pay for at-home nursing care

Friday night workshops were a regular event at the institute for 40 years – workshops involved live demonstrations of REBT with audience members as clients

Unfortunately, the board of trustees banned him from using the facilities at the institute for these workshops in 2005 and he was forced to relocate to a nearby rented building

Ellis sued the institute in 2005 after the board of trustees voted to remove him from the board and suspend him from all professional duties

Supreme Court concluded that Ellis should be returned to the board in 2006, but the trustees continued to limit his involvement and prevent his professional practice

Ellis eventually rejected the institute and claimed that the work of the institute no longer reflected his own mission statement

Despite threats from the institute to sue his advocates for trademark infringement, many fans of Ellis continued to teach and practise REBT according to his original guidelines

Family

Married three times (Ellis et al., 2005)

First marriage ended with an annulment

Second marriage ended with an amicable divorce

Third marriage to Debbie Joffe in 2004 lasted until his death

Debbie Joffe adopted the role of wife, caregiver and assistant, and she continued publicising REBT after his death (REBT Network, 2006)

No children

At least, no legitimate children . . .

Death

Died of natural causes at the age of 93 on 24th July 2007

Worked continually until his death

Until his final illness at the age of 92, he worked at least 16 hours every day (REBT Network, 2006)

One of his final messages to his supporters from his hospital bed that year was 'work harder'

Significant learnings

'Do, don't stew!' (Ellis, 1997)

'Nothing, yes nothing is awful, horrible. Or terrible, no matter how bad, inconvenient, and unfair it may actually be' (Ellis, 1999)

'Stop damning yourself and others by fully accepting the view that wrong, unethical, and foolish acts never can make you or them into bad or rotten people' (Ellis, 1999)

'There is no magic, no free lunch. Self-change, while almost always possible, requires persistent work and practice' (Ellis, 1999)

'Surrender your demand to be perfect' (attributed to Ellis, n.d.)

ABCDE model

ABC (Ellis, 1996)

REBT proposes that the ultimate goal for all humans is the attainment of happiness

> Goal is intrinsic to our nature, yet it is often blocked by the myriad problems encountered on the pathway through life

> Our responses to these blockages will depend on our beliefs about the world and ourselves

> Illustrated in the ABC framework

A-B-C

> Activating event (A)

>> An activating event (A) in the world may block the individual in their movement towards happiness

> Belief about the event (B)

>> The event will be followed by a belief (B) about the event, and this belief can be logically based on the given evidence or illogically based on prejudices and superstitions

> Emotional and behavioural consequences of belief (C)

>> This belief will influence the subsequent emotional and behavioural consequences (C), and these consequences can be psychologically healthy or unhealthy

> For example, Susan is made redundant (A) and believes that this is evidence that she is a failure (B), thus she does not begin looking for another job and feels depressed (C)

Belief mediates between event and consequence

> ABC model highlights the importance of belief as a mediating factor between an event and a consequence

>> Emotional disturbance is based on beliefs about events rather than the events themselves

>> Once you have gained this understanding, the locus of control is back in your hands

>> Although you may be unable to influence events, you are capable of changing your own beliefs about these events

> For example, Susan is not looking for another job and feels depressed (C) due to her belief about being a failure (B) rather than the redundancy itself (A) – if she could change her belief then she would alter the consequences

Irrational beliefs can lead to negative consequences

> Ellis did not propose that therapy should focus on how these irrational beliefs developed

Instead he argued that the therapist should focus on how the client is maintaining these beliefs and seek to dispute them

As a therapeutic response to the innate tendency towards irrationality, Ellis (1996) formulated two stages to be added to the original ABC framework

> Disputing beliefs (D)

> Effects of the new rational philosophy (E)

ABCDE (Ellis, 1996)

Model expanded to include D and E

Activating event (A)

> An activating event (A) in the world may block the individual in their movement towards happiness

Belief about the event (B)

> The event will be followed by a belief (B) about the event, and this belief can be logically based on the given evidence or illogically based on prejudices and superstitions

Emotional and behavioural consequences of belief (C)

LEARNING MY ABCS (AND MY DES)

Think of a negative experience in your own life and complete the following table to identify the ABCDE.

A. Activating event What was the negative event?	
B. Belief about the event What did you believe about the event?	
C. Consequences How did you feel and what did you do?	
D. Disputing the belief Could you believe something different about the event?	
E. Effects of the new rational philosophy How would this new belief make you feel and behave differently?	

This belief will influence the subsequent emotional and behavioural consequences (C), and these consequences can be psychologically healthy or unhealthy

Disputing the belief (D)

Therapy aims to identify, challenge and eventually dispute irrational beliefs through a process of questioning (D)

Effects of the new rational philosophy (E)

Disputed irrational beliefs will eventually give way to rational philosophies about the world and this will lead to fewer negative consequences in the future (E)

For example, Susan is made redundant (A) and believes that this is evidence that she is a failure (B), thus she does not begin looking for another job and feels depressed (C), but the therapeutic process helps her to question the belief that she is a failure by asking her to focus on other successes in her life (D) and she eventually accepts that she is not responsible for redundancies at her company, thus she is able to look towards the future with confidence and optimism (E)

Dangers of musturbation

'Neurosis-inciting musts' (Ellis, 1996)

Primary irrational beliefs usually involve irrational demands

Irrational demanding philosophy = must/ought/should/need

Rational preferential philosophy = like/want

Irrational demands are often absolutist

Individual cannot accept a world in which the demand is not met

Irrational beliefs can be defined as subconscious thought patterns about how the world must function based only on the consideration of the individual's own needs (Batte, 1996)

Derivatives of musts

Primary irrational beliefs (demands such as 'must') lead to an array of other secondary or derivative irrational beliefs (Ellis, 1995a)

Awfulising

Low frustration tolerance (I-can't-stand-it-itus)

Self/other/life downing

Three musts

Ellis (1996) identifies three 'neurosis-inciting musts' of irrational beliefs

Musts relating to the behaviour of the self

Musts relating to the behaviour of others

Musts relating to life

Musts relating to the behaviour of the self

> 'I must be thoroughly competent, adequate, achieving, and lovable at all times, or else I am an incompetent worthless person' (Ellis, 2003)

> This belief will lead to the unhealthy emotional consequences of depression and guilt followed by unhealthy behavioural consequences of risk avoidance and procrastination

Musts relating to the behaviour of others

> 'Other significant people in my life must treat me kindly and fairly at all times, or else I can't stand it, and they are bad, rotten, and evil persons who should be severely blamed, damned, and vindictively punished for their horrible treatment of me' (Ellis, 2003)

> This belief will lead to the unhealthy emotional consequences of rage and anger followed by the unhealthy behavioural consequences of violence and intolerance

> Ellis (2003) suggested that this can lead to extreme actions such as feuds, wars, fights, genocide, and ultimately, an atomic holocaust

Musts relating to life

> 'Things and conditions absolutely must be the way I want them to be and must never be too difficult or frustrating. Otherwise, life is awful, terrible, horrible, catastrophic and unbearable' (Ellis, 2003)

> This belief will lead to the unhealthy emotional consequences of self-pity and depression followed by the unhealthy behavioural consequences of procrastination and work avoidance

Musturbation is disputed in therapy (Table 6.1)

Disputing 'musts'

> We recognise the irrational nature of thoughts once we realise that there is no good reason why the world 'absolutely must' function in a certain way

> Disputed irrational beliefs will eventually give way to rational philosophies about the world and Ellis (1996) suggested that this will lead to a clearer insight into the main truths of the world

> > 'We upset ourselves by holding inflexible beliefs, we continue to feel upset by clinging to these irrational beliefs, and we need to work hard to change our beliefs' (Ellis, 1996)

> These insights allow us to fully accept all aspects of reality without conditions or assumptions

Disputing musts relating to the behaviour of the self

> Self-acceptance encourages us to view ourselves as fallible human beings who are equally worthy as every other human being

Disputing musts relating to the behaviour of others

> Other-acceptance encourages us to appreciate that other people are not obliged to treat people fairly, thus those who behave badly are equally worthy as every other human being

Disputing musts relating to life

> Life-acceptance encourages us to understand that life is rarely awful and almost always bearable irrespective of the fact that it might not always follow the path desired by the individual

TABLE 6.1 'I must' versus 'I would like'

Rephrase the following statements and consider the potential impact that the new expression might have on the speaker.

Demanding philosophy	Preferential philosophy	Impact on new philosophy
I must get an A in my exam		
My husband should be nice to me when I have a headache		
I need to win the lottery		
I ought to keep the house clean all of the time		
People should never cheat on their spouses		
I have to put my make-up on before I go out		
Everything has to go well in my interview tomorrow		
She should not treat me like that		
I have to lose two stone		
I must do better in the future		

Disputing irrational beliefs

Cognitive therapy focuses on cognitions

Cognitions are thoughts about the world

> Client is encouraged to correct faulty thoughts, but this can fail to address the underlying beliefs
>
>> Sometimes the cognition might not actually be faulty

REBT focuses on beliefs

Beliefs are deeper held values about the world

> Client is encouraged to detect potentially irrational beliefs, debate the rationality of these beliefs, discriminate between rational and irrational thought

Detect potentially irrational belief

> Client is helped to recognise their tendency towards the derivatives of irrational beliefs (awfulising, i-can't-stand-it-itus, damning)
>
> Client is then encouraged to reduce their problems by asking 'why is this so?' until s/he eventually arrives at one of the three neurosis-inciting musts

Debate the rationality of a belief

> Client is encouraged to test beliefs using logic, personal experience and therapeutic experimentation
>
> Logic can be used to determine whether the belief is essentially flawed or contradictive
>
> Personal experience can be used to test whether the belief has had support in the past
>
> Therapeutic experimentation can be used to test whether the belief is empirically true
>
> Discriminate between rational and irrational thought
>
> On the basis of the above debate, the client can determine whether the belief is rational or irrational

Irrational beliefs are discarded

Example of client with low self-esteem

> Client claims that she is so ugly that no one could ever love her
>
> Cognitive therapy would address only the cognition
>
>> Client has the potentially faulty cognition that 'people must be beautiful in order to be loved'
>>
>> Client is invited to debate the rationality of this cognition by using logic (can we think of anyone who is ugly but still in a positive relationship?), personal experience (were you loved by your mother?), and experiments (go to the park and count the number of people holding hands – are all of these people attractive?)

Client is asked to determine whether it is rational to believe that she is so ugly that no one could ever love her

Client discriminates between this irrational thought and the more rational thought that she could find love by putting more effort into meeting people

BUT what if the client really is very ugly?

It is true that some people might fail to find love because they are so unattractive

But is it true that a person absolutely must be loved?

REBT would also address the deep underlying belief

Accept the cognition and begin to ask 'so what is bad about that?'

Do not need to argue with the cognition (people can be very stubborn about cognitions)

Instead, assume that it is true and focus on exploring the underlying belief

Client is encouraged to recognise the derivatives of the irrational belief, such as I can't stand to be unloved, the world is an awful place if I am unloved, I am a horrible person if I am unloved

Client is taught to detect the underlying 'must', such as I must be loved

Client holds a must relating to self: 'I must be loved'

Client is invited to debate the rationality of this 'must' by using logic (you are surviving as an unloved person so is it true that you absolutely must be loved?), personal experience (have you ever had any happiness in your life, even though you are unloved?), and experiments (do something to make yourself happy thus proving that you do not have to be loved)

Client is encouraged to change her irrational demand 'I must be loved' to a rational preference 'I would like to be loved'

Client is then released from the pressure of something that absolutely definitely must happen or else the world will end

We tend to feel blocked and trapped by fear when the must is too large, so removal of this pressure can free the client

Client can now focus on doing something to meet her desire for love

Cognitive restructuring

Irrational faulty beliefs replaced with rational constructive beliefs

Client is taught to adapt self-talk (Spiegler, 2008)

Self-talk is the inner monologue operating within each individual

Positive self-talk can be motivating, inspiring, problem solving, etc.

Negative self-talk can be demotivating, depressing, self-defeating, etc.

Client is taught the dangers of musturbation and encouraged to avoid the use of these absolute terms in their own self-talk

For example, client might be encouraged to recognise that the inner thought 'I must do well in this exam' is an example of musturbation and would be better changed to 'I would like to do well in this exam'

It is less damaging to fail to get something that you would like to have than it is to fail to get something that you absolutely must have

Adaptive self-talk is realistic and rational, thus it can help the client to work towards success yet accept potential failure without devastating effects

Shame-attacking exercises

Shame and embarrassment are uncomfortable but not lethal

Acceptance of the fact that things are rarely unbearable can be difficult without evidence to show that you can survive apparently impossible situations

Shame-attacking exercises are designed to give the client an opportunity to experience and survive risky and embarrassing situations (Ellis, 1995b)

Clients may be asked to engage in public activities that would normally result in shame, such as singing loudly, walking in a strange way, approaching strangers, etc.

Once the client has survived the shame then s/he has learnt that it is possible to cope with feelings of embarrassment

Repeated exposure to controlled shame will desensitise the client so that s/he is no longer constrained by the fear of shame

Example of a shy client

Client is asked to sing loudly in public

Experience is embarrassing, but not damaging

Client learns that s/he can cope with embarrassment and becomes less shy as a result

Risks of shame-attacking exercises

Shame can be a powerful emotion

Rather than providing a learning opportunity to manage and reduce fear of shame, poorly managed exercises can increase fear in the client

Repeated experiences of shame can lead the client to engage in more avoidance strategies or confirm negative self-beliefs held by the client

It is essential that the clients remain in control throughout the exercises so that they know that they can withdraw at any point if the experience becomes overwhelming

Exercises should be closely followed by extensive debriefing in the form of discussions about the experience through a positive framework of how the client successfully managed to cope with the discomfort

ATTACK THE SHAME!

Think carefully about the things that make you most anxious and consider the underlying cause of that anxiety. In many cases, people fear the experience of shame. For example, the person who loathes public speaking may argue that they are afraid that they will mumble or blush or faint but these things are not terrifying experiences in themselves – fear comes from the shame associated with being negatively judged. One way to reduce the fear of shame is to actively engage in shame-inducing activities until you eventually become desensitised to the feeling of embarrassment.

Find something that makes you squirm with embarrassment. If you are struggling for ideas, consider the following: singing in a public place, going to a party without wearing make-up, walking down the street with food on your shirt, making a speech in front of strangers, asking someone out on a date, or wearing a silly costume to shop at the supermarket. Once you have identified a shame-inducing activity, try to answer the following questions.

1. Imagine that you saw a stranger doing the shameful activity. What would you think about him/her?
2. Imagine that your best friend was doing the shameful activity. What would you think about him/her?
3. Imagine doing the shameful activity yourself – close your eyes and visualise the whole experience. How do you look and sound? How are people reacting? Do you feel shame or embarrassment? How can you learn to cope with these feelings?

Now that you have imagined the experience, it is time to try it out. Choose a time and location that is safe and appropriate then test out your shame-inducing experience. The aim is for you to feel embarrassed so do not be deterred once the discomfort arises; instead, focus on how well you are coping with the embarrassment and remind yourself that it is a temporary state that will not do you any lasting harm.

IMPORTANT

Please consider legal, moral and safety parameters when selecting your shame-inducing activity. Do not engage in any activity that is illegal (for example, being naked in a public place) or unsafe (for example, starting an argument with a stranger). Remember that you are in control of this learning experience and you are free to stop at any time if it becomes overwhelming.

Possible exercises are constrained by legal, moral and safety guidelines

Some of the most shame-inducing activities should not be encouraged due to potential risks

For example, a woman who is embarrassed about her body should never be encouraged to strip naked in public to face her shame (but she could try wearing a bikini on the beach)

Shame is to be expected in certain situations and the experience of shame can motivate people to change their behaviour for the better under some conditions

Experience of shame is sometimes used as an expression of regret and this can provide an insight into the world of the client

These types of shame are not appropriate for a shame-inducing activity

For example, a man who is ashamed of his poor treatment of his wife should never be encouraged to attack this shame by repeating the behaviour

Case study demonstrating REBT

Sarah, 19, is a student at a local college and she decided to seek therapy after the unexpected end of her relationship with her girlfriend. She discovered that her girlfriend was having an affair with another woman when she found a romantic text on her phone. Although she tried to save the relationship, her partner left her two weeks later and moved in with the other woman. She is devastated by this loss and she is convinced that the affair happened because she has recently gained weight. She insists that she 'will never find love again'. The therapy was limited to eight sessions, as per the policy for the college counselling service.

In the following exchanges, therapist denotes therapist, client denotes Sarah. Confidentiality statement and the business contract have been discussed. The session is joined just after Sarah has explained her story.

Client: So now I don't know what to do. I keep thinking about getting her back. I mean, if I lost some weight and then maybe just ran into her at the library . . . I just can't believe that this has happened. I can't stand it. I keep expecting her to be in the flat when I get home. How could she do this to me?

Therapist: It sounds like you are feeling very angry with her.

Client: I am. How dare she treat me like this? You just don't hurt people like this.

Therapist: Who doesn't?

Client: People. Her. She's just a horrible person for doing this.

Therapist: So you are saying that she should not treat you like this?

Client: Yes. She shouldn't.

Therapist: Why not?

Client: Because . . . because I don't like it.

Therapist: Okay. I understand that you don't like it when you are treated badly. But does that mean that she absolutely must not treat you like that? Is it true that people must always treat you in the way that you want to be treated?

Client: Well . . . no . . . but it would be nice if they did.

Therapist: I agree, it would be nice if people treated us kindly. Perhaps that could be a better way of expressing it.

Client: You mean, I would like to be treated nicely?

Therapist: Yes. People do not absolutely have to treat you nicely, but it would be nice.

Client: (Sigh) I bet she would have treated me better if I were thinner.

Therapist: You believe that she would have been nicer to you if you were thinner?

Client: I think so, yes. I'm never gonna find anyone to love me while I look like this.

Therapist: And is it very important to you that you find someone to love you?

Client: Well, yes. Obviously.

Therapist: Why is that obvious?

Client: Because everybody needs love.

Therapist: Do they?

Client: Yes! If you don't have love then you go through life alone.

Therapist: And what is so bad about that?

Client: Well, it means that you are alone. You spend all of your time on your own.

Therapist: And what is so bad about that?

Client: Obviously it is bad to be alone. It means that no-one is there for you.

Therapist: I know that I am repeating myself, but I have to ask one more time. What is so bad about being independent and not having anyone there for you?

Client: I . . . It just is. I don't know. It is just bad.

Therapist: I see. So you absolutely must be loved?

Client: Well, no. I don't absolutely have to be loved. I could live without being loved. It would be nice though.

Therapist: Okay. So it would be nice to be loved and it would be nice if other people treated you kindly.

Client: Yes.

Therapist: So what happens if you do not get those 'nice' things? Is it bearable?

Client: I guess so. I would like to be loved by someone who treats me well, but I guess that I can cope if that doesn't happen.

Over the subsequent sessions, the therapist worked with Sarah to identify her musturbatory beliefs about the end of the relationship. She identified her own tendency towards the beliefs that she must be loved (self-must) otherwise life is awful (awfulising) and unbearable (low frustration tolerance) and that other people must be kind to her (other-must) otherwise they are horrible people (other-downing).

Sarah was eventually able to understand that her current distress was caused by her interpretation of the break-up, rather than the break-up itself. She acknowledged that an alternative interpretation would probably lead to more positive feelings and behaviours. She also recognised that her own low self-esteem might be contributing to her difficulties so she decided to join a local theatre group in order to tackle her fear of being negatively judged.

Sarah decided to end the counselling relationship after five sessions as she felt more confident and content in her life.

ANALYSING THE CASE STUDY

Try answering the following questions using information about rational emotive behaviour therapy.

- What were the activating event, belief about the event and emotional/behavioural consequences of this belief for Sarah?
- How did the therapist dispute the belief and what was the effect of the new rational philosophy?
- What 'neurosis-inciting musts' did Sarah demonstrate?
- What derivatives of musts did Sarah experience?
- How were these musts disputed and what was the effect of this?
- How did the therapist encourage Sarah to change her self-talk?
- What shame-attacking exercises could be recommended for Sarah?

SUMMARY

Cognitive and behavioural: rarely practised independently; REBT was one of the first integrations

Development: founded by Ellis as RT in the 1950s and changed to RET in 1961 then REBT in 1993; first type of cognitive-behaviour therapy

ABCDE: activating event (A), belief about the event (B), emotional and behavioural consequences of belief (C), disputing the belief (D), effects of the new rational philosophy (E); belief mediates between event and consequence, irrational beliefs can lead to negative consequences

Dangers of musturbation: irrational demanding philosophy = must/ought/should/need; rational preferential philosophy = like/want; three absolutist 'neurosis-inciting musts' of irrational beliefs, musts relating to the behaviour of the self, musts relating to the behaviour of others, musts relating to life; musturbation is disputed in therapy, self-acceptance, other-acceptance, life-acceptance

Disputing irrational beliefs: cognition versus belief; detect and debate

Cognitive restructuring: adaptive self-talk is realistic and rational

Shame-attacking exercises: embarrassment is uncomfortable but not lethal; exercises involve doing embarrassing things to accept that you can survive unpleasant experiences such as shame; risks associated with some of these exercises

COGNITIVE-BEHAVIOUR THERAPY

LEARNING OUTCOMES

After reading this section, you will be able to:

- explain that cognitive-behaviour therapy is an integrative therapy combining the cognitive and behavioural approaches
- discuss the history of cognitive-behaviour therapy with acknowledgement of the wide number of contributors spanning many different psychological fields
- explain how cognition drives emotional reactions to external events
- explain how assessment and formulation are utilised through the therapy
- discuss the combined application of cognitive therapy and behaviour therapy techniques
- outline the structure of the therapeutic sessions throughout the therapy
- discuss the empirical evidence evaluating therapeutic efficacy
- describe and evaluate the use of computerised cognitive-behaviour therapy
- describe some 'third wave' therapies emerging from cognitive-behaviour therapy, appreciate the application of cognitive-behaviour therapy in a therapeutic setting (case study)

Cognitive-behaviour therapy (CBT): cognitive and behavioural approaches

Cognitive-behaviour therapy is grounded in the cognitive and behavioural approaches

Integration of cognitive and behavioural therapies

Cognitive therapy and behavioural therapy are rarely practised independently any more

Instead, they are often integrated to produce a new form of therapy

Cognitive-behaviour therapy is one of these integrations

Development of cognitive-behaviour therapy

History of cognitive-behaviour therapy

Behaviour therapy developed in the early 1900s out of the work of the behavioural psychologists (Pavlov, Watson, Skinner)

> It was a challenge to and developed alongside the psychodynamic approach, which was particularly dominant in the early 20th century

> In contrast to the psychodynamic approach, with its emphasis on instinctual drives and unconscious processes, the behavioural approach focused on observable and measurable behaviours and learning processes

> This allowed a more scientific approach that could be supported by empirical evidence (criticism of the Freudian approach)

> Behavioural approach found to be effective working on a variety of client issues, particularly anxiety issues and phobias

> However, not all clients responded to the approach and it was accepted that focusing purely on behaviours meant that thought processes were largely ignored – clearly, people were influenced by their beliefs, their thoughts and by the mental images they created

Cognitive therapy developed in the mid-1900s out of the work of cognitive psychologists (Neisser, Beck)

> Cognitive interpretations of emotional disorders (particularly depression) were instrumental in shifting attention from behaviour to cognition

> This laid the foundation for the integration of the cognitive and behavioural approaches – cognitive-behaviour therapy (CBT)

Prevalence of CBT

> In the UK, the National Institute for Health and Clinical Excellence (NICE) stated that CBT should be the treatment of choice for individuals suffering from anxiety or depression (NICE guidelines, 2004, amended 2007)

> Likewise in the US, the American Psychiatric Association stated that CBT should be regarded as the primary psychotherapeutic approach for patients with anxiety or depression (APA, 2000)

> As a result of these guidelines for the NHS, the UK government highlighted CBT as the treatment of choice for those diagnosed with depression or anxiety and, in order to cement this recommendation, a budget of £170 million was promised in 2007 for the expansion of mental health therapies with the specific proviso that only evidence-based treatments such as CBT would be funded

> Announcement of this policy met with a mixed response

>> Those in favour argued that the additional funding would improve the likelihood of recovery from mental illness

>> Those against argued that the effectiveness of CBT is no better than other forms of therapy and so this proposal will limit patient choice

Over a decade on from the first NICE guidelines, CBT is still generally considered the best approach for dealing with anxiety and depression, and it is the most widely used therapeutic method within the NHS

Multiple contributors

No individuals regarded as 'founding fathers/mothers' of CBT

Instead, multiple key figures have contributed to the development of this approach

Since CBT is an integrative approach combining behavioural and cognitive approaches, key figures identified for each of these approaches could be regarded as contributors to the development of CBT (please refer to previous chapters for brief biographies of these contributors)

Pavlov
Thorndike
Watson
Skinner
Staats
Ellis
Bruner
Miller
Beck
Chomsky
Neisser

Donald Meichenbaum is perhaps the main contributor to the modern concept of CBT

Brief biography of Donald Meichenbaum (1940–current)

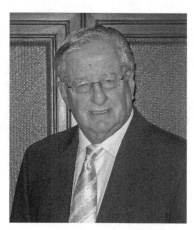

'Any advocate that says "This is the cure" or proposes a "revolutionary" approach does not deserve your attention, nor your money.'
—Meichenbaum (quoted in Howes, 2008)

Who is Donald Meichenbaum?

Focused on changing cognitions by modifying the 'inner dialogue' through psychotherapy

Integrated cognitive and behavioural theories to form cognitive-behaviour modification – original form of cognitive-behaviour therapy (alternative to REBT proposed by Ellis)

Early years

Born 10th June 1940 in New York

Education

Graduated with a degree in psychology at City College, New York

Completed postgraduate studies at Illinois University

Career

Originally intended to pursue a career in industry, but focused on clinical psychology instead after working as a research assistant in a psychiatric hospital

Professor at University of Waterloo, Ontario, from 1966 to 1998

Published *Cognitive-Behavior Modification: An Integrative Approach* in 1977 to combine the classical behavioural techniques with the newly emerging cognitive techniques in order to produce a novel integrative therapy

Voted one of the ten most influential psychotherapists of the 20th century in a survey of 800 clinical and counselling psychologists in 1982 (Smith, 1982)

Published *Stress Inoculation Training* in 1985

Retired in 1998

Significant learnings

'I have trained and supervised psychotherapists all over the world and the major challenge is that they DO NOT LISTEN to their clients. Instead, they act as what I call 'Surrogate Frontal Lobes' for their clients by giving explicit advice' (Meichenbaum, quoted in Howes, 2008)

'The art of questioning is the psychotherapist's most valuable tool. Mainly, these are HOW and WHAT questions' (Meichenbaum, quoted in Howes, 2008)

'Psychotherapy is a noble profession and I am honored to be a member of this community' (Meichenbaum, quoted in Howes, 2008)

Cognition-driven emotions

'The mind is its own place and in itself, can make a Heaven of Hell, a Hell of Heaven.'
—Milton (Paradise Lost, Book 1)

Clients often assume that events in their lives cause them to feel emotions

'The presentation made me anxious'

'I'm angry because he ignored me'

However, if it were the event itself that caused the emotional response then everybody would feel the same and this is clearly not the case

'I'm excited about the presentation'

'I'm fed up because he ignored me'

It is the cognition (thoughts, beliefs, interpretations) that we have of the event that leads to the emotional response

CBT uses a basic ABC model (Ellis, 1996)

A is the event

B is cognition (our interpretation) of the event

C is the emotional (and then behavioural) consequence of B

CBT considers clients' problems, in terms of both creation and maintenance, as an interaction between . . .

Cognition

Feelings

Behaviours

Physical sensations

Cognition is considered to be the starting point in this process

If a client has a core belief that s/he is worthless and useless in all areas of life . . .

When they have an exam looming, this core belief will lead to a dysfunctional assumption about being bad at exams in general, which will lead to a negative automatic thought about the forthcoming exam ('it will be awful')

CBT therapists work with clients to help them become more aware of these negative automatic thoughts and to replace them with more realistic thoughts

Therapy may also aim to change dysfunctional assumptions and core beliefs

These are harder to change but can lead to change that may affect many areas in the client's life

REBT, an alternative type of CBT, considers changing beliefs to be the focus of therapy, leading to a deeper and more fundamental change

Assessment and formulation

Collecting information about the client enables the therapist to make an assessment

Information gathering would focus on the following areas

Symptoms
Predisposing factors
Precipitating factors
Triggers
Beliefs and assumptions
Maintenance processes

Symptoms

> Thoughts, feelings, behaviours and physical sensations of the problem and how these interact

> It is how thoughts, feelings, physical sensations and behaviours interact with each other that show the client's individual way of approaching the problem

> Client has a problem in relation to the environment (external factors which influence the client)

> The greater the detail collected on these interactions, the better informed are the client and therapist about the nature and extent of the problem

> For example, a claustrophobic client may describe feelings of doom, increased heart rate and thoughts of death in response to being in a small room

Predisposing factors

> Aspects of the client's history that may be influencing the current problem

> Events in the client's past, especially in childhood, are likely to have influenced beliefs and assumptions about self, others, the world and the future

> While the main focus of CBT is on the present and the future, understanding of significant past events may help in the understanding of how the problem may be maintained in the present

> For example, an adult client experiencing depression may be able to identify early parental messages of being unloved

Precipitating factors

> What was happening in the client's life at the time that the problem started

> Past events may predispose a client to a problem, but this will not be triggered until a life event (or series of events) occurs

> For example, a client may have been unaware of early parental messages of being unloved until the breakdown of his marriage

Triggers

> What is happening in the client's life just before the problem occurs

> These are the current factors that have triggered the problem

> For example, seeing a spider might result in a phobic reaction

> This will be worse depending upon other factors (for example, the size and proximity of the spider)

Beliefs and assumptions

> What beliefs and assumptions the client holds about self, others and the future

> If we have rigid, irrational beliefs about self, others and the world then these are likely to create and maintain problems

> Dysfunctional assumptions also underpin our negative automatic thoughts

Maintenance processes or cycles

> What role the client plays in maintaining the problem

CBT focuses on how the client keeps the problem going

Some common maintenance processes are

> Avoidance: for example, someone with a fear of elevators will use the stairs

> Withdrawal: for example, if a person thinks that they will appear stupid if they give an opinion in a group then they are likely to withdraw and not contribute to the discussion

> Overvigilance: for example, someone who is scared of becoming ill is likely to be oversensitive to symptoms of illness and may misinterpret physical signs and symptoms

Much of this information will be collected in the first session with a client

> Further details are likely to be added as therapy progresses, but there will be enough information gained early on with a client to develop a basic formulation

Assessment forms the basis of the initial formulation (Figure 6.6)

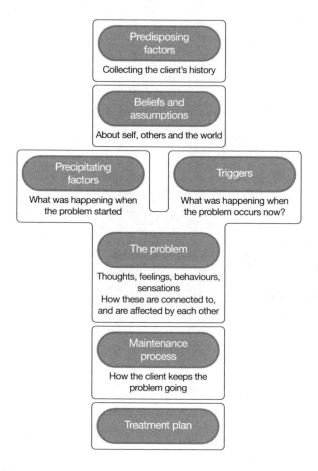

FIGURE 6.6 Formulation template.

'Formulation' is used to describe building up an understanding of the client's problem

> This includes how the problem developed, how it is maintained and how it can be treated

Formulation will draw together all the information gathered during the assessment to provide a full picture of the situation

FORMULATE YOUR PROBLEM

Think of a situation that may be a problem for you. This could be something like giving a presentation at work or going inside an elevator or travelling by airplane.

Spend a few minutes thinking about how you 'do' the problem. Try to complete your own formulation by answering the questions in the boxes below.

Symptoms What do you think, feel and do during the problem?	
Predisposing factors Can you think of anything in your past that might be contributing to the problem?	
Precipitating factors What was going on in your life at the time the problem started?	
Triggers What happens to start the problem?	
Beliefs and assumptions What do you believe about the problem?	
Maintenance processes What might you be doing to maintain the problem?	

Once you have a clearer understanding of the problem, you can begin to think what you can do about it (treatment).

Formulation will then add a treatment plan in order to give both the therapist and the client a good understanding of how the therapeutic process will progress

This basic outline of therapy will develop as more information is explored in future sessions

A useful method of representing all the information gathered during the assessment and the subsequent treatment plan is by using a formulation template

>This is a simple way of displaying all the key aspects of the client's problem

Application of cognitive therapy and behaviour therapy techniques

Cognitive-behaviour therapy is predominantly psychoeducational

The more the client knows about how the problem works and about the techniques to manage and overcome the problem, the more the client can become their own therapist

CBT for clients with mild depression or mild anxiety may encourage the client to use self-help guides or relevant books and manuals (bibliotherapy)

Another possibility is for clients to access computer-based CBT – this is one of the more recent developments of the approach

Wide variety of cognitive and behavioural techniques

CBT adopts a wide range of techniques from the fields of behaviourist psychology and cognitive psychology to provide an empirically based therapeutic approach to psychological disturbances such as depression and anxiety

Socratic questioning

Socratic questioning is an important technique that is used throughout the CBT therapeutic process

>It has been noted as one of the essential competencies for a CBT therapist (Roth & Pilling, 2007)

>Socratic questions can be asked at any stage in the process

Socratic questioning, named after the Greek philosopher Socrates, is a way of guiding a client to discover new perspectives by asking questions which she has the answer to but which may currently be outside her awareness

>Such questions help the client focus on aspects of her thoughts, feelings, physical sensations and behaviours in order to gain new cognitive insights, which can then be the basis for behavioural change

Examples of Socratic questions

>What were you thinking when . . . ?

>What are you thinking when you feel . . . ?

How did you feel when . . . ?

What would it mean to you if . . . ?

What else did you think/feel when . . . ?

What did you do when . . . ?

What was happening before . . . ?

Were you aware of any physical sensations when . . . ?

What else could you have done . . . ?

How useful is it to believe . . . ?

Socratic questions can be used to . . .

Gather information in the assessment and formulation stage

Make connections between thoughts, feelings, sensations and behaviours

Challenge irrational beliefs and negative thoughts

Explore solutions and resolve problems

A good Socratic question will leave the client feeling empowered, that she has arrived at an answer, rather than being told by the therapist.

Consider the difference between the following examples

Client: My four year old just started screaming and so I hit him. I can't believe I did that.

Therapist: You could have counted to 10 to give yourself time to think

Client: Yeah, I suppose so

SOCRATIC QUESTIONS IN ACTION

Think of three different Socratic questions for each of the following client statements.

'I don't know what to do'

'Well, you would feel angry, wouldn't you?'

'I just keep crying for no reason'

'It's hopeless'

'It all started about a year ago'

'I started panicking'

'I felt sick when I woke up on the morning of the presentation'

'I don't care one way or the other'

'She shouldn't treat me like that'

'How do you think it made me feel?'

In this first example, the therapist has made the suggestion and so the client has no ownership

> Client: My four year old just started screaming and so I hit him. I can't believe I did that.

> Therapist: What would have been a better thing to do?

> Client: I suppose I could have counted to 10 and . . .

In this second example, through the use of a Socratic question, the client comes up with her own answer

Identifying cognitive errors

Thoughts are connected to feelings

> Depression is linked to thoughts such as 'Nothing will ever change. I'm worthless and unlovable'

> Anger is linked to thoughts such as 'He shouldn't treat me like that'

> Anxiety is linked to thoughts such as 'It's going to be awful'

Socratic questions can help the client to link feelings and thoughts

> 'What are you thinking when you feel that?'

> 'When you feel like that, how does that affect your thoughts?'

> 'When you think that about yourself, how does that make you feel?'

> 'What feelings do you have when you say that to yourself?

We all have faulty thinking from time to time

> However, when people have problems these thinking errors are likely to be more frequent and more extreme

> Some thinking biases go together with specific problems

>> For example, people suffering with depression are more likely to focus on negative events and filter out positive events

There are many common thinking errors (Beck, 1975)

> All-or-nothing thinking

>> With this type of thinking there are no grey areas, only black or white

>> For example, 'If I don't get what I want now, I'll never get what I want'

> Catastrophising

>> Worst-case scenario thinking

>> For example, 'If I fail my driving test, I won't be able to drive and I'll never get that job. I'll end up on the scrap heap'

> Perfectionism

>> Setting standards that are unachievable

>> Often observed through the excessive use of 'should' and 'musts'

>> For example, 'I must do this perfectly or it will be/I am worthless'

Generalisations

> Taking one event and making a global statement

> For example, 'The car didn't start today. It always does that'

Focusing on negatives

> Focusing only on the negative elements of life

> Likely to become part of a process that reinforces depression

> For example, 'Nothing good ever happens to me. Ever'

Discounting positives

> Reducing the value or importance of the positive elements of life

> A common error, magnified when we have problems

> For example, 'He only complimented me because he wants something'

Mind reading

> Dysfunctional assumptions based on limited information (e.g. reading body language)

> For example, 'She's not speaking to me, that means she hates me'

Developing new perspectives

Once a client is aware of his thinking errors, there are techniques to help develop new perspectives and new ways of thinking

CBT therapists encourage clients to test the negative thoughts in order to identify errors

> Whenever a client has a negative thought, s/he can be challenged to justify the thought

> For example, 'Nothing good ever happens to me. Ever' could be tested by asking 'Has there ever been a time when something good did happen to you?'

> 'I must do this perfectly or it will be/I am worthless' could be tested by asking 'Who says you must do it perfectly?' or 'What would really happen if you didn't do it perfectly?'

Experimentation

Experiments can be used to empirically test potentially faulty negative cognitions

Experiments can be used to address actions that are maintaining negative behaviour

> Some clients may use avoidance as a maintenance process – for example, staying in the house to avoid the possibility of a panic attack

> What starts out as a logical strategy ('I had a panic attack yesterday, so I'll not risk it today') can turn into a major limitation (one day becomes two days, becomes a week, a month, a year . . .)

> Behavioural experiments involve graded tasks set as homework between sessions

For example:

Day 1	walk to front gate
Day 2	step outside front gate
Day 3	walk 10 paces from front gate, etc.

These tasks would be agreed between the client and the therapist

This is a simple desensitisation hierarchy but could be combined with some measurement to record thoughts and intensity and duration of feeling as the task was carried out

Relaxation techniques such as focusing on breathing or positive visualisation may also be integrated into the task

Changing self-talk from negative to positive

Cognitive-behaviour modification focuses on client's self-talk to change unwanted behaviours

Helps clients become more aware of their present internal dialogue, highlights how this dialogue affects emotion and behaviour, and demonstrates how to change negative self-talk to more useful, coping talk

Similar to Beck and Ellis in that it highlights that unhelpful emotions and unwanted behaviours are a result of dysfunctional, negative thoughts, but it is often less confrontational

Meichenbaum (1977) identified a three-phase change process

1.   Self-observation

Becoming more aware of emotions and behaviours and the internal dialogue that influences them

2.   Changing internal dialogue

Once we become aware of unhelpful internal dialogue, we can begin to change it

More positive dialogue will lead to more positive emotions and behaviours (which in turn reinforce the positive internal dialogue)

3.   New skills

Teaching clients more effective ways of coping in order for them to feel more in control

Homework tasks

CBT often involves setting the client homework tasks

Tasks will often involve collecting relevant data to 'measure' the problem, especially in the early stages of therapy

Collecting data is useful

Task engages the client in activity outside the session

Thoughts, feeling and behaviours noted as occurring at the time of the problem are likely to be more accurate than those reported in the session

Helpful to keep record of change because clients often forget how bad the problem was at the start of therapy by the time the changes have begun to take effect

Data serve as a therapeutic tool in itself as the client may benefit from focusing on what they are thinking when they become aware of the problem (mindfulness)

Measurements include . . .

Frequency (e.g. how often a client checks that the front door is locked)

Duration (e.g. how long does it take to get out of the house?)

Intensity (e.g. on a scale of 1 to 10 how bad did you feel?)

Methods of measurement include . . .

Rating scales

Thought diaries

Charts

COGNITIVE AND BEHAVIOUR TECHNIQUES IN THERAPY

Re-read the chapters on cognitive therapy (Chapter 5) and behaviour therapy (Chapter 4) then consider the following case studies. Try to identify the main issues for each client and outline a treatment plan incorporating both cognitive and behavioural techniques.

- Caroline is struggling with her dependency on alcohol after being made redundant. She is finding it difficult to get motivated to look for work and she feels that her only happy moments occur when she drinks wine in the evening.
- John is struggling to come to terms with the death of his dog. He has lived alone for most of his life and his dog has been his only companion over the last ten years. He feels like he does not want to continue living without his only friend.
- Janine has recently had a baby and she is terrified that the child is going to get sick or be injured. She tries not to go outside with the baby and she constantly checks on him at home. Although her husband tries to be supportive, her behaviour is having a major impact on their relationship.
- Drake is an excellent student but he has recently begun skipping classes and failing to submit assignments. He is terrified that he is going to fail his course and he regards any grade less than an A as a fail.
- Hazel suffers with acute social anxiety. She has a slight limp when she walks and she is extremely aware of this problem. She is convinced that people are laughing at her behind her back and she refuses to attend any public events in order to avoid being mocked.

Any measurements that the client is required to make should be . . .

Easy to carry out

Meaningful

Specific

Relevant

Done as close as possible to the event

Structure of therapeutic sessions

Structure of a session will depend upon where the client is in the process

Beginnings and endings of the process will have different formats, with more emphasis on the client taking responsibility as the process develops

However, during the main phase of therapy, a 50-minute session is likely to run as follows

Discussing the content of the session (5 minutes)

Discussion will include what both the therapist and client think would be useful to work on during that session

Checking the previous week (10 minutes)

Update on what has been happening over the last week and how the client managed with the previous homework tasks

Main content (25 minutes)

Specific work decided upon at the start of the session and including the application of CBT techniques

Setting tasks for the next week (5 minutes)

Homework agreed by therapist and client

CBT requires clients to work on tasks between sessions – as the process of therapy progresses, the client should take more responsibility for setting tasks and managing the change process

Review of the session (5minutes)

Checking out what the client thought was useful, and what was unhelpful, during the session

Empirical evidence for CBT

Due to the empirical nature of CBT, extensive research has been conducted to measure its impact on mental health

Findings suggest that CBT is effective in reducing the symptoms of depression and anxiety

Controlled trials exploring treatment outcomes in severely depressed outpatients have found that CBT is as effective as antidepressant medication in reducing symptoms (DeRubeis et al., 1999)

While research to date has provided a significant body of evidence to support the hypothesis that CBT is effective in treating depression and anxiety, there are a number of criticisms directed at this empirical approach to treatment

> One initial criticism relates to the fact that effectiveness is measured in accordance with the scores obtained in questionnaires before and after the treatment process

>> These questionnaire measures are subject to participant bias since many clients may feel obliged to indicate an improvement due to a sense of obligation to their therapist

> Another criticism is that clients will have been selected on the basis of their desire to work towards improved mental health

>> CBT is inappropriate for clients who refuse to engage with the mini-experiments, activities and homework

>> Clients presenting with depressive symptoms associated with poor motivation or an unwillingness to engage with therapy would not be prescribed CBT

>> A recent meta-analysis of ten controlled studies comparing CBT with treatment as usual indicates only a modest therapeutic benefit for sufferers of major depression and no therapeutic benefit for sufferers of bipolar depression (Lynch et al., 2010)

> Another criticism argues that the suggestion that it is the most effective method of treatment is based on a logical error

>> Cooper et al. (2008) state that the conclusions drawn from recent research are an example of a logical fallacy: as more researchers subscribe to the CBT approach, more research grants will be awarded and more studies will be published about the benefits of CBT

>> The large number of supporting studies is assumed to indicate the efficiency of CBT, but it could instead indicate the popularity of the method

Research that has attempted to control for these criticisms finds little difference between CBT and other therapeutic methods

> Patients receiving cognitive-behaviour therapy, psychodynamic therapy or person-centred therapy through the NHS primary care services were compared on the Clinical Outcomes in Routine Evaluation – Outcome Measure (CORE-OM) to reveal no significant differences between the three approaches (Stiles et al., 2005; successfully replicated by Stiles et al., 2008)

> Patients receiving non-directive counselling or cognitive-behaviour therapy were compared on treatment satisfaction measures to reveal no significant differences between the two approaches (Ward et al., 2000)

> These findings illustrate the equivalence paradox or the 'Dodo verdict', as they suggest that all treatment methods are approximately equivalent in terms of outcome

>> 'Everybody has won and all must have prizes' (Caroll, 1865/1946, as cited in Stiles et al., 2008)

On the basis of the evidence, it could be concluded that CBT has a positive impact on the symptoms of depression and anxiety

> However, positive effect of CBT is possibly no greater than any other therapeutic method

> CBT not suitable for all sufferers of depression and anxiety

>> CBT requires a collaborative relationship with both the therapist and the client working towards a positive change in mental health

>> Techniques often involve homework assignments and active experimentation in the world beyond the counselling room

>> Therefore, CBT requires the client to be motivated to change and engaged with the therapeutic process

>> Even if the client is motivated to engage with therapy, some individuals may not feel comfortable with the directive nature of this approach

>> As CBT is not appropriate for all sufferers of anxiety and depression, it is essential that there are alternative psychological therapies available

Computerised CBT

Computerised CBT (CCBT) is offered to people meeting the criteria for mild depression

> Programs allow people to work through a CBT-based computer program at their own pace

> There are a growing number of such programs available, most offering telephone supports, along with a comprehensive self-help program

> Testimonials from users of these programs indicate that they are very effective, life enhancing and life changing

>> However, by their very nature, testimonials are given by those who are motivated to engage with the programs – those who drop out of the program are unlikely to give feedback

Advantages of CCBT

Widening access to treatment

> This is particularly valuable in rural areas where access to a CBT therapist may be restricted

Cost effective

> One of the key arguments in favour of developing and implementing computerised packages is the low running cost due to the absence of counsellor wages

Convenient to use

> Individuals can work through the program at a time and pace that is appropriate to them

'Cost-utility and cost-effectiveness analyses tend to be in favour of CCBT. On balance, CCBT constitutes the most efficient treatment strategy, although all treatments showed low adherence rates and modest improvements in depression and quality of life' (Gerhards et al., 2010)

Disadvantages of CCBT

Requires self-motivation

>   This can be a problem, especially for those suffering with depression

>   Research highlights a high drop-out rate

Requires access to a computer and internet connection

>   Issues around equality of access are clearly present

>   While most people now have access to, and are confident in using, computers and the internet, this is not true for all

'Despite a short-term reduction in depression at post-treatment, the effect at long follow-up and the function improvement were not significant, with significantly high drop-out. Considering the risk of bias, our meta-analysis implied that the clinical usefulness of current CCBT for adult depression may need to be re-considered downwards in terms of practical implementation and methodological validity' (So et al., 2013)

Third wave cognitive-behaviour therapies

CBT continues to expand and develop

>   Recent developments include . . .

>>   Mindfulness-based cognitive therapy

>>   Acceptance and commitment therapy

>>   Dialectic behaviour therapy

Mindfulness-based cognitive therapy (MBCT)

MBCT was developed out of the work of Teasedale et al. (1995) when they challenged the assumption that CBT worked because it changed beliefs and replaced negative automatic thoughts with more positive thoughts

The alternative view offered was that it was the process of focusing on beliefs and thoughts

>   Stepping back from beliefs and thoughts (seeing them from a new perspective) was therapeutic

MBCT encourages clients to . . .

>   Focus on the here and now, be 'mindful' of the present, and not dwell upon past events or anticipate the future

>   Be non-judgemental about events in order to see them as neither good nor bad

>   Be aware that thoughts are not reality

By being in the here and now, clients cannot get into familiar cycles of avoidance, or of anticipatory anxiety

Mindfulness is about acceptance of our thoughts, rather than trying to enforce change

Acceptance and commitment therapy (ACT)

ACT is a mindfulness-based behavioural therapy developed out of relational frame theory (Barnes-Holmes et al., 2002)

Two parts to ACT

    Acceptance

        Rather than trying to change thoughts, clients are encouraged to accept them and to see them for what they are

        Thoughts influence the way we view the world (our representation of reality) but they are not in themselves reality

        Once we become more accepting, we will be less rigid and more flexible

    Commitment

        Client's commitment to make behavioural changes that are in keeping with the client's chosen values

To achieve a more fulfilling life, ACT identifies six core processes

    Contacting the present moment

        Client is aware of and present in the here and now

    Defusion

        Detaching from unhelpful thoughts and the worry or anxiety that they create

        By taking a new position to view these thoughts, the client can be more objective in 'observing' them

    Acceptance

        Once the client takes a different view of their thoughts, s/he can become more accepting of them

        This differs from CBT in that ACT does not try to change the thoughts, just become more aware and accepting of them

    Observing self

        With practice, the client can become more aware of their thoughts and feelings in the moment that they are having them

    Values

        Focuses on what things are truly important

        Big life questions: Who does the client want to be? What does the client want from life? What is significant and meaningful in the client's life?

    Committed action

        Client takes action to move towards his/her chosen goals in keeping with his/her chosen values

        Commitment to keep taking action even when that is difficult

Dialectical behaviour therapy (DBT)

Linehan (1993) developed DBT specifically for working with suicidal women who had been diagnosed with borderline personality disorder (BPD)

Four main areas of skills are taught (either individually or within a group setting)

Mindfulness

Observing what is happening in the here and now, being fully present, and being non-judgemental

Emotional regulation

Being able to identify and give a name to emotions

Being able to tolerate powerful, and at times overwhelming, emotions

Distress tolerance

Being able to distract oneself from powerful emotions

Being able to step back from these emotions and accept them for what they are

Interpersonal effectiveness

Having more effective communications to get what you need and want

Being assertive

Respecting and valuing self and others in relationships

These recent developments (or 'third wave') in CBT show that it is a flexible and changing approach; future developments will build upon this flexibility and show that this therapy is integrative in both practice and principle

Case study demonstrating cognitive-behaviour therapy

Margaret, 32, had come to counselling through a referral from her GP. The doctor simply stated 'generalised anxiety' as the reason for the referral. She described herself as 'sensitive' and 'emotional'. She had read up on CBT before coming and was hopeful that the course of therapy would 'sort her out'. The initial session was a counselling assessment in which the therapist sought to gather enough information to make a tentative formulation. It was agreed that there would be five further sessions and a review after the assessment session.

In the following exchanges, therapist denotes therapist, client denotes Margaret. Confidentiality statement and the business contract have been discussed. The session is joined as Margaret begins her story.

> Client: Well I suppose it started about a year ago, I was out shopping one day and I began to feel anxious, like nervous and panicky. It went away after a few minutes and I carried on doing the shopping. About two weeks later the same thing happened, only this time it was worse. I could really feel my heart beating fast and I thought I was going to pass out. It was awful. Ever since then it's been a real effort to go out. I have this kind of dread, and sometimes burst into tears for no reason. When it is bad like that I just have to get out of the shop – I leave my trolley full of food and escape . . . (*laughing*) . . . it's really embarrassing.

Therapist: Embarrassing when you were in the shop, or talking about it here?

Client: Both I guess.

Therapist: Okay, sometimes it is a little awkward to talk about things which we think are embarrassing, but it gives us some really useful information about how your anxiety happens. In CBT we like to understand how thoughts, feelings, behaviours and physical sensations interact with each other – how you *do* your problem, if you like.

Client: Yes, I remember reading that.

Therapist: The interesting thing is that two people could both get anxious about, say, shopping, but they might get anxious in very different ways. So let's concentrate on your way. Can you tell me in detail the most recent example of when this happened?

Client: Yes, just over a week ago, not long after I got the appointment with you for today, I was doing the weekly shop. I think I was already anxious even before I went out. Anyway, I was in the shop and I began to feel a bit breathless and nauseous. I held tight on to the trolley, and I remember thinking that it was so embarrassing, everybody looking at me and thinking I was so stupid. That's me, stupid.

Therapist: When you thought that, were you aware of any feelings?

Client: Well yes – I got this pain in my chest, I thought it was a heart attack but I remember reading about panic attacks and how people think they are going to die, so I told myself it was panic. That helped for about ten seconds, then I panicked again. I couldn't keep it all together, so I left the shop. After 10 minutes I went back in and finished the shopping.

Therapist: That sounds quite brave, going back in. How did you feel going back in?

Client: Yes, I was really proud of myself. I'd read a self-help guide on the internet, and I must have remembered it from there.

Therapist; And what did you tell yourself to help you go back in?

Client: I just said 'just pull yourself together – nobody cares, they're all too busy getting on with their own stuff'.

Therapist: Are you always this good at tackling the problem head on like that?

Client: Well no, that was the first time actually. Often if I'm feeling anxious before going out I just stay in. Why put yourself through all that?

Therapist: So sometimes you avoid the thing that gives you the anxiety. Makes sense in the moment, but actually can make it worse in the long run – if you avoid the problem you never challenge yourself to break the pattern. But last time you did, and felt really good because you managed.

In this exchange the client gives some detail to how she does the problem, and the therapist can begin to create the formulation. There is relevant information on:

Symptoms (thoughts, feelings, physical sensations and behaviours)

Triggers

Maintenance processes

There is also some useful information on management and possible treatment:

> Client is keen to read up

> Client broke the pattern of avoidance and felt 'proud' of her achievement

> This suggests that the client will be willing to carry out homework tasks and is keen to be active in the change process

During the subsequent sessions, the therapist covered other areas of assessment to add detail to the formulation

> What was happening in the client's life a year ago when the problem first started (precipitating factors)

> Some information about the client's childhood experiences (predisposing factors)

It was agreed at the end of the session that the client would . . .

> Keep a thought record for a week, noting when her thoughts were negative (frequency, duration and intensity)

> Go to the supermarket where the last occurrence happened each day

> Focus on breathing and positive self-talk whenever she felt anxious

> Read the self-help guide recommended by the therapist

Margaret finished therapy after five sessions in a much less anxious frame of mind. She was a good example of a client who comes into therapy ready for change and ready to work to make that change

ANALYSING THE CASE STUDY

Try answering the following questions using information about cognitive-behaviour therapy.

- What symptoms, triggers, and maintenance processes did Margaret report?
- What cognitive techniques could be/were used during work with Margaret?
- What behavioural techniques could be/were used during work with Margaret?

SUMMARY

Cognitive and behavioural: rarely practised independently, usually combined to form CBT

Development: behaviour therapy developed in early 1900s, cognitive therapy developed in mid-1900s, integration began in later 1900s when Meichenbaum introduced cognitive-behaviour modification; highly prevalent today, recommended by UK NHS and NICE

Cognition-driven emotions: ABC model (activating event, belief, consequence); cognition instigates subsequent emotions, behaviours, etc.

Assessment and formulation: information gathering during assessment focuses on symptoms, predisposing factors, precipitating factors, triggers, beliefs and assumptions, maintenance processes; assessment forms the basis of the initial formulation, formulation draws all information together and adds proposed treatment to create a full plan

Cognitive and behaviour therapy techniques: CBT is psychoeducational, wide variety of cognitive and behavioural techniques; Socratic questioning; identifying cognitive errors; experimentation; changing self-talk from negative to positive; homework tasks

Structure of therapeutic sessions: discuss upcoming session (5 mins), check previous session (10 mins), main content (25 mins), set tasks for next session (5 mins), review session (5 mins)

Empirical evidence for efficacy: evidence suggests CBT effective in reducing symptoms of depression and anxiety; critics argue that measures are subject to participant bias and client selection bias, and conclusions contain a logical error; some research finds little difference between therapies, relationship is the critical factor; conclude that CBT does have a positive effect but no more than other methods and not suitable for all clients

Computerised CBT: offered for mild depression; advantages include widened treatment access, cost effective, convenient to use; disadvantages include need for self-motivation, requires access to internet, lacks relationship connection

Third wave CBT: mindfulness-based cognitive therapy (MBCT); acceptance and commitment therapy (ACT); dialectic behaviour therapy (DBT)

MULTIMODAL THERAPY

LEARNING OUTCOMES

After reading this section, you will be able to:

* explain that multimodal therapy is an eclectic therapy adopting techniques from across the approaches
* discuss the history of multimodal therapy with a brief biography of Arnold Lazarus
* explain the origin of psychological problems
* outline the initial assessment process
* describe the seven modalities and associated interventions for the BASIC ID
* explain modality and structural profiles

- discuss the tracking of the firing order of modalities and explain how bridging helps clients move from one modality to another
- appreciate the application of multimodal therapy in a therapeutic setting (case study)

Multimodal therapy: eclectic

Multimodal therapy is an eclectic mix of theories and techniques from across the approaches

'Multimodal therapy ... provides Humanistic integration, systemization and a comprehensive "blueprint" for assessment and therapy. It deliberately avoids the pitfalls of *theoretical* eclecticism while underscoring the virtues of *technical* eclecticism' (Lazarus, 1981)

Multimodal therapy (MMT) is a structured and systematic approach that can be described as 'technically eclectic'

Eclecticism generally means to select techniques from a variety of therapies to meet the needs of the client, without subscribing to the theory that underpins the approach from which the technique is taken

MMT is pragmatic because it is prepared to use any technique that has been found to be effective

As long as there is a clear rationale and structure, the therapy can be designed specifically for each individual client

Developed by Lazarus on the basis of many years of experience from many different approaches (Lazarus, 1981)

'Aim of Multimodal Therapy is to reduce psychological suffering and to promote personal growth as rapidly and as durably as possible' (Lazarus, 1981)

Multimodal therapy adds established techniques to a positive relationship

Multimodal therapists accept the basic principles of developing an effective therapeutic relationship as identified by Carl Rogers

For example, therapist should provide the client with unconditional positive regards, congruence and empathy

Lazarus (1981) noted 'parity as a way of life' in which he stated that all people are equal to one another

Clients often consider the therapist to be the expert, thus starting the relationship in a 'one down' position

It is the job of the therapist to make the client an equal part of the therapeutic process

The therapist might have knowledge and techniques to impart (like teacher/ student) but the relationship itself is fundamentally one of equals

However, a range of techniques adopted from other therapeutic methods and tailored to specifically suit the individual client should supplement these core conditions

> Therapist must be flexible in meeting the relationship needs of the client

>> If the client wants a supportive, listening relationship, then the therapist can tailor the treatment to suit this need

>> Alternatively, if a client wants to focus on goals in an active and challenging relationship, then the therapist can alter the treatment to suit this need

Lazarus (1981) described being flexible and adaptable to meet the needs of individual clients as being an 'authentic chameleon'

Development of multimodal therapy

History of multimodal therapy

As a systematic eclectic therapy, multimodal therapy draws upon many different theories without taking on board the underlying principles of any one approach

> Lazarus, the founding father of the therapy, was trained in psychodynamic and humanistic approaches, attended seminars on behaviourism by Wolpe, experienced Adlerian therapy in London, and worked at Stanford University with social learning theorist Bandura

Initially focused purely on behavioural techniques, but later included cognitive techniques

> This integration increased success with clients and led to the idea that an eclectic mix of established techniques could be the most effective therapeutic method

Began to incorporate other elements, such as social learning theory (people influence, and are influenced by, others and may learn through conditioning and modelling)

Eventually, expanded to include many therapeutic elements and developed the multimodal approach based upon seven different dimensions

Brief biography of Arnold Lazarus (1932–2013)

> *'Remember, think well, act well, feel well, be well!'*
> —Lazarus (2010)

Who was Arnold Lazarus?

> Eclectic practitioner who sought to draw together successful elements of multiple therapies to create a new method of psychological treatment

> Founder of multimodal therapy

Early years

> Born 1932 in Johannesburg, South Africa

Education

Studied an Honours degree and Master's degree in psychology at Witwatersrand University, Johannesburg

Obtained a PhD in 1960

Worked in private practice and lectured part time at Witwatersrand Medical School

Training was primarily psychodynamic and humanistic

Attended seminars by behaviourist Wolpe to learn about theories of conditioning

Worked in the Marlborough Day Hospital in London for three months in 1957, encountering the Adlerian approach to psychotherapy

Career

Worked with Albert Bandura (famous for his work on social learning theory) as a visiting lecturer in psychology at Stanford University in 1963

Director of the Behavior Therapy Institute in Sausalito, California, in 1966

Published *New Methods in Psychotherapy: A Case Study* in 1958

First use of the terms 'behaviour therapy' and 'behaviour therapist' in an academic paper

In researching outcomes from behavioural therapy, he discovered that many clients relapsed over a period of time, but clients who had received cognitive as well as behavioural therapy had more successful outcomes over a period of time

Many influences in his education, career and research led him to explore a broader approach to therapy

He argued that no one single approach could provide a comprehensive understanding of a person's development or problems

Published *Broad Spectrum Behaviour Therapy and the Treatment of Agoraphobia* in 1966

Outlined a multidimensional approach to working with agoraphobics

Developed a systematic therapeutic intervention based on cognitive and behaviour techniques in the 1970s

Published *Behaviour Therapy and Beyond* in 1971 in which he advocated a broad approach to therapy

Influenced the development of cognitive-behaviour therapy

Published *Multimodal Behaviour Therapy: Treating the 'Basic ID'* in 1973

Introduced the concept of the BASIC ID and outlined multimodal methods to address the various components of the BASIC ID

Published *The Practice of Multimodal Therapy* in 1981

Outlined the process of multimodal therapy and presented the therapy without the 'Behaviour' title

Family

Married in 1955

Raised two children

Death

Died on 1st October 2013, in Princeton, South Africa

Significant learnings

'We firmly believe that therapy is education rather than healing; that it is growth rather than treatment' (attributed to Lazarus, n.d.)

'My basic approach to therapy is very much that of problem solving. I see that people come into therapy with a whole myriad of different problems, and yet do not know how to solve some simple ones. And quite often simple solutions can have a tremendous, reverberating, positive effect' (Lazarus, n.d.)

'The therapist is on the client's payroll, and if one is not satisfied with what he or she is saying or doing, pull the plug' (Lazarus, 2010)

Basis of psychological problems

Psychological problems stem from numerous influences (Lazarus, 1981)

Misinformation

Incorrect beliefs and assumptions internalised from parents and significant others

For example, 'the world is a dangerous place', 'I must be perfect in all that I do', 'I must do for others', 'others should treat me well at all times'

Specific misinformation provided by others

For example, we may have been incorrectly informed that there is a long waiting list for referrals to a local agency to help with drink or drug addiction

Missing information

Lack of all of the pertinent information relating to the topic

For example, we may not know how to prepare for examinations

Defensive reactions

Avoiding situations that trigger negative feelings (such as anxiety)

This is understandable, but it does not help to challenge the anxiety

For example, a man with an anxiety about bridges will avoid bridges but this does not help him to deal with the underlying anxiety

Lack of self-acceptance

Drawing inappropriate conclusions from experiences based on beliefs about the self

For example, a woman goes for a job interview but is unsuccessful at getting the job, so she concludes that she is useless and will never get the job that she wants

Experience is assumed to be representative of the entire life, when it would often be better to look at the experience objectively in order to see what aspects could be improved

For example, the woman who failed to get a job could consider which aspects of the interview process could be improved so that she is better prepared for the next interview

Assessment process

Initial assessment is extremely important

Similar to most other approaches

> Developing relationship
>
> Establishing rapport
>
> Gathering information
>
> Assessing and determining a sense of direction

Lazarus (1981) identifies 12 areas that the therapist should be aware of during the first session

> Signs of psychosis
>
> Presenting problem and main antecedents
>
> Risk of harm to self or others, attitude towards self
>
> The way the client presented (appearance, body language, etc.)
>
> Key points in the client's history
>
> Maintenance factors (e.g. behaviours) that keep the problem going
>
> Goals that the client wishes to achieve
>
> Indication of particular therapeutic style appropriate for the client
>
> Suitability of therapy or the need to refer
>
> Client's strengths and resources
>
> Reason for engaging in therapy now
>
> Client's motivation and sense of hope

Multimodal life inventory

At the end of the first session (or, if there is a gap between initial contact and the first session, prior to the first session) the client will be asked to complete a multimodal life inventory

Detailed questionnaire that covers:

> Relevant aspects of the client's history, early relationships, etc.
>
> Details of the problem that the client is bringing to therapy
>
> Expectations of therapy
>
> Questions on each of the modalities

Inventory will provide the therapist with comprehensive information for the BASIC ID (Lazarus, 1973)

BASIC ID

BASIC ID is an acronym for seven modalities of human experiencing and functioning (Lazarus, 1973)

> As individuals we think, feel, behave, have physical sensations, create images, interact with others and have biological functions – these are our modalities

>> The acronym covers these seven core modalities

>>> Behaviour
>>> Affect
>>> Sensation
>>> Images
>>> Cognition
>>> Interpersonal
>>> Drugs

Behaviour

> How we act and react in relation to self, others and events

> Behaviour can be a reaction to change in another modality

>> For example, we become angry so we take action

Affect

> Our feelings about self, others and events

> Emotions are managed through one or more of the other modalities

>> For example, we reduce anxiety by using coping imagery

Sensation

> Physical feelings and how our senses experience the world

> Sensation and affect are closely connected

>> For example, we sense butterflies in the stomach so we feel excited

> Sensation is influenced by other modalities

>> For example, we practise mindfulness so we feel relaxed

Images

> Visual, auditory and kinaesthetic creations

> Images influence other modalities

>> For example, flashbacks can create strong physical sensations and panic reactions

Cognition

> Thoughts, values, attitudes and beliefs

> These can be positive and life enhancing or negative and limiting

> Cognition influences our feelings and behaviours

> For example, if a person thinks 'I must always be in control' they will behave in ways to ensure they can be

Interpersonal

> Relationships with significant others

> These will influence the way we feel and behave

>> For example, we have an argument so we might feel angry and slam a door

Drugs/biology

> This should be **B** for biology, but BASIC ID is more memorable than BASIC IB

> Not only does it include drugs and medication, but also all that we take in, nutrition, exercise, fitness, hygiene, etc.

> This modality influences and is influenced by other modalities

>> For example, we eat more healthily, we feel fitter and happier; we have a health scare, we stop smoking and drinking

As these seven modalities cover all aspects of the human experience, all need to be considered when assessing a problem

> Failure to address one of the modalities may result in an important aspect of the problem being missed

> Each modality influences, and is influenced by, other modalities so it is essential to understand each modality in the context of the other modalities

IDENTIFYING MODALITIES

Think of a problem that you have experienced in your life and identify all of the modalities associated with that event.

For example, you have a car accident (Behaviour), you get upset (Affect), replay the incident in your head (Interpersonal) and tell yourself 'I'm lucky to be alive' (Cognition) and feel sick (Sensation).

Look for examples in yourself and others throughout the next day – we can become very skilled at identifying modalities with practice.

Therapeutic interventions can be directed at specific parts of the BASIC ID

> Therapy can apply any technique that has been found to improve client wellbeing in empirical studies to address specific problems in the BASIC ID

> Interventions directed at Behaviour include . . .

>> Behaviour rehearsal

>>> Therapist takes the role of the person to whom the client needs to speak

Client practises the communication until he feels confident enough to speak to the person directly

Modelling

Therapist takes the role of client to show the client how to deal with a specific situation

Client can then practise the behaviour having had it modelled by the therapist

Exposure

Client is encouraged to face a feared situation

Client could engage with a gradual, systematic exposure

For example, with a phobia of spiders, the client could be gradually introduced to spiders

Alternatively, client could be 'flooded' with the stimulus

For example, a client with a fear of bridges could be taken onto a bridge to stay there until anxiety reduces

Recording and monitoring

Client will keep records and monitor thoughts and feelings

For example, a client who gets angry with his children may keep records of how often he gets angry, the triggers preceding the anger, the intensity of the anger, etc.

Positive reinforcement

Client is encouraged to reward him/herself for achieving goals

Interventions directed at Affect include . . .

Raising awareness of feelings

Client is helped to expand his feelings vocabulary and to be clearer about labelling feelings accurately

Anxiety management

Teaching the client elements of relaxation training and coping strategies

Client can then either utilise these in actual situations that create anxiety or practise these by imagining anxiety-provoking situations within the therapeutic setting

Interventions directed at Sensation include . . .

Relaxation training

Muscular relaxation training helps the client focus on the main muscle groups in the body, by tensing, holding and relaxing each muscle group in turn

Alternatively, the client may focus on specific muscle groups, for example the neck and shoulders, to manage a specific sensation

Mindfulness

> Helps the client focus and raises here-and-now awareness

> There are connections between mindfulness and meditation

Focusing on felt sense

> Client is encouraged to relax and then to 'go inside' and pay attention to bodily sensations

> Client can then be asked to stay with the sensation and label it appropriately

Interventions directed at Imagery include . . .

Coping imagery

> Clients imagine a situation in which they think they will not cope and go through the process step by step

> At each point, they focus on how they are coping, despite any negative feelings that they see themselves experiencing

Rational emotive imagery

> Client imagines the worst-case scenario, experiences unhealthy negative emotions (e.g. fear) and, while keeping the negative image, changes the feelings to healthier emotions (e.g. concern)

Changing the structure of the image

> Technique to change the submodalities of a mental image (how the image is constructed)

> For example, a mental image in colour and moving like a video can be changed to a black and white photograph

> Emotional reactions to mental images will change when the structure of the mental image is changed

Interventions directed at Cognition include . . .

Challenging negative automatic thoughts

> Looking for evidence can challenge negative automatic thoughts

> For example, a client may be anxious about going to the local shop because he believes that people will laugh at him so the challenge could be 'What is the evidence that people laugh at you in shops?'

> If there is evidence that it has happened in the past, then the client can be challenged with the likelihood that it will happen again in the future

> A more positive thought would be 'It has happened in the past but it is unlikely to happen again – however, if it did, it would not be the end of the world, and I could cope with it'

Disputing irrational beliefs

    Negative automatic thoughts may be underpinned by irrational beliefs

    These beliefs are absolute statements of 'shoulds' and 'musts'

    These can be disputed and replaced with more flexible rational beliefs

    For example, 'They must treat me well at all times' can be disputed and replaced with 'I would prefer them to treat me well, but they don't absolutely *have* to and, if they don't, I can cope'

Positive self-statements

    Positive self-statements may be about coping in stressful situations

    For example, 'I am a loving and lovable person'

Correcting misinformation

    People often maintain their problems because they do not update and correct misinformation

    This may be incorrect factual information or statements about the self that were originally introjected in childhood but no longer apply in adulthood

Interventions directed at Interpersonal include . . .

Assertiveness training

    Clients who are passive in their communications with others benefit from assertiveness training

    Assertiveness training may assist clients in learning to say 'no', asking for what they want, and demanding their rights

    Role-play to rehearse situations would be used as part of assertiveness training

Communication training

    Clients can learn about effective communications (e.g. TA ego-state model to explore transactions)

    Modelling and role-play would be used so that clients can practise starting and ending conversations

Interventions directed at Drugs/biology include . . .

Smoking cessation programmes

Alcohol/drug reduction programmes

Nutrition awareness programmes

Weight reduction programmes

Exercise programmes

Various other techniques designed to motivate and maintain progress towards achieving realistic goals

Profiling

Modality profiling

Modality profile is a chart drawn up to outline the presenting problem in the seven modalities

Profile remains open to change as more information is revealed and the therapy develops

Profile identifies interventions that may be used to deal with each aspect of the problem

MODALITY PROFILE

Below is an example of a modality profile for a student with examination anxiety. This modality profile is a work in progress and will be updated in response to the development of the therapy.

Modality	Problem	Intervention
Behaviour	Procrastination in revising Problems sleeping Avoiding lecturers	Realistic revision timetable Relaxation techniques Behaviour rehearsal
Affect	Anxiety Panic Anger	Anxiety management Breathing exercises Anger expression
Sensation	Nausea Headaches Palpitations Tension in shoulders and neck	Dietary information Relaxation techniques Breathing exercises Muscular relaxation training
Imagery	Negative image of self in exam Images of not coping Images of being unable to write	Positive self-talk Coping imagery Changing the structure of the image
Cognition	'I am going to fail' 'I will let my parents down' 'People will think I'm stupid' 'I am worthless'	Coping statements Challenging negative thoughts Disputing irrational beliefs Practising rational beliefs
Interpersonal	Avoiding friends Angry outbursts with family	Social skills training Strategies for coping
Drugs/biology	Missing meals Drinking lots of coffee	Nutrition education Information giving about effects of too much caffeine

Second-order profiling

Sometimes a client may be stuck in one area of the modality profile

> In these cases, a second modality profile may be drawn up specifically for that area (Lazarus, 1973)

> For example, the above client may become increasingly concerned about the palpitations he is having so a second-order profile about the palpitations might identify the following problems associated with this specific modality

Behaviour	Sits still for a while
Affect	Panic
Sensation	Shallow breathing
Images	Imagining having a heart attack
Cognition	I am going to die
Interpersonal	Withdrawal from friends
Drugs/biology	Not seeking medical advice

> In this case, a new issue has emerged that needs to be explored – client is avoiding going to his doctor for fear of what might be discovered

> This issue clearly impacts upon his presenting problem, and is likely to be resolved easily by correcting his misinformation and providing the relevant medical information with a visit to his GP

> Therapy can then return to the presenting problem

PROFILING THE SOAPS

Take a character from a TV programme (soaps are a rich source of people with problems) and draw up a BASIC ID modality profile for their problem. Identify some possible interventions that would be appropriate for each of the seven dimensions

Structural profiling

Structural profile is how the client perceives him/herself in relation to each of the seven modalities (Lazarus, 2005)

> Some people consider themselves to be 'thinkers', while others see themselves as 'doers'

> Some people spend a lot of time creating images (daydreaming or visually planning), while others consider themselves as emotional, in touch with their feelings

Clients are asked to rate themselves for each of the dimensions (Lazarus, 1981) in response to questions such as:

B   How active are you in getting things done?

Do you procrastinate?

A   How much are you in touch with your feelings?

How emotional are you?

S   How aware are you of bodily sensations?

How much do you focus on your senses in the here and now?

I   Are you a daydreamer?

Do you consider yourself to be an imaginative person?

C   How much of a thinker are you?

Do you like to think things through before acting?

I   How important are other people to you?

How would you rate yourself as a social person?

D   How healthy are you?

How much do you exercise and pay attention to nutrition?

Clients are then asked to rate themselves on a scale of 1 to 10 (Lazarus, 1981)

For example, the client who sees himself as very active would score 10 for D whereas the client who sees himself as overweight and taking no exercise would score 0 for D; this would then represent his current structural profile

Client could then be asked to draw up a preferred profile, and the differences between the two would indicate some areas to work on

For example, if a client wants to lose weight, have a better diet and become healthier, then his preferred D score may be close to 10; this would identify some work to be done on weight reduction and exercise planning

Any differences in the modality score for the current and preferred structural profile would indicate areas to focus on in the therapy

MY STRUCTURAL PROFILE

Spend a few minutes to think about yourself in relation to the seven dimensions of BASIC ID to draw up a current structural profile. Then think about how you would like to be to draw up a preferred structural profile. Note the differences between the two profiles and think of ways to start the change in the direction of the preferred profile.

Tracking and bridging

Tracking the firing order of the modalities (Lazarus, 2005)

Everyone has their own way of 'doing' their problem

This can be explored in the specific modality sequence (or order) in which the problem occurs

For example, two people who get anxious before going into a social situation may respond to the situation in very different ways

One person may become aware of feeling nauseous (S), label the feeling 'anxiety' (A), thinks 'It'll be an awful evening' (C), and decides to have a glass or two of wine to relax before going (B); this person has a firing order of S-A-C-B

Alternatively, another person may remember 'I've got that party tonight, I'm going to hate it' (C), visualises who will be there and sees herself being cornered by people she thinks are overbearing (I), feels 'anxious' (A), and senses the start of a headache (S); this person has a firing order of C-I-A-S

There are interventions for each of these modalities and in order to tailor the therapy to the individual, it is best to use the techniques in the same order as the modality firing order

For example, in the case given above, taking tablets for the headache may be appropriate but this does not stop the person from the negative thought, the negative image and the labelling of the feeling – it is dealing with the S of the C-I-A-S sequence

It would be better to deal with the modality that starts the sequence (Cognitive)

If the negative thought can be changed (e.g. 'I've got that party tonight and I'm not looking forward to it, but I can always leave early') then the other problem modalities may not follow (there may be a more positive image, no identifiable anxiety and no resulting headache)

Bridging between modalities (Lazarus, 2005)

As noted in the structural profile above, individuals have preferred modalities

We often hear expressions such as 'I'm a doer, not a thinker', 'She's very into her emotions', 'He's always daydreaming'

Individuals will also have least preferred modalities

Many people find it difficult to access and express their own feelings and they may answer feeling-questions with cognitions

However, in order to explore all areas of a problem, the therapist will need to help the client access some of the less preferred modalities

For example, a client may often answer Affect questions with Cognition response

'How did that make you feel?' (Affect question)

'I felt it was really unfair' ('unfair' is a thought, not a feeling)

In order to help the client access Affect, the therapist could stay with the same line of questions until the client gets to a feeling

'And how did you feel when you thought it was unfair?'

'Well, it's not right to be treated like that'

'And the feeling you were left with?'

'Well, angry I suppose'

These directed questions help the client move from Cognition to Affect

Bridging is an alternative way of engaging the client to help him/her access other modalities

For example, a client may often answer Affect questions with Cognition response

'How did that make you feel?' (Affect question)

'I felt it was really unfair' ('unfair' is a thought, not a feeling)

Therapist might note the Cognition response and ask the client about Sensations as a bridge to Affect

'What sensations were you aware of as this was happening?'

'Well, my breathing got shallower and faster and my heart started pounding'

'And how would you label that feeling?'

'Anger'

This uses the Sensation bridge to move the client from Cognition to Affect

Not only does bridging help the client access all modalities (and therefore become more fully connected to all aspects of self), it also helps build rapport between therapist and client

Case study demonstrating multimodal therapy

Carl, 17, was advised by his tutor to visit the therapist at his college. Although he is a good student, he struggled with his mock exams and he is becoming increasingly anxious about his final exams. His final maths exam will take place in two weeks time, but he has not yet begun to do any revision at all.

The first session was an initial assessment in which the therapist sought to find out the reason for attending therapy and establish a therapeutic relationship. It was agreed that there would be three further sessions after the assessment session. Carl was asked to complete the life inventory in order for the therapist to begin working with him to produce modality and structural profiles.

In the following exchanges, therapist denotes therapist, client denotes Carl. Confidentiality statement and the business contract have been discussed. The session is joined as the therapist begins to create the modality profile.

Therapist: Okay Carl, can you perhaps tell me a little bit about the revision problem?

Client: It's hard to explain really. I have always done so well at school, but I am just struggling with these exams. None of the information seems to stay in my head and

I think that I am going to fail everything and not get into university. I'm the only one in my family to go to university and my mum is so excited. She would be so angry . . . no, not angry . . . she would be so disappointed in me if I failed. But I just can't face doing the work at the moment.

Therapist: So can you tell me what happens when you come to do your work?

Client: Well, I decide that I am going to do it. But then I start to feel all hot and I keep imagining my mum's face when I get my failed results through the post and I feel sick so I have to just get away from my books for a while. So I play on the computer. And then another day passes and I haven't started revising yet.

Therapist: In multimodal therapy, we try to work out something called your BASIC ID. This is a profile of your problem so that we can really start to explore it fully. And you have already told me quite a lot that can fit in this profile. Let's write each bit down so that we can see it all together. So the B is behaviour and it sounds like your behaviour is procrastinating?

Client: Yeah. I play on my computer instead of revising.

Therapist: And the S is sensation and you said that you feel hot and sick?

Client: I do, yeah. All of my skin gets hot and I start to sweat then I get butterflies in my stomach and I start to feel sick. Sometimes my head starts to hurt too and I have to lie down for a while.

Therapist: You also mentioned an image and that is one of the I's.

Client: My mum's face. I keep picturing it when she reads the letter with my results.

Therapist: And the other I is interpersonal and that one focuses on your relationships with other people. I guess that the significant one here would be your mum?

Client: Mainly, yeah. But also my tutor. Mr Roberts has been so good to me and I don't want to let him down.

Therapist: So it sounds like your thoughts about the problem are that you are going to fail and your mum and your tutor will be disappointed in you? That would be the C for Cognition.

Client: They're gonna think that I'm stupid and that they shouldn't have wasted their time on me.

Therapist: Okay, so we have got most of the BASIC ID for your problem. But now that I am looking at it, I notice that there is something missing. The A is for affect or feelings. How do you feel about this problem?

Client: I just told you. I feel like my mum will be disappointed in me.

Therapist: And so you get butterflies and start to feel sick?

Client: Yes.

Therapist: So what name could you give to the feeling behind that sickness?

Client: Erm, I don't know. Worry, maybe?

Therapist: I guess worry sounds quite mild to me, but your feelings sound quite strong.

Client: Yeah, you're right. Not worry. Fear.

Therapist: Okay, so our A for affect would be fear?

Client: Yeah, that's it.

Therapist: Okay, so the last part of the BASIC ID is D for drugs.

Client: (quickly) I'm not on drugs!

Therapist: No, it doesn't really mean that. It means biology. Do you eat healthily and exercise?

Client: Oh. No, not really. I guess I eat a lot of rubbish at the moment. I haven't put any weight on, but I'm really sluggish and tired all of the time. I used to play football on a weekend, but I haven't done that for months. I keep saying that it's because I'm too busy revising, but I just sit on the computer and don't revise either.

Therapist: I think that gives us a lot to work with. Would you like to look over your BASIC ID profile? (*both look at the profile together*) One of the interesting things about problems is that everybody does them differently. Two people might seem to have the same problem, but they might feel very different or think in completely different ways. For example, two people might share a fear of dogs, but one might start the fear by shaking while another might start the fear by thinking that the dog is going to bite. So I am just wondering how you do your problem? Which bit of this BASIC ID comes first for you when you sit down to start working?

Client: Do you mean, which one do I feel first? Well, I guess that I feel hot first. Because I start thinking that I will never get through all of my work and I am going to fail and I picture my mum's face.

Therapist: So do you feel hot and then think that you are going to fail? Or do you think that you are going to fail and then feel hot?

Client: Erm, I guess that thinking comes first. I think that I'm gonna fail and then I picture my mum's face and then I feel hot.

Therapist: And when does the fear start?

Client: As soon as I think that I'm gonna fail.

Therapist: So you think that you are going to fail and then you feel fear and then you picture your mum's face and then you feel hot and sick?

Client: Yeah, that's exactly right.

In this exchange, the therapist successfully formulated an entire BASIC ID modality profile. In the next stage, the therapist works on designing interventions to address the modalities. Since Carl's firing order begins with Cognition, they decide to devise an intervention to tackle this area. The therapist plans to begin working on the structural profile in the next session, but Carl does not return to therapy.

Carl only ever attended this single session (he cancelled his next sessions by telephone), but he sent the therapist an email at the end of the academic year. The email thanked the therapist for helping him to understand his problem and said that he had been able to start revising straight after the session. His delay in starting work cost him in his final grades, but he did successfully pass all of his exams and he was accepted to study biology at university.

ANALYSING THE CASE STUDY

Try answering the following questions using information about multimodal therapy.

* What was the BASIC ID structural profile for Carl and which interventions could be used for each modality?
* How did the therapist use bridging in the session?
* How did the therapist track the firing order of the modalities?
* What would be expected in an actual and preferred structural profile for Carl?

SUMMARY

Eclecticism: technical eclecticism across multiple therapies, structured and systematic method, highlights importance of therapeutic relationship but also adds empirically supported techniques tailored to the individual

Development: Lazarus drew on many approaches to form this therapy, including humanistic, psychodynamic, behavioural, cognitive, etc.; therapy was introduced in a book by Lazarus published in 1973

Basis of psychological problems: all problems stem from misinformation, missing information, defensive reactions and lack of self-acceptance

Assessment process: initial assessment is crucial for developing the therapeutic relationship; multimodal life inventory provides information for the BASIC ID

BASIC ID: Behaviour, Affect, Sensation, Images, Cognition, Interpersonal, Drugs/biology; therapeutic interventions directed at specific parts of the BASIC ID: Behaviour (rehearsal, modelling, exposure, recording and monitoring, positive reinforcement), Affect (raising awareness of feelings, anxiety management), Sensation (relaxation training, mindfulness, focusing on felt sense), Imagery (coping imagery, rational emotive imagery, changing structure of image), Cognition (challenge negative automatic thoughts, dispute irrational beliefs, positive self-statements, correcting misinformation), Interpersonal (assertiveness training, communication training), Drugs/biology (health programmes)

Profiling: modality profile is a chart drawn up to outline the presenting problems and proposed intervention in the seven modalities; second-order profile involves profiling the seven modalities within one of the original modalities; structural profile is how the client perceives him/herself in relation to each of the seven modalities

Tracking: everyone has their own way of 'doing' their problem, can be explored in the specific modality sequence (or order) in which the problem occurs;

tracking the firing order of the modalities allows the treatment to focus on the original problem rather than later symptoms

Bridging: some clients will have most preferred (often Cognition) and least preferred (often Affect) modalities; bridging uses other modalities to move the client from the preferred modality to the least preferred modality

NEUROLINGUISTIC PROGRAMMING

LEARNING OUTCOMES

After reading this section, you will be able to:

* explain that neurolinguistic programming is an eclectic therapy adopting techniques from across the approaches

* discuss the history of neurolinguistic programming with brief biographies of Richard Bandler and John Grinder

* describe and evaluate representation systems in terms of sensory modalities and submodalities

* describe and evaluate the meta model with specific focus on faulty thought patterns involving distortions, deletions and generalisations

* discuss the techniques of anchoring and swishing

* discuss the controversies associated with neurolinguistic programming

* appreciate the application of neurolinguistic programming in a therapeutic setting (case study)

Neurolinguistic programming: eclectic

Neurolinguistic Programming (NLP) draws from a range of different therapies

Aims to unite all of the successful techniques and approaches in different therapies in order to establish a successful method of psychological change

NLP focuses on the use of language to make changes in the brain

Since therapy is known as the 'talking cure', it is logical that language should form the basis of the treatment and evidence suggests that language does influence thoughts and feelings

However, some practitioners have taken it a step too far by making excessive claims about the potential for NLP

Development of neurolinguistic programming

History of neurolinguistic programming

Bandler and Grinder (1975) introduced neurolinguistic programming as a method of psychotherapy designed to instil fast and effective change in those individuals experiencing psychological discomfort (such as phobias, depression, anxiety disorders, etc.)

  This therapy was established following a review of current practices in psychotherapy to determine common methods yielding the greatest levels of success across many different approaches

  Bandler and Grinder highlighted three highly successful therapeutic approaches: family therapy, Gestalt therapy and hypnotherapy

Family therapy

  Bandler and Grinder were inspired to develop the meta model by the work of family therapist Virginia Satir

    Satir argued that change is possible following the disruption of the status quo and subsequent conversion towards an improved state would only be possible if the foreign element creating the disruption could be effectively integrated into the life of the individual

Gestalt therapy

  Bandler and Grinder were inspired to develop the meta model by the work of Gestalt therapist Fritz Perls

  Perls focused on the concept of personal responsibility to devise the Gestalt Prayer:

    'I do my thing and you do your thing; I am not in this world to live up to your expectations; and you are not in this world to live up to mine; you are you, and I am I, and if by chance we find each other, it's beautiful; if not, it can't be helped'

    This prayer summarises the idea that the individual should focus on his or her own needs without projecting these needs onto others or allowing these needs to be influenced by the projections of others

Hypnotherapy

  Bandler and Grinder were inspired to develop meta model by the work of hypnotherapist Milton Erikson

  Erikson adopted an unconventional approach to psychotherapy using therapeutic metaphor and hypnotic suggestion to influence behavioural and emotional change in his clients

Brief biography of Richard Bandler (1950–current)

  'We take the very best of what people do, synthesise it down, make it learnable and share it with each other – and that is what the real future of what NLP will be and it's gonna stay that way!'
  —Attributed to Bandler (n.d.)

Who is Richard Bandler?

Co-founder of NLP

Early years

Born on 24th February 1950 in the US

Education

Graduated with a degree in philosophy and psychology from the University of California in 1973 and an MA in psychology from Lone Mountain College in San Francisco in 1975 (Clancy & Yorkshire, 1989)

Career

Ran a Gestalt group at the University of California in Santa Cruz

Worked with linguistic professor John Grinder in therapy sessions

Published *The Structure of Magic Volume 1* in 1975 and *Volume 2* in 1976 with John Grinder

Introduced the concept of NLP for effective therapeutic change

Published *Frogs into Princes* with John Grinder in 1979

Transcript of a seminar outlining the practice of NLP in therapy

Bandler and Grinder stopped working together in the 1980s

Rumour suggests that the separation was acrimonious (Renton, 2009)

Published *Using your Brain for a Change* with Steve and Connirae Andreas in 1985

Focused on the concept of manipulating submodalities to promote positive personality changes

Bandler filed a lawsuit for trademark infringement against Grinder in 2000 based on the claim that Bandler was the original creator and legal owner of the term 'neurolinguistic programming' (Wong, 2000)

Eventually both parties agreed to accept that they were co-creators of NLP and all claims were settled in 2000 (Grinder & Bostic St Clair, 2001)

Developed a new system of therapy called design human engineering

Ran a series of seminars on this new approach in 2000

Family

Reportedly abused alcohol and cocaine throughout his life (Clancy & Yorkshire, 1989)

Acquitted of the murder of Corine Christensen (Clancy & Yorkshire, 1989)

Corine Christensen was shot dead in her home in 1986

She lived with James Marino (convicted burglar and drug dealer) who was a friend of Bandler

Marino and Bandler were seen leaving the house after the shooting and Bandler's shirt was covered in her blood

In court, Bandler claimed that Marino shot his girlfriend because he believed that she was trying to have him murdered – in contrast, Marino claimed that

Bandler shot her because he believed that she was having a lesbian affair with his girlfriend

Bandler was acquitted in 1988

Significant learnings

'Most people plan by disaster. They think of what can go wrong and then they master it' (Bandler quoted in Bandler & Fitzpatrick, 2009)

'You can't just be happy, but you can learn to do things happily. Living happily entails paying attention to and enjoying the process of doing whatever it is you happen to be doing' (Bandler, 2010)

'Simply put, the meaning of life is the meaning you ascribe to it. What you believe is what you'll see, hear and feel; therefore it makes sense to pay special attention to the beliefs you hold' (Bandler quoted in Bandler & Thomson, 2011)

'In life you are given a bag of moments. You don't know how many of those moments you have. My courses are about learning how to maximize those moments' (Bandler, n.d.)

Brief biography of John Grinder (1940–current)

'Control is a fiction – a seductive illusion – choice is the point.'
—Grinder (2001)

Who is John Grinder?

Co-founder of neurolinguistic programming

Early years

Born on 10th January 1940 in the US

Education

Graduated with a degree in psychology from the University of San Francisco and a PhD in linguistics in 1961 (Preube, 2013)

Career

Served as a captain in the Special Forces (Preube, 2013)

Worked for the US Intelligence Agency (Preube, 2013)

Linguistics professor at University of California in Santa Cruz

Worked with psychology student and Gestalt practitioner Richard Bandler in therapy sessions and became interested in the effective use of language in therapy

Published *The Structure of Magic Volume 1* in 1975 and *Volume 2* in 1976 with Richard Bandler

Introduced the concept of NLP for effective therapeutic change

Published *Frogs into Princes* with Richard Bandler in 1979

Transcript of a seminar outlining the practice of NLP in therapy

Bandler and Grinder stopped working together in the 1980s

Rumour suggests that the separation was acrimonious (Renton, 2009)

Published *Turtles All The Way Down* with Judith DeLozier in 1987

Developed a New Code of NLP

Bandler filed a lawsuit for trademark infringement against Grinder in 2000 based on the claim that Bandler was the original creator and legal owner of the term 'neurolinguistic programming' (Wong, 2000)

Eventually both parties agreed to accept that they were co-creators of NLP and all claims were settled in 2000 (Grinder, 2001)

Published *Whispering in the Wind* with partner Carmen Bostic St Clair in 2001

Theoretical guide to the New Code of NLP with a specific set of recommendations, including focus on modelling as a critical component of NLP

Significant learnings

'Surely, if there is one thing all of us who have extended experiences inducing change with human beings (ourselves included, of course) through the application of NLP patterning can agree on, it is the futility of thinking in terms of controlling anything in the realm of human activity' (Grinder quoted in Grinder & Bostic St Clair, 2001)

Representation systems

Three sensory modalities

The human mind will represent information in accordance with particular senses

Visual

Auditory

Kinaesthetic

For example, an individual may process information by seeing internal images (visual), hearing an internal voice (auditory) or focusing on internal feelings (kinaesthetic)

These methods of internal representation of information are known as sensory modalities

Visual sensory modality

Visual individuals will focus on how something looks

They will think about things in picture form and may be more likely to recall information that has been presented in pictures

They are less distracted by noise but will have difficulties following verbal instructions

Visual people are often organised and orderly, and they will have a high regard for physical appearances

Auditory sensory modality

> Auditory individuals will focus on how something sounds

> They will think about things through an inner voice and may even talk to themselves or move their lips when thinking about a particular issue

> They are more likely to recall verbal information, but they can be easily distracted by noise

> Auditory people are often sequential, and they are more likely to respond to verbal instructions that have been worded in an appropriate way and delivered in a suitable tone

Kinaesthetic sensory modality

> Kinaesthetic individuals will focus on how something feels

> They will think about things in terms of feeling

> They are more likely to learn by doing and will recall information if they have physically experienced an associated activity

> Kinaesthetic people are usually tactile, and may respond well to physical rewards

Detecting preferred sensory modalities

Most people will have a preferred sensory modality indicating the way that their own mind structures and organises information (Bandler & Grinder, 1979)

Preferred sensory modalities will often be revealed through verbal cues

> An individual with a particular preference for a distinct modality will often exhibit this preference by describing their world in those terms

Preference for visual sensory modality

> An individual may display a visual preference by exclaiming that they can 'see' themselves trapped inside a cage or describing something confusing as 'misty' or 'cloudy'

Preference for auditory sensory modality

> An individual may display an auditory preference by stating that they feel like the world is 'shouting' at them or that they cannot concentrate because they are 'surrounded by noise'

Preference for kinaesthetic sensory modality

> An individual may display a kinaesthetic preference by explaining that they feel that there is a 'weight on their shoulders' or they are concerned that they cannot get a 'grasp' on their problem

Matching language

> Effective therapists should strive to recognise the sensory modalities preferred by the client and match the language in order to build rapport

> Bandler and Grinder (1979) illustrated the importance of matching language in accordance with the client's representational system

They present a comical imaginary dialogue between the client and the therapist to highlight the difficulties associated with these language conflicts

For example, the client states 'things feel really heavy in my life . . . I can't handle it' and the therapist responds with 'I can see that'

An observant therapist would have noticed that the client is demonstrating a kinaesthetic preference and would have responded accordingly

Therapists can enhance the effectiveness of their treatment by matching their language to the preferred sensory modality of the client

DETECTING SENSORY MODALITIES

Record yourself during conversation – try letting the recorder run for a long time to ensure that the discussion is natural. Now listen carefully to your own use of language. Do you use visual terms ('I see what you mean') or auditory terms ('I hear you') or kinaesthetic terms ('I get that feeling')? Try to identify your own preferred sensory modality.

Once you have experienced detecting sensory language, try to identify the preferred modalities of the people around you. Listen carefully to their use of language, particularly when they are using metaphors or analogies. Think about how you could match your own language to their preferred sensory modalities – see what happens when you intentionally mismatch and match language.

Submodalities

Human mind represents information in accordance with particular senses and these methods of internal representation of information are known as sensory modalities

Each of these sensory modalities can be further divided into submodalities in accordance with the specific representational system

Visual submodalities

Framed/panoramic
2D/3D
Colour/monochrome
Brightness
Sharpness
Focus
Location
Size
Shape
Style
Contrast

Clarity

Movement

Auditory submodalities

Mono/stereo

Volume

Pitch

Tone

Variations

Location

Range

Clarity

Voice

Kinaesthetic submodalities

Intensity

Texture

Pressure

Heat

Weight

Location

Movement

Submodalities are closely linked to emotional perception

Our emotional responses to a memory will be associated with certain submodalities

For example, an individual may visualise a negative event in monochrome with a dark frame

Submodalities can be used to explore feelings about a particular issue and, more importantly, alter feelings if required

For example, the above individual could improve their feelings about the negative event by mentally replacing the dark frame with a light frame and adding colour to the memory

Meta model

The meta model can encourage the client to address deeper issues

Set of questions designed to challenge and expand the client's internal model of the world (Grinder & Bandler, 1981)

Meta model focuses on the translation of three faulty thought patterns

Distortions

Deletions

Generalisations

Distortions refer to inaccuracies or assumptions

Mind-reading distortions

> Client claims to know the thoughts of another person

> For example, 'he hates me'

> We can challenge this distortion by asking the client how they know this information

Lost performance distortions

> Client makes value judgements without identifying the source

> For example, 'it is important to be liked'

> We can challenge this distortion by asking the client who has made this judgement

Cause-and-effect distortions

> Client assumes that one thing will cause another

> For example, 'I will be miserable if he goes away'

> We can challenge this distortion by highlighting the assumption and asking the client how or why one thing causes the other

Complex equivalence distortions

> Client assumes that two things are synonymous

> For example, 'I didn't get a good grade in this exam, I am rubbish at everything'

> We can challenge this distortion by highlighting the assumption and asking the client if there are any cases when these two things are not synonymous

Presupposition distortions

> Client assumes that something is true

> For example, 'I am worried that my new boyfriend will be as unreasonable as my old boyfriend'

> We can challenge this distortion by highlighting the assumptions and questioning their validity

Deletions refer to the exclusion of certain information

Simple deletions

> Client omits certain information

> For example, 'I am unhappy'

> We can challenge this deletion by requesting further information

Lack of referential index deletions

> Client fails to specify the relevant person or thing

> For example, 'they are mean to me'

> We can challenge this deletion by requesting further information

Comparative deletions

> Client makes an unspecified comparison using general terms like 'best', 'worse', etc.
>
> For example, 'he is a better person'
>
> We can challenge this deletion by asking the client to define the terms

Unspecified verb deletions

> Client uses a verb without specifying the details of the action
>
> For example, 'she rejected me'
>
> We can challenge this deletion by asking the client to define the verb in more detail

Nominalisation deletions

> Client changes a verb into a noun
>
> For example, 'he values his freedom'
>
> We can challenge this deletion by asking the client to define the verb in more detail

Generalisations refer to the use of absolute sweeping statements

Universal quantifier generalisations

> Client uses global terms such as 'all', 'every', 'never', etc.
>
> For example, 'everyone thinks he is wonderful'
>
> We can challenge this generalisation by highlighting the global term and then asking the client to consider exceptions and counter-examples

Modal operators of necessity

> Client uses a verb implying obligations ('should', 'must', 'need to', etc.) to describe a verb
>
> For example, 'I have to do it'
>
> We can challenge this generalisation by asking the client to consider the effect of not meeting the obligation

Modal operators of possibility/impossibility

> Client uses a verb implying prospects ('can/can't', 'possible/impossible', 'will/won't', etc.) to describe a verb
>
> For example, 'I can't do it'
>
> We can challenge this generalisation by asking the client to explain why these prospects exist

Dangers of challenging

Although this model could be helpful in highlighting faulty thinking, it is important to ensure that any challenges or confrontations with the client are handled delicately as they could make the client feel defensive

Therapists who have established a good rapport with a client could use these challenging questions to successfully help the client to understand their deeper feelings about problem issues, but care must be taken at all times

Anchoring and swishing

Anchoring

Anchors are based on the principles of classical conditioning

> Classical conditioning occurs naturally in many of our interactions: we might feel good when we hear a song that was in the charts during our happy childhood or we might feel bad when we smell a perfume that was worn by a teacher during our unhappy teenage years

Anchors use the same principles as conditioning to forge a link between a physical act (such as touching thumb to forefinger) and a desired emotional response (such as a feeling of calm) (Bandler & Grinder, 1979)

> Client visualises a positive scene in order to induce the desired emotion

>> For example, imagining relaxing by the sea in order to induce a feeling of calm

> Client performs the physical act as the feeling is ascending towards a peak

>> For example, touches certain part of the hand

Anchors can be established effectively by ensuring that certain key behaviours are completed during this process (Bandler & Grinder, 1979)

> First key to anchoring is that the desired emotional state should have a high intensity

>> Intense relaxation is more easily anchored than mild relaxation

> Second key to anchoring is that the physical act is unique to the anchor

>> Waving is not an appropriate act as it is too often fired unintentionally thus leading to the extinction of the association

> Third key to anchoring is that the physical act is easily replicable

>> It is unreasonable to expect a person to complete a complex difficult action in order to elicit the positive emotion

> Fourth key to anchoring is that the anchor is set a significant number of times

>> Process of setting the anchor should initially be repeated several times and this stacking of the anchor should be regularly refreshed

> Final, and perhaps most important, key to anchoring is that the physical act is precisely timed to coincide with the peak of the emotional experience

>> Anchor should always be set as the state is nearing the peak in the ascendancy to ensure that the physical act is not inadvertently associated with a diminishing emotion

Once anchor has been fixed, client can induce the desired emotion during negative situations by simply completing the physical act

> For example, the nervous student could induce a feeling of calm during an exam by simply touching thumb to forefinger

ANCHORING POSITIVITY

Try out the anchoring technique for yourself. Identify a positive emotion and then work to create that emotion within yourself. As the emotion reaches the peak, make a simple hand gesture. Repeat this process several times to ensure that the positive emotion is firmly anchored to the action. Once you have anchored the gesture, try it out when you are in a less positive frame of mind – does the gesture recreate the positivity?

Swishing

Swish pattern technique is used to redirect thoughts and behaviours from negative patterns to positive patterns (Masters et al., 1991)

Client is instructed to visualise the problem state from a fully associated position with the solution state in the left-hand corner of the problem image

> Swish is then completed by simultaneously switching the locations of the two images: the problem image shrinks and recedes to a distant point while the solution image explodes into view

> Swish between the two images is further supported by the use of submodalities: for example, the problem image may fade to monochrome while the solution image develops bright colours

Swish is repeated several times until it becomes difficult to visualise the problem image

> At the point when the problem image is difficult to visualise effectively, the swish pattern should be ceased in order to encourage the establishment of the new desired state

> Irrespective of alterations in the visualisation of the problem image, the swish should not be repeated more than ten times in any one session

SWISH AWAY NEGATIVITY

Try out the swishing technique for yourself. Identify a negative habit and then imagine yourself doing the behaviour on a big screen. Picture the alternative desired behaviour in the bottom left-hand corner. For example, if your negative habit is biting your nails, you might create a mental picture of your own hand with ragged fingernails coming up towards your mouth. Remember, you must be fully integrated into the image – you should not be observing as though it is happening to someone else. You could then imagine a pair of beautiful hands with long nails in the left-hand corner. Swish between these two images several times until it becomes more difficult to imagine the problem. What impact does this activity have on your subsequent behaviour?

Controversies in NLP

NLP is arguably the most controversial therapy in this textbook

> Some therapists regard it as pseudoscientific and consider it an unprofessional method of engaging with clients

> Some researchers have highlighted the exaggerated claims of proponents as evidence of weak theoretical foundations

Preferred representation systems

Little evidence for the use of preferred sensory modalities (Sharpley, 1984)

Eye movements were found to have no relation to the recall of visual, auditory and kinaesthetic stimuli (Wertheim et al., 1986)

No theoretical foundation or evidence

Roderique-Davies (2009) concluded that, despite three decades of use across thousands of organisations, there is little empirical evidence to support NLP techniques and no credible theoretical basis for NLP that is not strictly anecdotal

Tosey and Mathison (2007) argued 'the pragmatic and often anti-theoretical stance by the founders has left a legacy of little engagement between practitioner and academic communities'

Plagiarism?

Sharpley (1987) noted that several 'NLP' techniques are actually modifications of previous techniques from other therapies – they are marginally effective but cannot be classed as original

> But is therapy ever truly original? Or do all theories simply build on the previous theories? NLP is an eclectic therapy and has always admitted to borrowing successful techniques from other approaches

Despite the controversies surrounding this approach, there are some interesting and engaging techniques and these can be useful for the eclectic therapist

Case study demonstrating neurolinguistic programming

Laura, 26, has been struggling to reduce her weight for the last three years. Her doctor has advised her that she is experiencing many health difficulties relating to her diabetes because she is clinically obese yet continues to binge on sugary foods. She craves sweet things all of the time and regularly consumes six times the recommended daily allowance of sugar. She has visited an NLP therapist in the hope of finding a technique to control her eating habits. She is hoping to attend for only one session, but she is willing to attend a top-up session in the future.

In the following exchanges, therapist denotes therapist, client denotes Laura. Confidentiality statement and the business contract have been discussed. The session is joined just after Laura is completing her story.

Client: So I know that it is going to kill me, but I just can't stop. I picture food in my head all the time and I'm miserable on a diet. It feels like life isn't really worth living anyway if I have to be miserable. I just can't see myself ever being happy on salads.

Therapist: I can see your point, but could there be a compromise?

Client: Maybe. I guess. If I just ate a little bit less of everything, maybe.

Therapist: I get how that could work, but can you picture yourself stopping after only eating a little bit?

Client: (sighs) No. Once I start, I can't stop.

Therapist: Okay, so what if we come at this problem from another angle? Instead of stopping after starting, what if you just avoid some things altogether?

Client: I don't know. Like what?

Therapist: What is your favourite food? Absolute most favourite?

Client: Erm, probably chocolate biscuits. No, wait, chocolate cake.

Therapist: So let's leave that one alone. But what is your second favourite?

Client: Chocolate biscuits.

Therapist: So let's work with that one and our aim is for you to not eat chocolate biscuits at all. First of all, can you picture a plate of chocolate biscuits?

Client: Yes.

Therapist: Good. Try to make the picture in your head really vibrant. Make it bright and colourful. Now describe it to me – describe the whole picture including the plate.

Client: There are six biscuits and they are really rich and brown. They are on a bright red plate. One of the biscuits is broken and there is melting chocolate in the middle and it is oozing out onto the plate.

Therapist: And the colours are very rich?

Client: Yes. And it is really close to me. Just within reach. And they are really big.

Therapist: Gosh, they sound delicious! I feel hungry now!

Client: (laughs) They look delicious!

Therapist: Okay, now I would like you to work on changing that mental image. Let's start with the colour. Can you make the colours duller? Maybe less rich and more grey?

Client: (frowning) Yes, I guess so.

Therapist: You don't sound too happy about that?

Client: Well they look so delicious. I don't want to spoil them.

Therapist: That's good. Spoiling them is exactly what we are trying to do. If we spoil your mental image of them then you are less likely to want to eat them. Now try making the colour even greyer. And move the image away from you. Move it back and shrink it a little. How do they look now?

Client: A bit pointless really. I don't know why I was so interested in them. It seems stupid that these little grey things are more important to me than my health.

Therapist: Let's talk a little bit more about your health. What does being healthy mean to you?

Client: I'd quite like to run a marathon. (laughs) But no, seriously, I know that is never going to happen. It would be good to be able to play with the kids though. I could maybe see myself doing that.

Therapist: Tell me about that image.

Client: Well, I guess that I can see myself at the park, pushing Karen on the swings, and maybe kicking a ball about with Jay. Not getting exhausted and needing to sit down all the time.

Therapist: Is that an easy image for you to create?

Client: No. It seems impossible at the moment.

Therapist: Now I want you to go back to that image of the biscuits – the first image – all big and bright. Imagine that this picture is on a huge television screen right in front of you. Have you got that?

Client: Yes.

Therapist: Okay, now imagine that there is a tiny little box in the bottom left corner of the screen. Inside that box is the image of you at the park, running around with Jay, pushing Karen on the swings. Try to make this image grey and fuzzy and small inside that little box.

Client: Okay, that's easy because it's hard to imagine me doing that anyway.

Therapist: Right, but now comes the tricky bit. On my word, you are going to do something called a swish. You are going to make the two images swop places. That big bright image of the biscuits will shrink to the little grey fuzzy image in the left corner. And the little grey image of you at the park will fill the screen in bright colours. Can you do that?

Client: I think so. I'll try.

Therapist: Okay, and SWISH.

In this exchange, the therapist has identified a preferred modality and begun working within that modality to introduce interventions. The rest of the session involves focus on the faulty thought patterns held by Laura. The session finishes with a repeat of the swish exercise. Laura found this session very helpful and she was able to reduce her craving for biscuits by repeating this technique at home. When she returned for a top-up session, she asked to focus on her desire for all sweet food and she has since been able to eliminate sugary treats from her diet.

ANALYSING THE CASE STUDY

Try answering the following questions using information about neurolinguistic programming.

- What was Laura's preferred sensory modality and how did the therapist detect this?
- What submodalities were used during this session and how might this have impacted on Laura's feelings about food?
- How was swishing used in this session?
- Could anchoring help Laura to overcome her problems with food?
- Can you anticipate any potential problems in the methods used by this therapist?

SUMMARY

Eclecticism: mix of techniques across multiple therapies; focuses on the use of language to make changes in the brain; very controversial and some proponents have taken the claims too far

Development: developed by Bandler and Grinder in 1975 as a therapeutic method of instilling fast effective change using the best techniques from a range of therapies; eclectic blend of family therapy, Gestalt therapy and hypnotherapy

Representation systems: sensory modalities (visual, auditory, kinaesthetic), detecting preferred modalities, matching language to representation system; submodalities, nature of the visual/auditory/kinaesthetic experience, closely linked to emotional perception, emotions can be manipulated by changing submodalities

Meta model: faulty thoughts; distortions (mind reading, lost performance, cause and effect, complex equivalence, presupposition); deletions (simple, lack of referential index, comparative, unspecified verb, nominalisation); generalisations (universal quantifier, modal operators of necessity, modal operators of possibility)

Anchoring: classical conditioning; anchor a physical act (such as touching thumb to forefinger) to a desired emotional response (such as a feeling of calm); keys to anchoring success, desired state should have high intensity, physical action should be unique and easily replicated, anchor is set a number of times, physical action is timed to coincide with peak emotion

Swishing: cognitive visualisation to redirect thoughts and behaviours from negative patterns to positive patterns; visualise vibrant problem state on a big screen with the dull solution state in the left-hand corner of the problem image then switch between the two

Controversies: questionable empirical evidence for preferred representation systems; limited theoretical foundation; accusations of plagiarism

REFERENCES AND BIBLIOGRAPHY

Albert Ellis Institute (2012) *Ellis Biography.* Retrieved from http://albertellis.org/about-albert-ellis-phd/

American Psychiatric Association (APA) (2000) Practice guidelines for the treatment of patients with major depressive disorder. Retrieved from http://psychiatryonline.org/content.aspx?bookid= 28&sectionid=1667485

Bandler, R. (2010) *Richard Bandler's Guide to Trance-Formation.* Florida: Health Communications.

Bandler, R. & Fitzpatrick, O. (2009) *Conversations: Freedom is Everything and Love is All the Rest.* Florida: HCI Books.

Bandler, R. & Grinder, J. (1975) *The Structure of Magic, Volume 1.* Palo Alto, CA: Science and Behavior Books.

Bandler, R. & Grinder, J. (1976) *The Structure of Magic, Volume 2.* Palo Alto, CA: Science and Behavior Books.

Bandler, R. & Grinder, J. (1979) *Frogs into Princes: Neuro Linguistic Programming.* Colorado: Real People Press.

Bandler, R. & Thomson, G. (2011) *The Secrets of Being Happy.* Massachusetts: IM Press Inc.

Bandler, R., Andreas, S. & Andreas, C. (1985) *Using your Brain for a Change.* Boulder, CO: Real People Press.

Barnes-Holmes, Y., Hayes, S.C., Barnes-Holmes, D. & Roche, B. (2002) Relational frame theory: a post-Skinnerian account of human language and cognition. *Advances in Child Development and Behavior,* 28, 101–138.

Batte, M. (1996) ABCs of rational living. Retrieved from www.thejoveinstitute.org/

Beck, A.T. (1967) *Depression: Clinical, Experimental, and Theoretical Aspects.* Philadelphia, PA: University of Pennsylvania Press.

Beck, A.T. (1975) *Cognitive Therapy and the Emotional Disorders.* Oxford: International Universities Press.

Beisser, A.R. (1970) The paradoxical theory of change. In: Fagan, J. & Shepherd, I. (eds) *Gestalt Therapy Now.* Palo Alto, CA: Science and Behavior.

Berne, E. (1961) *Transactional Analysis in Psychotherapy.* New York: Grove Press.

Berne, E. (1964) *Games People Play.* New York: Ballantine Books.

Berne, E. (1966) *Games People Play – The Theory Video.* National Education Television.

Berne, E. (1972) *What Do You Say After You Say Hello?* New York: Grove Press.

Clancy, F. & Yorkshire, H. (1989) The Bandler Method. *Mother Jones Magazine.* Retrieved from www.american-buddha.com/bandler.method.htm

Clarkson, P. (1989) *Gestalt Counselling in Action.* London: Sage Publications.

Cooper, M., Elliott, R., Stiles, W.B. & Bohart, A. (2008) CBT superiority questioned at conference [Press release]. Retrieved from www.uea.ac.uk/mac/comm/media/press/2008/july/CBT +superiority+questioned+at+conference

DeLozier, J. & Grinder, J. (1987) *Turtles All The Way Down.* California: Grinder, DeLozier and Associates.

DeRubeis. R.J., Gelfand. L.A., Tang. T.Z. & Simons, A.D. (1999) Medications versus cognitive behavior therapy for severely depressed outpatients: mega-analysis of four randomized comparisons. *American Journal of Psychiatry*, 156, 1007–1013.

Ellis, A. (1946) The validity of personality questionnaires. *Psychological Bulletin*, 43(5), 385.

Ellis, A. (1957) Rational psychotherapy and individual psychology. *Journal of Individual Psychology*, 13(1), 38–44.

Ellis, A. (1962) *Reason and Emotion in Psychotherapy*. Oxford: Lyle Stuart.

Ellis, A. (1995a) Thinking processes involved in irrational beliefs and their disturbed consequences. *Journal of Cognitive Psychotherapy*, 9(2), 105–116.

Ellis, A. (1995b) Fundamentals of rational emotive behavior therapy for the 1990s. In: Dryden, W. (ed) *Rational Emotive Behavior Therapy: A Reader*. London: Sage Publications, pp.1–30.

Ellis, A. (1995c) Changing rational-emotive therapy (RET) to rational emotive behavior therapy (REBT). *Journal of Rational-Emotive and Cognitive-Behavior Therapy*, 13(2), 85–89.

Ellis, A. (1996) *Better, Deeper, and More Enduring Brief Therapy: The Rational Emotive Behaviour Therapy Approach*. New York: Brunner/Mazel.

Ellis, A. (1997) The evolution of Albert Ellis and rational emotive behavior therapy. In: Zeig, J.K. (ed.) *The Evolution of Psychotherapy: The Third Conference*. New York: Brunner/Mazel.

Ellis, A. (1999) *How to Make Yourself Happy and Remarkably Less Disturbable*. San Luis Obispo, CA: Impact Publishers.

Ellis, A. (2003) Early theories and practices of rational emotive behavior therapy and how they have been augmented and revised during the last three decades. *Journal of Rational-Emotive and Cognitive-Behavior Therapy*, 21(3), 219–243.

Ellis, A., Abrams, M. & Abrams, L. (2005) Biography of Dr Albert Ellis. Retrieved from www.rebt.ws/albertellisbiography.html

Gerhards, S.A., de Graaf, L.E., Jacobs, L.E., et al. (2010) Economic evaluation of online computerised cognitive-behavioural therapy without support for depression in primary care: randomised trial. *British Journal of Psychiatry*, 196(4), 310–318.

Goulding, M. & Goulding, R. (1979) *Changing Lives Through Redecision Therapy*. New York: Brunner Mazel.

Grinder, J. & Bandler, R. (1981) *Trance-formations*. Boulder, CO: Real People Press.

Grinder, J. & Bostic St Clair, C. (2001) *Whispering in the Wind*. California: J & C Enterprises.

Harris, T. (1967) *I'm OK, You're OK*. New York: Grove Press.

Hayes, S.C. & Strosahl, K.D. (2004) *A Practical Guide to Acceptance and Commitment Therapy*. New York: Springer.

Howes, R. (2008) Seven questions for Donald Meichenbaum. Retrieved from www.psychologytoday.com/blog/in-therapy/200812/seven-questions-donald-meichenbaum

International Transactional Analysis Association (2013) Retrieved from www.itaaworld.org/

Kahler, T. (1978) *Transactional Analysis Revisited*. Little Rock, AR: Human Development Publications.

Karpman, S. (1968) Fairytales and script drama analysis. *Transactional Analysis Bulletin*, 7(26), 39–43.

Lazarus, A.A. (1958) New methods in psychotherapy: a case study. *South African Medical Journal*, 32, 660–664.

Lazarus, A.A. (1966) Broad spectrum Behaviour Therapy and the treatment of agoraphobia. *Behaviour Research and Therapy*, 4, 95–97.

Lazarus, A.A. (1971) *Behavior Therapy and Beyond*. New York: McGraw-Hill.

Lazarus, A.A. (1973) Multimodal behavior therapy: treating the 'Basic Id'. *Journal of Nervous and Mental Disease*, 156(6), 404–411.

Lazarus, A.A. (1981) *The Practice of Multimodal Therapy: Systematic, Comprehensive and Effective Psychotherapy*. New York: McGraw-Hill.

Lazarus, A.A. (2005) Multimodal therapy. *Handbook of Psychotherapy Integration*, 2, 105–120.

Lazarus, A.A. (2010) When to fire your therapist. Retrieved from www.psychologytoday.com/blog/think-well/201008/when-fire-your-therapist

Lazarus, A.A. (n.d.) Live case consultation. Retrieved from www.psychotherapy.net/video/lazarus-live-consultation

Leibig, A. (1990) Laura Posner Perls in memory. Retrieved from www.gestalt.org/laura.htm

Lewin, K. (1943) Defining the field at a given time. *Psychological Review*, 50(3), 292.

Linehan, M.M. (1993) *Cognitive-Behavioural Treatment for Borderline Personality Disorder: The Dialectics of Effective Treatment*. New York: Guilford Press.

Lister-Ford, C. (2002) *Skills in TA Counselling and Psychotherapy*. London: Sage Publications.

Lynch, D., Laws, K.R. & McKenna, P.J. (2010) Cognitive behavioural therapy for major psychiatric disorder: does it really work? A meta-analytical review of well-controlled trials. *Psychological Medicine*, 40, 9–24.

Masters, B.J., Rawlins, M.E., Rawlins, L.D. & Weidner, J. (1991) The NLP swish pattern: an innovative visualizing technique. *Journal of Mental Health Counseling*, 13(1), 79–90.

Meichenbaum, D. (1977) *Cognitive Behavior Modification: An Integrative Approach*. New York: Plenum.

Meichenbaum, D. (1985) *Stress Inoculation Training*. New York: Pergamon Press.

National Institute for Health and Clinical Excellence (NICE) (2004, amended 2007) *Clinical Guidelines for Depression in Adults*. Retrieved from www.nice.org.uk/cg90

Padesky, C.A. & Greenberger, D. (1995) *Clinician's Guide to Mind Over Mood*. New York: Guilford Press.

Perls, F. (1942) *Ego, Hunger, and Aggression: The Beginning of Gestalt Therapy*. New York: Random House.

Perls, F. (1969) *Gestalt Therapy Verbatim*. Boulder, CO: Real People Press.

Perls, F. (1970) Four lectures. In: Fagan, J. & Shepherd, I. (eds) *Gestalt Therapy Now*. Palo Alto, CA: Science and Behavior.

Perls, F., Hefferline, R.F. & Goodman, P. (1951) *Gestalt Therapy: Excitement and Growth in the Human Personality*. New York: Julian Press.

Perls, L. (1990) A talk for the 25th anniversary. *Gestalt Journal*, 13(2), 15–22.

Perls, L. (1992) Conceptions and misconceptions in Gestalt therapy. In: Smith, E. (ed.) *Gestalt Voices*. New York: Ablex Publishing.

Polsner, E. & Polsner, M. (1988) *Gestalt Therapy Integrated*. New York: Random House.

Preube, I. (2013) John Grinder and the history of neurolinguistic programming. Retrieved from http://smokingcessationguide.blogspot.co.uk/2009/10/john-grinder-and-history-of-neuro.html

REBT Network (2006) Dr. Albert Ellis, Creator of psychology's cognitive revolution. Retrieved from www.rebtnetwork.org/updates/obituary_albert_ellis.html

Renton, J. (2009) *Coaching and Mentoring: What They are and How to Make the Most of Them*, Vol. 21. London: Profile Books.

Roderique-Davies, G. (2009) Neuro-linguistic programming: cargo cult psychology? *Journal of Applied Research in Higher Education*, 1(2), 58–63.

Roth, A. & Pilling, S. (2007) *The Competencies Required to Deliver Effective Cognitive and Behaviour Therapy for People with Depression and Anxiety disorder*. London: Department of Health.

Rubin, E. (1915) *Synsoplevede Figurer. Studier i psykologisk Analyse*. Copenhagen: Gyldenhal.

Sharpley, C.F. (1984) Predicate matching in NLP: a review of research on the preferred representational system. *Journal of Counseling Psychology*, 31(2), 238.

Smith, D. (1982) Trends in counseling and psychotherapy. *American Psychologist*, 37(7), 802.

So, M., Yamaguchi, S., Hashimoto, S., Sado, M., Furukawa, T.A. & McCrone, P. (2013) Is computerised CBT really helpful for adult depression? A meta-analytic re-evaluation of CCBT for adult depression in terms of clinical implementation and methodological validity. *BMC Psychiatry*, 13(1), 113.

Spiegler, M.D. (2008) Behavior therapy II: cognitive-behavioral therapy. In: Frew, J. & Spiegler, M.D. (eds) *Contemporary Psychotherapies for a Diverse World*. Boston, MA: Lahaska Press.

Steiner, C. (1966) Script and counterscript. *Transactional Analysis Bulletin*, 5(18), 133–135.

Steiner, C. (1974) *Scripts People Live: Transactional Analysis of Life Scripts*. New York: Grove.

Stewart, I. & Joines, V. (1987) *TA Today: A New Introduction to Transactional Analysis*. Nottingham: Lifespace.

Stiles, W.B., Barkham, M., Twigg, E., Mellor-Clark, J. & Cooper, M. (2005) Effectiveness of cognitive-behavioural, person-centred, and psychodynamic therapies as practiced in National Health Service settings. *Psychological Medicine*, 36, 555–566.

Stiles, W.B., Barkham, M., Mellor-Clark, J. & Connell, J. (2008) Effectiveness of cognitive-behavioural, person-centred, and psychodynamic therapies in UK primary-care routine practice: replication in a larger sample. *Psychological Medicine*, 38(5), 677–688.

Teasdale, J.D., Segal, Z.V. & Williams, J.M. (1995) How does cognitive therapy prevent depressive relapse and why should attention control (mindfulness) training help? *Behaviour Research and Therapy*, 33, 25–39.

Tosey, P. & Mathison, J. (2007) Fabulous Creatures of HRD: A Critical Natural History of Neuro-Linguistic Programming. 8th International Conference on Human Resource Development Research and Practice across Europe, Oxford Brookes Business School.

Ward, E., King, M., Lloyd, M., et al. (2000) Randomised controlled trial of non-directive counselling, cognitive-behaviour therapy, and usual general practitioner care for patients with depression. *BMJ*, 321, 1383–1388.

Wertheim, E.H., Habib, C. & Gumming, G. (1986) Test of the neurolinguistic programming hypothesis that eye-movements relate to processing imagery. *Perceptual and Motor Skills*, 62(2), 523–529.

Woldt, A.L. & Toman, S.M. (2005) *Gestalt Therapy: History, Theory and Practice*. London: Sage.

Wong, M. (2000) Former suspect in notorious murder trial is back in town – and back in court. Retrieved from http://web.archive.org/web/20071009061842/ http://www.santacruzsentinel.com/archive/2000/February/02/local/stories/1local.htm

Yalom, I.D. (1980) *Existential Psychotherapy*. New York: Basic Books.

Yontef, G. (1993) *Awareness, Dialogue and Process: Essays on Gestalt Therapy*. New York: Gestalt Therapy Press.

Conclusion

This book aimed to provide a comprehensive guide to the four main psychological approaches (three forces and a revolution). This guide to the psychological approaches and the main associated therapies was the primary focus of Chapters 2–5.

- Third force: humanistic approach and person-centred therapy
    - Development of the humanistic approach
    - Personal and professional biographies of Rogers and Maslow
    - Humanistic theories of human nature and personality
    - Therapeutic relationship in person-centred therapy
    - Therapeutic techniques in person-centred therapy
    - Case study demonstrating person-centred therapy

- Second force: psychodynamic approach and psychoanalytic therapy
    - Development of the psychodynamic approach
    - Personal and professional biographies of Freud and Klein
    - Psychodynamic theories of human nature and personality
    - Therapeutic relationship in psychoanalytic therapy
    - Therapeutic techniques in psychoanalytic therapy
    - Case study demonstrating psychoanalytic therapy

- First force: behavioural approach and behaviour therapy
    - Development of the behavioural approach
    - Personal and professional biographies of Pavlov, Watson and Skinner
    - Behavioural theories of human nature and personality
    - Therapeutic relationship in behaviour therapy
    - Therapeutic techniques in behaviour therapy
    - Case study demonstrating behaviour therapy

- Revolution: cognitive approach and cognitive therapy
    - Development of the cognitive approach
    - Personal and professional biographies of Neisser and Beck
    - Cognitive theories of human nature and personality
    - Therapeutic relationship in cognitive therapy
    - Therapeutic techniques in cognitive therapy
    - Case study demonstrating behaviour therapy

This book also aimed to introduce you to a range of modern integrative and eclectic therapies and this was the primary focus of Chapter 6.

*   Gestalt therapy
*   Transactional analysis
*   Rational emotive behaviour therapy (REBT)
*   Cognitive-behaviour therapy (CBT)
*   Multimodal therapy (MMT)
*   Neurolinguistic programming (NLP)

We said at the end of our introduction that we hoped that this textbook would serve as a knowledgeable guide on your journey through the fascinating subject of counselling and psychotherapy. Now that you have reached the end of this book, please take a moment to reflect on what you have learnt. If you have gained a little insight into some of the concepts discussed in this book to the extent that you are able to appreciate the approaches and evaluate the therapies, then we can be happy that we have achieved our goal. More importantly, if you now recognise that you have only just begun your therapeutic education and have been inspired to read further into these fascinating approaches and therapies, then we are thrilled to have exceeded our goal and delighted that we were able to offer some signposts at the start of your journey. We hope that you are able to apply your new understanding of counselling and psychotherapy in your professional and personal life, and we are confident that your deeper appreciation of human nature will benefit you in all aspects of your life.

If we have succeeded in motivating you to study this topic further, please log into our website to access further materials to support and enhance your learning experience. You will find all of the following available online:

*   Glossary of key words as a reference guide
*   Key word clouds to summarise content of textbook
*   Mindmaps to support associative links between concepts
*   Multiple choice questions to test recall of factual content
*   Short answer questions to test understanding of material
*   Essay questions to test critical appreciation of approaches and therapies
*   List of resources (including films, books, documentaries, poems, songs and websites) to improve understanding and expand appreciation of the topics

We would like to take this opportunity to thank you for allowing us to join you on your educational journey and wish you lots of luck for your further travels in the future.

> '*I am not a teacher; only a fellow traveller of whom*
> *you asked the way.*'
> —George Bernard Shaw (1856–1950)

Index

Note: Page numbers in **bold** are for figures.